PUBLIC HEALTH: PRACTICES, METHODS AND POLICIES

THE COVID-19 PANDEMIC

A TRIBUTE TO THE CORONA WHISTLEBLOWERS

PUBLIC HEALTH: PRACTICES, METHODS AND POLICIES

JOAV MERRICK - SERIES EDITOR

MEDICAL DIRECTOR, HEALTH SERVICES, DIVISION FOR INTELLECTUAL AND DEVELOPMENTAL DISABILITIES, MINISTRY OF SOCIAL AFFAIRS AND SOCIAL SERVICES, JERUSALEM, ISRAEL

The COVID-19 Pandemic: A Tribute to the Corona Whistleblowers
Joav Merrick, Søren Ventegodt and Niels Jørgen Andersen (Authors)
2020. ISBN: 978-1-53618-146-3 (Hardcover)
2020 ISBN: 978-1-53618-236-1 (e-book)

Advances in Chinese Children, Adolescent and Family Research
Ariel Tenenbaum, Daniel T.L. Shek, Moon YM Law and Joav Merrick (Editors)
2020. ISBN: 978-1-53617-870-8 (Hardcover)
2020. ISBN. 978-1-53617-871-5 (e-book)

Child Environmental Health Disparities: Looking at the Present and Facing the Future
I. Leslie Rubin and Joav Merrick (Editors)
2020. ISBN: 978-1-53617-823-4 (Hardcover)
2020. ISBN. 978-1-53617-824-1 (e-book)

Positive Youth Development: Digital Game-Based Learning
Ty Lee, Daniel T.L. Shek, Sarah Sw Lee, and Joav Merrick (Editors)
2020. ISBN: 978-1-53617-795-4 (Hardcover)
2020. ISBN. 978-1-53617-796-1 (e-book)

Service Leadership Education in an Era of Service Economy
Daniel TL Shek, Xiaoqin Zhu, and Joav Merrick (Editors)
2020. ISBN: 978-1-53617-514-1 (Hardcover)
2020. ISBN: 978-1-53617-515-8 (e-book)

Parenting and Family Life in a Chinese Society
Daniel TL Shek, Moon YM Law, Joav Merrick (Editors)
2020. ISBN: 978-1-53616-705-4 (Softcover)
2020. ISBN: 978-1-53616-706-1 (e-book)

Public Health: Topics, Themes and Trends
Satesh Bidaisee, Sadik Uddin Emmanuel Keku, Joav Merrick (Editors)
2020. ISBN: 978-1-53616-655-2 (Softcover)
2020. ISBN: 978-1-53616-656-9

Public Health: Environment and Child Health in a Changing World
I. Leslie Rubin and Joav Merrick (Editors)
2019. ISBN: 978-1-53615-394-1 (Hardcover)
2019. ISBN: 978-1-53615395-8 (e-book)

Service Leadership: Tools to Assess Knowledge, Attitude and Behavior
Daniel TL Shek, Xiaoqin Zhu, Li Lin and Joav Merrick (Editors)
2019. ISBN: 978-1-53614-852-7 (Hardcover)
2019. ISBN: 978-1-53614-853-4 (e-book)

Public Health Yearbook 2017
Joav Merrick (Editor)
2018. ISBN: 978-1-53613-792-7 (Hardcover)
2018. ISBN: 978-1-53613-793-4 (e-book)

Resilience and Health: A Potent Dynamic
I Leslie Rubin and Joav Merrick (Editors)
2018. ISBN: 978-1-53613-412-4 (Hardcover)
2018. ISBN: 978-1-53613-413-1 (e-book)

Medical History: Some Perspectives Second Edition
Donald E. Greydanus and Joav Merrick, (Editors)
2018. ISBN: 978-1-53613-319-6 (Hardcover)
2018. ISBN: 978-1-53613-320-2 (e-book)

University Students: Promotion of Holistic Development in Hong Kong
Daniel TL Shek, Lu Yu and Joav Merrick (Editors)
2017. ISBN: 978-1-53612-535-1 (Hardcover)
2017. ISBN: 978-1-53612-537-5 (e-book)

Alzheimer's Disease: Awareness among Young Adults
Ronald Chow, Drew Hollenberg, Michael Borean and Joav Merrick (Editors)
2017. ISBN: 978-1-53612-456-9 (Softcover)
2017. ISBN: 978-1-53612-457-6 (e-book)

Service Leadership Education for University Students
Daniel TL Shek, Po Chung, Li Lin and Joav Merrick (Editors)
2017. ISBN: 978-1-53611-949-7 (Hardcover)
2017. ISBN: 978-1-53611-969-5 (e-book)

Leadership: Promoting Leadership and Intrapersonal Development in University Students
Daniel TL Shek, Cecilia MS Ma and Joav Merrick (Editors)
2017. ISBN: 978-1-53611-950-3 (Hardcover)
2017. ISBN: 978-1-53611-970-1 (e-book)

Caribbean Adolescents: Misuse and Abuse of Alcohol
Cecilia Hegamin-Younger and Joav Merrick (Editors)
2017. ISBN: 978-1-63485-880-9 (Hardcover)
2016. ISBN: 978-1-63485-894-6 (e-book)

Public Health: An Ecological Framework for Child Environmental Health Interventions
I. Leslie Rubin and Joav Merrick (Editors)
2017. ISBN: 978-1-53610-700-5 (Hardcover)
2017. ISBN: 978-1-53610-714-2 (e-book)

Diabetes Mellitus: A Medical History Journey
Donald E. Greydanus and Joav Merrick
2016. ISBN: 978-1-53610-094-5 (Softcover)
2016. ISBN: 978-1-53610-103-4 (e-book)

Education in Hong Kong: Service Leadership for University Students
Daniel TL Shek, Cecilia MS Ma, Li Lin and Joav Merrick (Editors)
2016. ISBN: 978-1-63484-928-9 (Hardcover)
2016. ISBN: 978-1-63484-960-9 (e-book)

Environmental Health Disparities: Costs and Benefits of Breaking the Cycle
I. Leslie Rubin and Joav Merrick (Editors)
2016. ISBN: 978-1-63484-211-2 (Hardcover)
2016. ISBN: 978-1-63484-212-9 (e-book)

Higher Education in Hong Kong: Nurturing Students to be Caring Service Leaders
Daniel TL Shek, Andrew MH Siu, Hildie Leung and Joav Merrick (Editors)
2016. ISBN: 978-1-63484-980-7 (Hardcover)
2016. ISBN: 978-1-63485-009-4 (e-book)

Measles: Epidemiology and Control of Measles in the Gweru Urban District in Zimbabwe
Tawanda Marufu, Seter Siziya, Mazyanga L. Mazaba and Joav Merrick (Editors)
2016. ISBN: 978-1-63485-559-4 (Hardcover)
2016. ISBN: 978-1-63485-573-0 (e-book)

Medical History: Some Perspectives
Donald E. Greydanus and Joav Merrick
2016. ISBN: 978-1-63484-747-6 (Hardcover)
2016. ISBN: 978-1-63484-849-7 (e-book)

Public Health: Some International Aspects
Joav Merrick (Editor)
2016. ISBN: 978-1-63484-612-7 (Hardcover)
2016. ISBN: 978-1-63484-630-1 (e-book)

Public Health: International Aspects on Environment and Health
I. Leslie Rubin and Joav Merrick (Editors)
2016. ISBN: 978-1-63484-834-3 (Hardcover)
2016. ISBN: 978-1-63484-849-7 (e-book)

Smoking and Adolescence: International Public Health Experiences
Mazyanga L. Mazaba, Seter Siziya and Joav Merrick (Editors)
2016. ISBN: 978-1-63484-311-9 (Hardcover)
2016. ISBN: 978-1-63484-312-6 (e-book)

Arbovirus: Public Health Experience from Zambia
Seter Siziya, Mazyanga L. Mazaba, and Joav Merrick (Editors)
2015. ISBN: 978-1-63463-601-8 (Hardcover)
2015. ISBN: 978-1-63463-618-6 (e-book)

Health Issues in Diverse Cultures
Cecilia Obeng, Samuel Gyasi Obeng and Joav Merrick (Editors)
2015. ISBN: 978-1-63463-613-1 (Hardcover)
2015. ISBN: 978-1-63463-619-3 (e-book)

Public Health, Social Work and Health Inequalities
Bruce D. Friedman and Joav Merrick (Editors)
2015. ISBN: 978-1-63482-838-3 (Hardcover)
2015. ISBN: 978-1-63482-850-5 (e-book)

Patient Dumping: Background, Protections, and the Mentally Ill
Tabitha E. Rivers (Editor)
2015. ISBN: 978-1-63483-726-2 (Hardcover)
2015. ISBN: 978-1-63483-727-9 (e-book)

Tomorrow's Leaders: Service Leadership and Holistic Development in Chinese University Students
Daniel TL Shek, Andrew MH Siu and Joav Merrick (Editors)
2015. ISBN: 978-1-63321-880-2 (Hardcover)
2014. ISBN: 978-1-63321-943-4 (e-book)

Environment and Public Health: Environmental Health, Law and International Perspectives
I. Leslie Rubin and Joav Merrick (Editors)
2014. ISBN: 978-1-63463-167-9 (Hardcover)
2014. ISBN: 978-1-63463-189-1 (e-book)

PUBLIC HEALTH: PRACTICES, METHODS AND POLICIES

THE COVID-19 PANDEMIC

A TRIBUTE TO THE CORONA WHISTLEBLOWERS

SØREN VENTEGODT, MD

NIELS JØRGEN ANDERSEN, MSC

AND

JOAV MERRICK, MD, MMEDSCI, DMSC

nova science publishers
New York

NOTICE TO THE READER

The Publisher has taken reasonable care in the preparation of this book, but makes no expressed or implied warranty of any kind and assumes no responsibility for any errors or omissions. No liability is assumed for incidental or consequential damages in connection with or arising out of information contained in this book. The Publisher shall not be liable for any special, consequential, or exemplary damages resulting, in whole or in part, from the readers' use of, or reliance upon, this material. Any parts of this book based on government reports are so indicated and copyright is claimed for those parts to the extent applicable to compilations of such works.

Independent verification should be sought for any data, advice or recommendations contained in this book. In addition, no responsibility is assumed by the Publisher for any injury and/or damage to persons or property arising from any methods, products, instructions, ideas or otherwise contained in this publication.

This publication is designed to provide accurate and authoritative information with regard to the subject matter covered herein. It is sold with the clear understanding that the Publisher is not engaged in rendering legal or any other professional services. If legal or any other expert assistance is required, the services of a competent person should be sought. FROM A DECLARATION OF PARTICIPANTS JOINTLY ADOPTED BY A COMMITTEE OF THE AMERICAN BAR ASSOCIATION AND A COMMITTEE OF PUBLISHERS.

Additional color graphics may be available in the e-book version of this book.

Library of Congress Cataloging-in-Publication Data

ISBN: 978-1-53618-146-3

Published by Nova Science Publishers, Inc. † New York

CONTENTS

Preface		**xi**
Introduction		**1**
Chapter 1	Corona COVID-19 pandemic: Do we have a crazy dangerous new virus, or just a common cold?	**3**
Section one: A tribute to the Corona COVID-19 whistleblowers		**13**
Chapter 2	A tribute to the Corona virus COVID-19 (SARS-CoV-2) whistle-blowers	**15**
Chapter 3	The media and the Corona pandemic	**103**
Chapter 4	World Health Organization (WHO), health and the Swine flu	**111**
Chapter 5	Drug and treatment guidance	**127**
Chapter 6	A review of World Health Organization's recommendations in "WHO's model list of essential medicines": Who provides the data for the drug register?	**133**

Section two: Psycho-immunology and sustainability in medicine **161**

Chapter 7 The psychosomatic work of Dean Ornish: The power of mind in disease **163**

Chapter 8 Brain and consciousness **175**

Chapter 9 Our immune system **195**

Chapter 10 Practical psycho-immunology **211**

Chapter 11 The traditional Hippocratic holistic mind-body medicine **215**

Chapter 12 The strengths and weaknesses of ten major medical systems **233**

Chapter 13 The authors' epilogue: What now? **291**

Section three: Acknowledgments **299**

Chapter 14 About the authors **301**

Chapter 15 About the Quality of Life Research Center in Copenhagen, Denmark **305**

Chapter 16 About the National Institute of Child Health and Human Development in Israel **313**

Section four: Index **317**

Index **319**

PREFACE

We are living in a time of change. It is easy to assume that we live in a safe and stabile world, but the Corona COVID-19 pandemic has shown the whole world that this is not the case. Mighty forces change our way of living, thinking and things changes fast.

It is difficult to understand what is happening, for you need to be an expert in many different fields in order to really get it: medicine, economy and politics. You even need psychology, sociology and maybe even consciousness-research to fully comprehend what we are dealing with in the 2019-2020 Corona pandemic.

OUR INTENTION

This book tries to give you sufficient background in different areas to at least get an idea of what is happening.

We start by sharing the Corona whistleblowers perspective on the present crisis: Three of leading figures in virology tells us what they know and what they think, and the conclusion is that there is no dangerous threat to our existence behind the Corona COVID-19 pandemic.

The craziness comes from politicians who senselessly and un-reflected follows advises from the World Health Organization (WHO), instead of consulting the scientists that for years have done research in the field. The protest against what is happening comes from these scientists who with one voice question the figures of the Corona mortality rate that comes from the WHO.

WHO says that 3.4% of infected people will die from the infection, making the COVID-19 pandemic the worst pandemic the world has seen till this day, threatening to kill millions of people world-wide. The whistle-blowing experts say the mortality rate is 0.01%, 340 times less than what the WHO claims. 340 times, that is an enormous difference. The difference is hard to comprehend. It is the difference between global disaster – and a common cold. And a common cold is what we are dealing with here, according to the scientists.

But this is obviously not the case. Clinicians report that patients coming with a positive test for Corona COVID-19 feel bad, very bad indeed. They are often confused, anxious, exhausted, in deep trouble. So it must be a new virus, for the common cold has never looked like this. No, it hasn't.

So what is happening?

We have a complex situation. Politicians are acting in despair, they are following advice they do not understand, for problems they do not understand. They create a panic and the media are much too happy to follow. Small stories become big stories, sensational stories and horrible pictures of dying and dead people fill the tabloid papers and the TV programs every single day. Restaurants closes, borders closes, work places closes, shops have lines to separate the customers. The streets are empty, people are told to stay home. Doctors are seen in space-suits, streets are disinfected. The world has gone crazy. Three billion people are under lock-down. Countries like the Czech Republic make laws to force everybody to carry facemasks. In Denmark people are fined if they are more than 10 people together publicly – each gets a fine of 200 Euro!

The global economy breaks down, countless companies go bankrupt, and hundreds of thousand workers are sent home. The presidents of China and USA are discussing it. It is on the agenda, every day, in every country. That is a big thing.

WE ARE SOCIAL BEINGS AND WE NEED CLOSENESS FOR HAPPINESS AND HEALTH

The true problem of the political interventions is that the belief that we are spreading a deadly virus to each other lead to a whole set of behaviors and beliefs about the necessity of staying away from each other, keeping distance, minimalizing social contact, closeness, intimacy, touch, kisses and hugs. The whole thing becomes horribly antisocial. Other people are contagious, their mere existence and presence threaten your life. This class of ideas is horribly destructive and goes right against our most important need as human beings: the need for love.

We are social beings, and we need contact, love, touch, intimacy. We need to feel safe with each other, we need to be able to relax together. The whole event about COVID-19 and its mortal danger, all the social distancing, all the sterilization and disinfection, all the rules of no-touch, no closeness, no-visits, no-going-out, not meeting in public space and more are infusing massive antisocial ideas and behaviors into our culture that is doing incredible harm, and will stay with us for years to come. The whole Corona scare campaign have already done billions of people harm, and if we are not extremely careful to undo the brainwashing of the billions of citizens the politicians and authorities have been working on for month, we will have to change the whole culture in the direction of alienation, horror of other people, fear of strangers, and insecurity about travelling, dating, dancing, meeting people, even studying or working together in teams.

What we see in the Corona COVID-19 pandemic is mass-hysteria, and this time a mass hysteria that involves the whole planet. Mankind has gone crazy! It is time to wake up, and understand the importance of love and social contact, closeness, intimacy and touch – it helps you to get healthy, it heals you, it strengthens your immune system, it makes you resistant to infections and can prevent cancer and heart diseases. We beg all politicians in the world to understand this.

UNDERSTANDING PSYCHOSOMATICS IN COVID-19 AND MEDICINE

It seem that the Corona COVID-19 infection, which still is the common cold, gives stronger symptoms and becomes more dangerous when in fear. This is very inconvenient as fear is the hallmark of the COVID-19 pandemic. In this book we try to explain why emotions and negative beliefs can enhance symptoms of infectious diseases and also the danger of an infection.

Psychosomatics and psycho-immunology are so very difficult subjects, which we after researching the subject for 20 years still are puzzled about it, and we cannot expect lay people or even our own collogues to understand all aspects of it.

In this book we give a glimpse into the magical and wonderful universe of what you could call "deep biology" – the still little understood side of biology that is about biological information, and biological fields explaining the connection between body and psyche, or more precisely between consciousness and biological order. It is really a quantum thing, and even scientists to not understand it well. But that should not stop us from studying it and learning about it, as it is extremely important. This understanding is the basis for understanding medicine and healing. In the end of the book we show that psychosomatic medicine might be the only sustainable medicine, and therefore the medicine we should research in and aim to develop so we can have sustainable, safe and before anything else – effective – medicine in the future.

How can we understand it?

We need to understand the ways and culture of the large industries, especially the pharmaceutical industry. We need to understand how WHO operates, and we need to know who controls the WHO. So we need to know about WHOs history and here the 2009 Swine flu pandemic is very informative.

We need to understand money, corruption, business strategy. And we need to understand biology. Not only to understand virology, but also how psychosomatic issues works. We need to understand the brain, and the immune system. We need to understand psycho-immunology, and psychosomatics. We need to understand sociology to the extent where phenomena like mass-hysteria make sense for us.

There is so much to know. It is not easy. But it is not impossible either. It seems a matter of the highest importance that you understand it well enough to make up your mind and form your own opinion. Not based on what people, politicians, doctors and other authorities are telling you, but based on your own common sense, you own feeling, experience and understanding.

We cannot make this a neutral and objective book. We are also human beings and we have our own opinions about things. So we have chosen to be transparent in what we believe and think, in what the experts we quote and portrait know and think. And we hope that you will be clear and wise enough to take what is true for you, and use for your own final conclusion about what is happening in the world.

It shall be no secret that we are very much concerned about the state of the world, especially the issue of sustainability. We firmly believe that the global ecosystem is in a major crisis caused by the extreme number of people on the planet, and the uninhibited consumption of the surface of the Earth.

We need to find sustainable ways to live in the future. We are researchers in medicine so of course we focus on what we know in this field. In the end of the book we bring a deep analysis of the different kinds of medicine we know, and look into how effective, safe and sustainable they are, to point to the direction we should take medicine, if we want it to be sustainable and help mankind to survive in the future.

It is not a secret either that we to some extent find chemical medicine, pharmaceutical medicine, too ineffective, too harmful, and definitely not sustainable, so this is also why we are chocked to see a whole world following the WHO in this mad move, that could lead to an explosive use of pharmaceutical medicine, vaccines, tests and more in the future.

Many people have a tendency to think: Medicine – we need that. Yes, we do, but the right kind of medicine. Again, please orient yourself in the many different possibilities, please come to know what there is to know, before you make up your mind. You might end up very surprised, because you did not know much of the wonderful and amazing things we are going to share with you in this book.

It is about a disaster, a global catastrophe, caused by massive misinformation. But the learning is sweat and beautiful. There is so much to be learned from this, so many things to think about and look into, that we believe that the whole Corona pandemic in the end will serve mankind.

May this work serve all living beings.

Søren Ventegodt,
Niels Jørgen Andersen
and Joav Merrick

INTRODUCTION

Chapter 1

CORONA COVID-19 PANDEMIC: DO WE HAVE A CRAZY DANGEROUS NEW VIRUS, OR JUST A COMMON COLD?

In the Corona COVID-19 infection, if you really come to believe that you have attracted a mortal new virus, the common cold you normally would experience, becomes a terrible disease that is threatening your life. Are the symptoms exhaustion, disorientation, malaise, as we see it described from clinicians, what we would expect in this situation? Yes, exactly. And why?

- Exhaustion, because it takes a lot of energy from your body to worry.
- Disorientation because there is a fundamental mismatch between what you believe and what you actually feel.
- Malaise, because you feel miserable due to the circumstances, and your beliefs and fear, but are unable to put a finger precisely to the problem.

The Corona hype, the Corona panic, has manifested the common cold as a brand new disease. What we present here is the psychosomatic hypothesis for COVID-19.

We are living in a time of change. It is easy to assume that we live in a safe and stabile world, but the Corona COVID-19 pandemic has shown the whole world that this is not the case. Mighty forces changes our way of living, thinking and things changes fast. It is difficult to understand what is happening, for you need to be an expert in many different fields in order to really get it: medicine, economy and politics. You even need psychology, sociology and maybe even consciousness-research to fully comprehend what we are dealing with in the 2019-2020 Corona pandemic. This book tries to give you sufficient background in different areas to at least get an idea of what is happening around us in all parts of the world.

INTRODUCTION

What is unique about the human being is before anything else the human brain. Consciousness seems to be in all living being, but only humans are able to make a mental model of the world, that allows us to use language, use tools, build complicated civilizations, and with intelligence and acquired knowledge conquer all corners of the planet, from the coldest, icy North to the hottest jungle.

Our model of the world is shared between individuals, and inherited from generation to generation. Is has amazing features, and it gives us a feeling that we know the world. Often we forget that what we perceive is our own description much more than it is the reality in front of us. We are *interpreters*, and this is both our strength and our weakness.

It is a strength, because it means that we only need a sign to get a meaning; we see very little and we already know a lot. It is a weakness, because we come to believe that we know a lot when we just see a little. You can say that we guess a lot from what we know.

So mind gives us a world to live in; a world that is very different from reality. Every human being lives in its own world; and this world can be sweet, if the mental map, the mental description of live is sweet, or it can be painful, and full of fear, disappointments, regrets and self-pity. Most people live in fear. Fear is a natural ting which comes together with the fight for survival all children has to win, to grow up. Ideally, when we are adult, we become independent, self-confident, and autonomous, and fear is replaced with a deep-rooted joy of existence, inner peace and happiness.

To grow up you encounter challenges, troubles, suffering and from this you learn. If your upbringing is too easy, if life is without challenges, you will not learn enough to be free, independent and autonomous. You will never be happy, but stay worried, scared and small. Your inner child is still with you, and it takes a lot of space. You didn't grow up psychologically. And that is the problem in many parts of the civilized world, where stability and wealth have substituted the poverty and insecurity, and the necessity to fight for your life, we had in most of the world just a century ago.

So the dark side of our modern, rich, materialistic society is that people are becoming dependent, immature and in some way you can say, naïve.

We do not really grow up psychologically; we do not reach the fully mature, free, and happy state. Therefore, we become dependent on authorities.

Unfortunately, such a dependency is often making people easy prey for manipulation and abuse of authority. The media becomes powerful; commercials effective, politicians words more important. The modern democracy has an inborn problem: People are too easily misled. The COVID-19 Pandemic is an example of where this can take us.

Experiencing Physical Health: Why Well-Being Can Be Compromised by Fear, Negative Emotions and Beliefs

Because we interpret the world through our description of the world we carry in our brain-mind, our experience becomes very sensitive to what we believe. We experience our partner through our beliefs about love and the opposite sex; we experience work through our beliefs about work and our own talents; we experience other people through our social understanding, which defines our social skills and ability. Out whole experience of life comes from our beliefs about other people and the world.

Moreover, we experience our bodies through our beliefs about health, sex and body. So, if we buy a belief that we are infected with a deadly virus, we will already there start to change our experience of our own body. We will start to shiver and fear, and all signs of disease we have heard about will start to appear, and real symptoms will be enhanced, all symptoms will be worsened. If you have some capacity of self-suggestion, the expected symptoms of a disease will be felt the moment you know or just suspect that you have attracted a certain infection, and before the infection have had time to manifested clinically (i.e., before the incubation time).

In the Corona COVID-19 infection, if you really come to believe that you have attracted a mortal new virus, the common cold you normally would experience, becomes a terrible disease that is threatening your life. Are the symptoms exhaustion, disorientation, malaise, as we see it described from clinicians? Yes, as mentioned above, exhaustion comes from losing your energy to worries, disorientation from the mismatch between what you believe and what you actually feel, and malaise - you feel miserable, but you are unable to put a finger precisely to the physical problem.

The Corona hype, the Corona panic, has manifested the common cold as a brand new disease. That is our psychosomatic hypothesis for COVID-19.

Psycho-Immunology: How Can a Thought Disturb the Body's Self-Nonself Regulation?

Unfortunately, it does not stop here. In a confused, disoriented, exhausted and troubled state of mind, your immune system stops working precisely. The connection between psyche and immunology has been a deep mystery for science, but a matter of intensive scientific investigation fort the last three decades.

To understand this connection between psyche and immune system, you need both a deep understanding of the human brain, and a deep understanding of what is called the self-nonself discrimination in biology; this mechanism is one of the oldest, most fundamental and most surprising capabilities of biological systems. The mystery of how the brain and the immune system are connected has only recently been solved and many questions remain unanswered.

The theoretical solution seems to be an information field that both give us mind and body; it is a unified field of the biological organism that works through the highest level of the organism; a level we could call consciousness. The reason why many questions remain unanswered is that nobody has been able to explain or model the phenomena of consciousness on a mechanical level – meaning the chemical or physical substratum of consciousness is not known.

This might seem like a farfetched statement; many people will take the position that if chemistry and physics has not been able to explain it, then it might be that it does not exist at all. If physics cannot explain consciousness, maybe consciousness does not exist. It is a reasonable argument, except – I am!

We cannot deny that we are conscious. So the informational field that both lent itself to the brain-mind and to the body as the "morphological field", mystical as it is, makes a strong connection between psyche and immune system.

The field of psycho-neuro-immunology is full of wonderful and strange experiments, where it is proven that the connection is not humoral – carried by hormones or signal drugs – as you maybe would expect. One example is an experiment with hypnosis on people with warts, where the hypnotist manages to make the warts disappear on one side of the body – the left or the right hand – and not on the other. Not only warts can disappear; surprising experiments have been done with cancer, coronary artery stenosis in heart diseases, and other serious diseases have shown to react dramatically on change of state of mind and revision of the patient's belief system.

Some of the most convincing studies of this have been done in California, United States, where Professor Dean Ornish has been able to cure heart patients and cancer patients with a psychosomatic therapy program (1, see also below). Dean Ornish alternative cures have been accepted as a part of the health care offered to US citizens as part of the public health care offer (Patient Protection and Affordable Care Act also called "Obamacare"). And the core teaching in Ornish psychosomatic medicine, that cures people is, that we need to be close to each other, we need to feel and express love, we need to live intimately close to each other. That is the key to health!

AUTONOMY AND SLAVERY: THE IDEAL OF FREEDOM, AND HOW TO GET THERE

In every classical culture, there have been an ideal of a free and happy person. In Buddhism, this person is enlightened; in India he is a yogi; in the Native American cultures, this man or woman is a shaman; in the Australian aboriginal cultures this free man is a healer. In the Samic cultures, as in the Eskimo culture, he or she a child of the spirits. In the classical Greek society, he was philosopher. In many other cultures, the ideal man was artist, poet, leader, warier, holy, a priest, a sage.......

If you ask what all these ideals have in common, is it to be present in life, with freedom of mind – or rather, the freedom from mind. The perfect one is... one with what is, real, one with reality, the ocean of life, the source of love and wisdom.......

The ideal man is free; he is happy, independent and knowledgeable. He is intelligent, strong, responsible, caring and loving. These qualities are always there in the hero, in the good one, independent of the continent, the time or the culture. And this seems to be an amazing thing. This point to the possibility we have as human beings to break free of mind, free of our conditioning and upbringing, to find truth and autonomy.

The opposite of freedom is slavery. The opposite of freedom of mind is illusion. The illusion takes the form of a dream of life, which turns into a nightmare. Illusion is the father of suffering. Illusion is the mother of deception, abuse, and misguidance.

Another thing that always comes with the highest state of being, the happy, conscious state, is *physical and mental health.* An old Indian saying amongst yogis is "Perfection of the body shall be your last and final triumph" In the Native American cultures, the shaman is also healer of all physical and mental disease and suffering. Hippocrates, the father of medicine, was Asclepiad, i.e., priest-healer.

SPIRITUALITY, FREEDOM, AND HEALTH HAVE ALWAYS BEEN CONNECTED IN ALL PRE-MODERN CULTURES

The opposite of spirituality is materialism. Today, materialism - money and material wealth - has been the religion of modern societies. The problem of this is that the spirit is not developed; it is hardly known anymore. People fall into sweet slumber, and forget to grow and learn. Out of this comes illusion, slavery and suffering.

What we have seen in the COVID-19 pandemic, where the whole world has bought into the illusion of a horrible new virus that has come to sweep mankind off the planet – a pandemic of a danger that according to the world's leading experts in medicine, virology, and infectious biology does not exist – is the price we collectively have to pay for our unconscious and dependent state of mind and existence. It is time for the people of the world to wake up and be responsible, present beings, so this great deception of the whole planet cannot repeat itself.

Sustainability and the Medicine We Need for Surviving the Future

The planet is in trouble; the global eco-system is breaking down under the weight of 10 billion human beings and their senseless (ab)use of nature and resources. In all aspect, from the food we eat, to the things we use and the culture we have, we need to integrate concern for the environment.

The biggest burden for the planet comes from the huge industries, like the chemical industries. Amongst these the pharmaceutical industry is the biggest and the most burdensome for our global climate.

The World Health Organization (WHO) actions seems to create a craving for more pharmaceutical medicine, more tests and machines, more vaccines and drugs. If this is intended, is not yet known, but the close bond between the WHO and the pharmaceutical industry makes it a likely scenario. We need to think deeply about what medicine we must have in the future, to save the planet from destruction.

There are many kinds of medicine, and each of these have different profiles of effect, harm and sustainability. In our analysis of the world's medicine we have tried to find a medicine for the world in the future, which is safe, effective and sustainable.

Psalms 91 (Prayer of Moses the man of God)

> Verse 1:
>
> He who dwells in the shelter of the Most High will rest in the shadow of the Almighty
>
> Verse 5-6:
>
> You will not fear the terror of the night, nor the arrow that flies by day,
> Nor the pestilence that stalks in the darkness,
> Nor the plague that stalks at midday.

Verse 7:
A thousand may fall at your side,
Ten thousand at your right hand,
But it will not come near you

REFERENCES

[1] Ventegodt S, Merrick J. A citizen's guide to survive Corona COVID-19 (SARS-CoV-2). Copenhagen: Quality-of-Life Research Center Press, 2020.

SECTION ONE:
A TRIBUTE TO THE CORONA COVID-19 WHISTLEBLOWERS

Chapter 2

A TRIBUTE TO THE CORONA VIRUS COVID-19 (SARS-COV-2) WHISTLE-BLOWERS

We are at this moment of writing in the middle of the Corona COVID-19 (SARS-CoV-2) pandemic facing a global disaster, which seemingly is caused by a new deadly virus the whole world is trying to cope with after warning from the World Health Organization (WHO) about a mortality of 3.4%. Three leading experts in infectious diseases, Wolfgang Wodarg, Sucharit Bhakdi and John PA Ioannidis on the other hand hold the position that we are misinterpreting the statistics and instead facing a misinformation campaign, not a dangerous new virus. The WHO is counting the death-numbers wrongly, ignoring large dark numbers of infected, and ignoring both all we know about the Corona virus already, and all the statistics on the common cold and flu we have access to, and the statistics on mortality in the population we also have access to, thus creating an image of a mortal pandemic. Unfortunately, the politicians of the world have reacted to the WHO campaign as if it was true, creating massive fear in the population, which now has come to believe that we are facing a deathly new infection. Massive fear boosts the symptoms of Corona patients strongly in susceptible individual for psychosomatic reasons: If you believe you have a mortal infection, and everybody, including your own doctor and the hospital affirms you in this belief, it is only natural that you feel miserable. If you feel bad at the hospital, you will get treated. Hospitalization, ventilators, and drugs can give hospital infections, side effects, and increase mortality. In this way, the world has affirmed itself in the illusion of a mortal pandemic, which simply does not exist to begin with. COVID-19 has a mortality of around 0.01%, in accordance with the death statistics from many countries. Recent studies where all patients that died WITH Corona had an autopsy showed that not one single patient has died BY Corona. Based on this the Corona COVID-19 mortality rate is found to be ≤0.001%.

KEY POINTS

Three Corona COVID-19 (SARS-CoV-2) whistle-blowers, Wodarg, Bhakdi, and Ioannidis agrees on:

- The new Corona virus is just the harmless, common cold.
- The mortality rate is 0.01%, ten times less than influenza.
- WHO exaggerates the mortality 340 times, saying the COVID-19 has a mortality rate of 3.4%. This high number comes from the *case fatality rate*, which has nothing to do with the mortality rate!
- Doctors overreact, burdening the health care sector.
- Politicians overreact, limit personal freedom, compromise quality of life, harm the economy, and shorten life expectancy.

We find:

- Fear boosts the symptoms psychosomatically, *making COVID-19 look like a new disease.*
- The non-specific immune system is primarily responsible for people's general immunity to Corona COVID 19 (the "herd immunity"). The non-specific immune system is cell-mediated and do not use antibodies. Corona COVID-19 tests based on antibodies are therefore not able to detect Corona COVID-19 in people infected but did not have symptoms, which is about 99% of the infected.

Introduction

At the moment of writing the whole world is closing down under the pressure of a deadly new Corona virus, the COVID-19, which is reported to kill thousands of people. Every day the media is giving us new numbers of the dead by Corona from each country. Emergency laws are passed daily everywhere, and most European countries have closed the borders, closed schools, workplaces, restaurants and public meeting places, almost stopped production, and send millions of workers home. Over two billion people have been quarantined worldwide. People are suffering, economy is suffering, personal freedom limited overall. That is the sad state of the world March 26th 2020.

According to the German lung specialist Wolfgang Wodarg the new SARS-CoV-2 virus is harmless and just another common cold (1-9). The only reason we know about this virus is a new Corona-test, which recently came into use, making the spread of virus tractable. But it is a test, which has not been scientifically validated and it seems to be seriously flawed, unspecific and not precise. Nevertheless science agree that a novel Corona virus, COVID-19, is spreading over the world.

But there are always new viruses spreading, which is not a problem if it is not dangerous. Leading researchers in medicine and infection biology, like Professor Bhakdi (10-15), Professor John PA Ioannidis (16-20), and Professor Jay Bhattacharya (21, 22) all say the same: There is no scientific evidence to back the claim that the new Corona COVID-19 should be dangerous; therefore we must assume, that it is just as harmless as the common cold we had last year, and the year before, and the year before that, and every year since forever. That is the logic of science: If you do not know anything specific, you have to go with the simplest explanation, which is that what you are facing today is just the normal thing, the same as yesterday. This follows from the famous principle of Occam's razor (23).

If this is true, what about the horrible statistics you see every day in the media? Are all these death counts not documenting the horrible viral mortality? No, says Wodarg, Bhakdi, and Ioannidis, again in perfect agreement: these horrible numbers are scary, but when you look closer they are just a product of the wrong way the statistics are made, the poor quality of data collected, and of severely manipulated interpretations of the statistics (1-22).

All normal scientific indicators of common cold and flu, which are still available in most countries, show that there is no signs of any abnormal virus attacking us. There is no documented over-mortality, not even in Italy, where the Corona reports say that 7% of the Corona infected have died (19). When Wodarg, Bhakdi, and Ioannidis calculated the mortality rate from the available numbers, they all found the same low mortality rate for Corona COVID-19 of 0.01% (1-22). This is 10 times less than a normal flu. Nothing to worry about at all!

The information about a deadly COVID-19 pandemic comes from the World Health Organization (WHO), claiming that the new virus has a mortality of 3.4% (24, 25) and from the national statistics, which WHO have been guiding the making of (26). WHO has warned the world that we are facing the medical catastrophe of the century. Politicians all over the world have taken WHO's warning very seriously and reacted accordingly. "Better safe than sorry" has been the motto.

If that was the whole story, it would be understandable what is happening, maybe even reasonable. The problem is that there have been enormous problems with the information coming from WHO about pandemics already. Anybody who remembers the Swine flu scandal from 2009 will immediately have this reaction (27-70): But can we trust WHO in this?

SWINE FLU

In the 2009 H1N1 influenza "Swine flu" pandemic, WHO was making the flu much worse than it was; in the end the Swine flu turned out to be one of the mildest influenzas we have ever had. The problem was that WHO pushed the Swine flu vaccine to such an extent that almost all countries bought unnecessary vaccine, which later had to be send to destruction. Vaccine for billions of dollars (27-70).

Journalists researched the WHO and found a much too close cooperation with the pharmaceutical industry, leading the researching journalists to conclude that WHO had fallen victim to corruption: the pharmaceutical industry had placed its own people in the WHO advising committee, and in this way the industry could control WHO (27-70). The corruption of WHO was condemned by many countries and by many national and international organisations ((27-70).

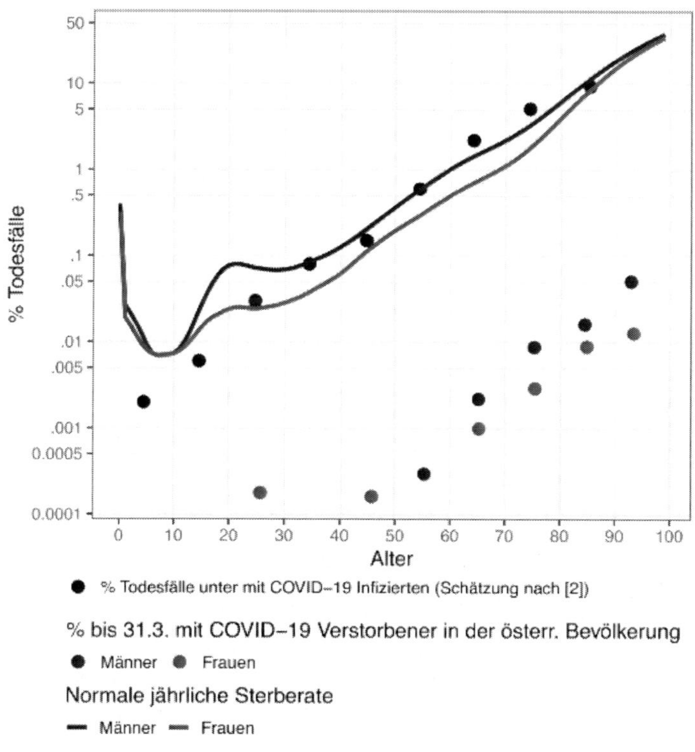

Figure 1. A new study on Corona COVID-19 mortality in Austria (72) has looked into the difference in mortality for persons with and without a positive Corona COVID 19 test; the study shows no difference at all in mortality, no matter how old you are! The finding is in accordance with the estimate of Wodarg, Bhakdi and Ioannidis of a mortality rate of 0.01% for COVID-19.

Wolfgang Wodarg was chairman of the PACE Health Committee during the Swine flu pandemic and said then: "The WHO's "false pandemic" flu campaign is one of the greatest medicine scandals of the century" (37). In 2010 he also stated that: "The definition of an alarming pandemic must not be under the influence of drug-sellers" (37).

When Wodarg, Bhakdi, Ioannidis say that the mortality rate of Corona COVID-19 is very low, about 0.01%, they backed it up with recent mortality statistics from the USA (17), Denmark (71), Austria (72) (see figure 1), the Czech Republic and Italy (2, 8) – which all shows, that there is no over-mortality this spring in any of these countries. If there was a harmful virus spreading, there should be somebody dying from it, which is not the case according to these statistics. So this becomes a strange story, where WHO claims the COVID-19 to be a factor 340 times more deadly than what Wodarg, Bhakdi, Ioannidis says. The difference between these two estimates is extreme, so who is right and who is wrong here?

AGAIN, THE PICTURE IS MORE COMPLEX

Many clinicians have unusual, strong symptoms from patients infected with Corona COVID-19; the symptoms look strangely like symptoms from the brain, not from the body; they look like neurological symptoms (73, 74). A general pattern is that the patients can feel very miserable; in some cases, COVID-19 may present as malaise, disorientation, or exhaustion (73). That is not a part of the common cold as we know it, so are we dealing with a new dangerous virus after all? The vast number of seemingly neurological symptoms is likely to be psychological symptoms; and these points to the strangeness of the clinical picture of COVID.-19, which is definitely different from the normal common cold.

Here we present a *psychosomatic hypothesis* for COVID-19. We suggest that the massive misinformation by the media, constantly repeating misinterpretations of poorly made statistics on the Corona mortality, and the general alarm about the Corona virus, in our societies and especially in all parts of the health care sectors, makes people *believe* that COVID-19 is a deadly new disease.

Dramatic precautions made in many countries to prevent the spread of the Corina infection create a state of public panic, which has an extremely strong impact on vulnerable, suggestible souls, which is exactly what is needed to make a common cold look clinically like a serious disease in these people.

This is in accordance with the reported polarity the COVID-19 patients have shown (73, 74), where most people do not even notice the infection, because it is subclinical, and many people who do get symptoms only get mild symptoms, while others have wild and extreme reactions, where they go fast into a severe clinical state with many strong symptoms, many of which seem to come from the brain/mind, and not from the body.

The theory is that the people who have a mild reaction simple recognize the infection as another harmless, common cold, and react according the their prior experience with common cold. The sensitive and susceptible people add their fear of dead and a general tendency to worry, to their infected state, and they therefore react strongly, when they realize that they are infected with Corona. These people are very attentive to all symptoms, making them stronger. The fear and disorientation is seen to come from the infection but is really coming from the mind as a reaction to the situation, where they believe that they have caught a mortal infection.

Amongst the latter are the people who are too willingly to follow their doctor's idea of treatment and hospitalization, and even a group of people, also younger people, who insist on going straight to intensive care, in the bleak hope that they will survive this horrible, deadly COVID-19 infection they already have heard so much about.

If Wodarg, Bhakdi, and Ioannidis are right and the novel Corona COVID 19 is as harmless as any other common cold, the new Corona COVID-19 can still look clinically like a new, much more serious disease than the common cold, because of the extreme circumstances. This is very important to point out.

SOMETHING STRANGE IS HAPPENING

Something very strange and unusual is definitely going on in the COVID-19 pandemic. People behind the WHO and the research in Corona virus vaccines, like Bill Gates, who has invested billions of dollars into the vaccine industry (75, 76), has publicly stated that viruses are a bigger threat to health than nuclear war (76) and thus the new threat of mankind.

According to Wodarg, Bhakdi, and Ioannidis it is not true that we are facing a new deadly virus, and it is also extremely unlikely that a Corona virus will mutate into a dangerous virus, because our body is so familiar with this type of viruses that it has extremely good immunity to them. This is why most infected people do not even notice that they are infected.

Instead, we are facing a "Corona hype", which might very well just be another gigantic WHO-scare-campaign, with dire consequences for the whole, global community, but this time done so well that we cannot so easily call the bluff. If that is the case, you can say that WHO learned from its mistake in 2009. Meaning that there is no vaccine ready to buy; this is a smart thing and the connection to the pharmaceutical industry is more hidden. Or is it? WHO's agenda with exaggerating the Corona virus mortality is not so clear, because there are many interests impacting the WHO.

SOMETHING TO THINK ABOUT

The obvious hypothesis is, that we face a scare-campaign intended to once again make the whole world buy unnecessary vaccines for billions or trillions of dollars, as a cure for the new "deadly" COVID-19 virus and many, many dangerous viruses yet to come. This suspicion is logical as it already happened in 2009 with the Swine flu scandal (27-70).

An alternative hypothesis is that WHO, now functioning as a private institution, simply is after more funding and more power for itself, and therefore make interpretations and guide the fabrication of statistics that documents its own importance. President Trump in the United States had seen this and stopped a yearly funding of WHO for 400 million dollars.

A third hypothesis is that the problem is not so much WHO itself, but that it is the politicians, who are naively relying on the WHO, instead of following the world's leading experts in science, for their knowledge and understanding of diseases and there cures, that create the problem. It is very strange that politicians follow the WHO in the light of the former Swine flu scandal. We have seen all over the world, that politicians have been very fast to claim and use the absolute power, which the fear of a new super-deadly pandemic gives them; the problem might simply be that politicians in general love to step into the limelight and play heroes, saving the world from a deadly pandemic. Politicians might love this play so much that they fail to analyse the situation carefully, and they obviously also fail to analyse the dire consequences of their actions. Basically, in the heat of the day, the politicians fail to step back and see, that the whole thing about the Corona virus is about saving the very sick, old people from dying on average a few weeks earlier than expected. Because that is what we are talking about.

You might know that the average age of people in the "dead by Corona COVID-19 statistics", even in Italy, the country said to suffer most from the novel Corona virus, is 81 years old, and that 99% of the dead patients had 1, 2 or even 3 serious diseases (co-morbidity) already (8, 10, 18-22).

Could it be that the industry has its people everywhere to help the politicians look towards WHO? Is what we see in the COVID-19 pandemic simply the influence of cooperating pharmaceutical industries (called "Big Pharma")? We know that the pharmaceutical industry is employing millions of people all over the world; with a yearly turnover of about two trillion dollars, they are becoming more powerful than even some national states. Due to size, accumulation of money, bought academic status, and other assets, combined with massive marketing, and worldwide lobbyism, they have an enormous influence. The pharmaceutical industry acts through the doctors, that benefit from the cooperation in many ways and the critique of the industry's use of doctors in the medico-industrial complex is nothing new (77). Maybe the Corona hype is not about WHO at all, but about hidden and ubiquitous actions of Big Pharma?

Maybe it is not the pharmaceutical industry that is behind this, but people with interest, like Bill Gates, who has invested billions of dollars in the vaccine industry and at the same time gives billions of dollars to the WHO? What we see these days might be a New World Order where big commercial interest and single people with endless amounts of money, and not common sense and democratic processes, controls the world?

What are we trying to say?

In this paper we will take a brief look into many of the aspects mentioned above. It is simply impossible in a single paper to go deep; what we hope to do is to start a debate and encourage investigation into the many unknown and unclear things we are facing.

The analyses of Wodarg, Bhakdi and Ioannidis stay with the science; they do not talk about politics. But they all strongly criticize the WHO for saying that COVID-19 is dangerous, with a mortality rate of 3.4%, without having any scientific support of this statement at all. Their analyses are clear and relevant and their conclusion seems in agreement with each other: We are all totally overreacting – people, patients, doctors, and politicians. The whole world has entered a state of hysteria; what sociologists and psychologists call *mass hysteria* or *mass psychosis* (78). That was what we also saw in 2009 (31, 32).

In this phenomenon, collective illusions of threats, whether real or imaginary, are transmitted through a population in society as a result of rumours and fear. In medicine, the term is used to describe the spontaneous manifestation of the same or similar hysterical physical symptoms by more than one person; a common type of mass hysteria occurs when a group of people believe they are suffering from a similar disease or ailment; this has been seen countless times through history (78). Such beliefs often have some base in reality, which makes it much harder to realize the illusionary nature of the mass hysteria, as in this case of the Corona virus.

The three whistle-blowers we have chosen to focus on in this article are not alone with the message that we are making a scary monster out of a harmless common cold; a large number of doctors and academics in many countries are saying the same. We have chosen these three people because of their clarity of speech, excellence in scientific skills, and their bravery in talking straight against the opinion of a whole world in panic.

Please keep in mind that the protest against what is happening worldwide in the Corona COVID-19 pandemic is not coming from a few crazy scientists, but from a substantial fraction of the scientific community. Many more could talk, but do not dare. As we shall see, even in our modern democracy, talking against the politicians can easily cost your job.

In this paper, we first look into what the whistle-blowers are saying, and after that we discuss some of the many questions this brings up.

WOLFGANG WODARG (1)

Wolfgang Wodarg (see figure 2) (born March 2, 1947) is a German physician specialized in lung diseases with a subspecialty in virology. He is also a politician for SPD (Sozialdemokratische Partei Deutschlands), the Social Democratic Party in Germany. As chair of the Parliamentary Assembly of the Council of Europe Health Committee Wodarg co-signed a proposed resolution on December 18, 2009, which was discussed January 2010 in an emergency debate ("faked pandemics, a threat to health. PACE Plenary session social affairs Council of Europe to investigate WHO Jan 25-29, 2010"). Wodarg called at that time for an inquiry into alleged undue influence exerted by pharmaceutical companies on the World Health Organization's global H1N1 flu campaign (27, 28, 37).

Education and profession (1, 3-8)

Wodarg is from Schleswig-Holstein. He studied medicine in Berlin and Hamburg and got his physician's licence in 1973, and in 1974 he received his Dr Med doctorate degree from the University of Hamburg. Since 1983 he has held the position of Amtsarzt (regional medical director) at the Health Department of Flensburg and a lecturer at the University of Flensburg. Wodarg has given courses at the Charité Berlin and at other European universities on the topics of research and ethics, European policy, healthcare and sociological issues in healthcare, politics and science.

He is a lung specialist, a doctor in the state health system, occupational physician and former head of the Health Department of the city of Flensburg, where he was head of the Department of Pulmonary and Bronchial Medicine. He was a member of the examination boards of the Schleswig Holstein Medical Association for environmental medicine, pulmonary and bronchial medicine and for social medicine. In 1991, Wolfgang Wodarg received a scholarship to study epidemiology and health economics at Johns Hopkins University in Baltimore, United States.

Party affiliation (1)

Wodarg has been a member of the Social Democratic Party (SPD) since 1988. From 1992 to 2002 he was the head of the SPD's Schleswig-Flensburg district. From November 19, 2005 to December 1, 2007 Wodarg was chairman of the SPD district of Flensburg. Since 1990 Wodarg has been member of the executive committee of the national Association of Social Democrats in the Health Sector, and since 1994 the federal deputy chairman, and in 2002 he became elected chairman of the federal Committee.

Member of Parliament (1)

From 1986 to 1998 Wodarg belonged to the parish council of his native Nieby. From 1994 to 2009 he has been a member of the Bundestag. Here Wodarg was spokesman from 2003 to 2005 of the SPD caucus in the inquiry commission *ethics and law of modern medicine.* Since 1999 Wodarg has also belonged to the Parliamentary Assembly of the Council of Europe. Since 2002 he has been vice chairman of the Socialist Group, and since 2006 president of the German social democrats and deputy head of the German delegation. Some of his famous quotes:

> "The WHO's "false pandemic" flu campaign is one of the greatest medicine scandals of the century" (37).

> "The definition of an alarming pandemic must not be under the influence of drug-sellers" (37).

WHAT IS WOLFGANG WODARG SAYING ABOUT THE CORONA COVID-19 PANDEMIC?

According to Local Today (Lokalheute) (March 17 2020), Wodarg takes a clear stand regarding the Corona COVID-19 pandemic, here is the text following a video where Wodarg presents his viewpoints (8):

> "The current panic has nothing to do with illness or epidemics." claims Dr Wolfgang Wodarg - not a conspiracy theorist, but as a pulmonologist and former head of a health department with his own monitoring system for flu diseases, someone who knows what he is talking about. He is convinced that: "All flu watch indicators only show normal values. No exceptional cases of serious illness are registered in China, Italy or anywhere else."

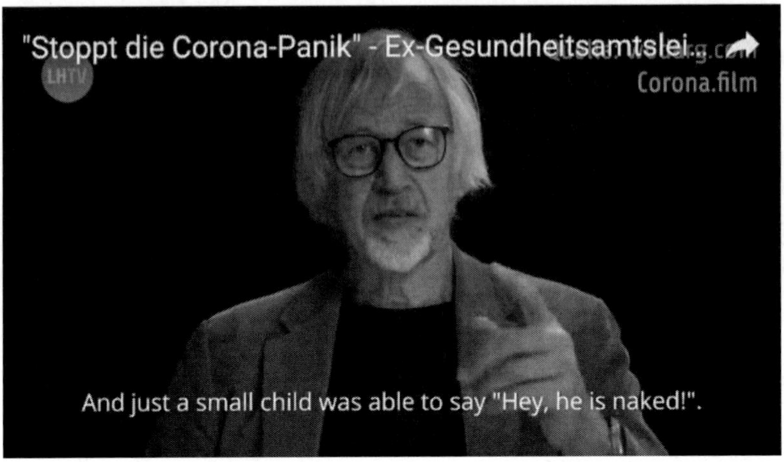

Figure 2. Wolfgang Wodarg compares the Corona situation to Hans Christian Andersen's story about the Emperor who was tricked to believe he has cloth on, by two smart hustlers. First when a small child says: "The emperor is naked" can everybody see the fraud. Wodarg obviously sees himself as the small child (8).

The doctor from Kiel is asking questions and seeking to understand why the perception [of the disease] is different in politics and in the society. He is not one of those who want to play down Covid-19 - like many other viruses it should not be underestimated.

China shocked its people in Wuhan for only two months and demonstrated to the world how to track down an epidemic, hype it up, and then fight it using authority. European countries are now following this theatre and isolating each other. In Europe, the economy is collapsing and human rights are being forgotten, while China has just finished these useless COVID-19 tests and has quickly declared the crisis to be a foreign problem", said the pulmonologist. Covid-19 - a real danger or have we all just gotten blind? Form your own opinion on LOKALHEUTE.TV.

It is then noted that "Local Today is not taking side, neither pro or contra, nor are we talking against any presumed necessary precautionary measures - we lack the specialist knowledge. But of course we have verified the statements".

WODARG'S HOMEPAGE (2)

Wolfgang Wodarg also communicates to the public via his webpage (2). Here he has the following statements about the Corona COVID-19 Pandemic:

Health assessment: There is no valid data and no evidence of exceptional health threats.

Undisputed facts: The official mortality statistics, which are still available, and various national flu monitoring institutes show the normal course of the curves.

The seasonal "flu" is as usual.

Corona viruses are and have always been there. Corona viruses, influenza viruses and other viruses have to change continuously. So "new" viruses are normal.

The significance and application of the [Corona COVID-19] PCR tests: The tests used have not been officially validated, but have only been approved by cooperating institutes. The tests are often selective (Wuhan and Italy), e.g., applied to critically ill people anyway and are then useless for the assessment of a disease risk. Without the tests, which are questionable in terms of their informative value, and gives a misleading picture of the situation, there would be no indication for emergency measures.

Other risks of wrong interpretations:

WHO is financially dependent on the Gates Foundation.

The non-verifiable pandemic scenarios are images used to scare the public.

Wuhan and Italy are used to produce scary pictures.

Even in Italy, without the new tests, you would only see the annual flu damage.

On this website you will find numerous documents and sources to support his statements above.

Wodarg on the radio (6)

In a radio interview in Radio München March 27 2020, "Covid 19 - Test ist unspezifisch - Dr. Wolfgang Wodarg" Wodarg further explain his hypothesis, that if we did not have the new Corona test, we would not notice anything about the Corona virus COVID-19 at all. This year's global Corona infection would just be another common cold with a harmless virus.

The problems with the test is that it is un-specific; if anybody had a corona infection in the past it will be positive, and often the tested will have three different corona viruses reacting to the test. The inventor of the test made a protocol that was submitted to the WHO; everybody can download it. The protocol shows that the test finds all Asian SARS, not only one. The test only shows that the tested people at some point had contact with one of these SARS viruses.

Wodarg is also here pointing to the fact that in Italy, the country where the Corona is said to kill most people, 99% of the patients who were tested positive for Corona and died, already suffered from several severe diseases and disabilities, which is the true cause of death, not the Corona virus (10-12). There are not more people dying in Italy this year than at the same time last year, so there is no deadly pandemic, not even in Italy (2-8). The horrible mortality numbers comes from the way the statistics are made; it has nothing to do with a dangerous infection.

About the people dying from Corona in the statistics, without having a dangerous disease before the infection, Wodarg explains that Spain, Italy and Greece are known for having a very high antibiotic resistance. In hospitals, these countries have very high rates of hospital infections. If you go to a hospital in Italy, you are in life-danger. If you are lung-ventilated, the risk for getting such a hospital infection is again much higher. Wodarg is stressing the fact, that most infections are subclinical, because Corona viruses are so common that almost all people have good immunological resistance to them. Wodarg is worried that he finds the same researchers names involved in the new Corona research as in the research, which was used by the WHO to create the Swine flu scandal. The text to the Radio program says:

> "Corona – COVID-19: No topic has brought society to [such an extreme] level of action and at the same time to a standstill in the shortest possible time like this little virus. The climate crisis has not done it, terrorist attacks have not done it... Everybody is coming together against this new enemy. One of the first to take a public stand against the panic was Dr Wolfgang Wodarg and was accordingly treated badly in the media. Hardly any controversy about his theses remained factual and above the belt. So here is a list of his expertise… ."

CAN WE TRUST WOLFGANG WODARG?

The fact that Wodarg is also a politician makes it necessary to ask this question as political interests could bias his views. Wodarg seems to have his science right, and he is as a lung specialist talking within his area of expertise. The question is if he as a politician is going for the limelight with an intended controversial position on the Corona COVID-19 pandemic. Wodarg's position that the whole thing is a "hype", not a dangerous virus, seems to be a very difficult position to hold in the public space, where so many people are genuinely worried because of the information they have received from the media and the German health officials, that the Corona virus has a very high mortality rate.

Wodarg is an experienced politician, with many years in the German parliament. Also, he is 73 years old. Therefore, it does not seem likely that he is after quick fame and popularity, and a career boost. The position Wodarg hold is not a new position either; he had the same position in 2009 with the Swine Flu pandemic, where it turned out that he was right.

He is not an extremist in any way, but a politician close to the political center; therefore, we have no reason to believe that he has a predilection for extreme positions. All in all, we find Wodarg trustworthy.

SUCHARIT BHAKDI (9)

Professor Sucharit Bhakdi, is a microbiologists and researcher, who has made substantial scientific contributions to our knowledge of the proteins, our immune system, our blood complement system, bacteriology and pathology. Bhakdi is one of the most-cited medical researchers in Germany. Bhakdi, born 1st November 1946 in Washington DC, United States, is son of Thai parents in the diplomatic service, studied human medicine at the University of Bonn from 1963 to 1970, from 1966 to 1970 as a fellow of the German Academic Exchange Service. In February 1971 he received his PhD. From 1972 to 1974, he received a scholarship from the Max Planck Society, at the Max Planck Institute for Immunobiology in Freiburg. From 1974 to 1976 he received a scholarship from the Alexander-von-Humboldt Foundation at the Max Planck Institute for Immunobiology in Freiburg. After a one-year stay at the University of Copenhagen, he worked from 1977 to 1990 at the Institute of Medical Microbiology of the Justus-Liebig-University in Giessen, Germany. He was appointed C2 Professor in 1982 and 1987 as C3 Professor of Medical Microbiology, before being called to the University of Mainz in 1990.

From 1991 he taught as a professor at the Institute of Medical Microbiology and Hygiene. Bhakdi was a member of the Special Research Area of the German Research Community "Proteins as Tools in Biology" at the University of Giessen (1987-1909), Deputy Speaker of the Special Research Area "Immunopathogenesis" (1990-1999) and Speaker of the Special Infection Area in Mainz (2000–2011).

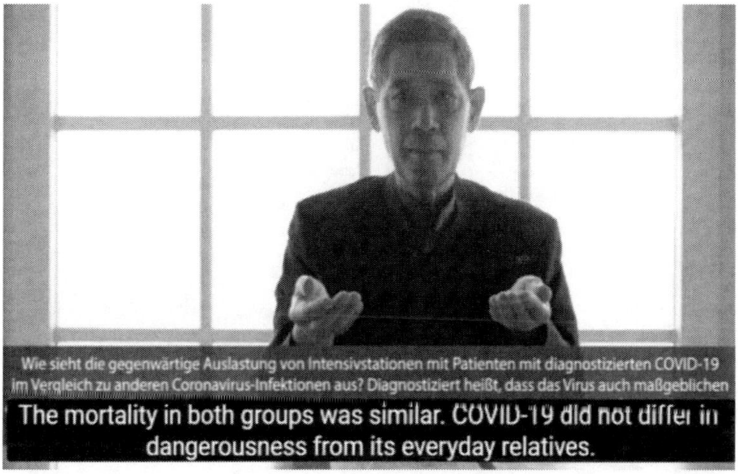
Wie sieht die gegenwärtige Auslastung von Intensivstationen mit Patienten mit diagnostizierten COVID-19
im Vergleich zu anderen Coronavirus-Infektionen aus? Diagnostiziert heißt, dass das Virus auch maßgeblichen
The mortality in both groups was similar. COVID-19 did not differ in
dangerousness from its everyday relatives.

Figure 3. Bhakti tells us that COVID-19 is not dangerous at all.

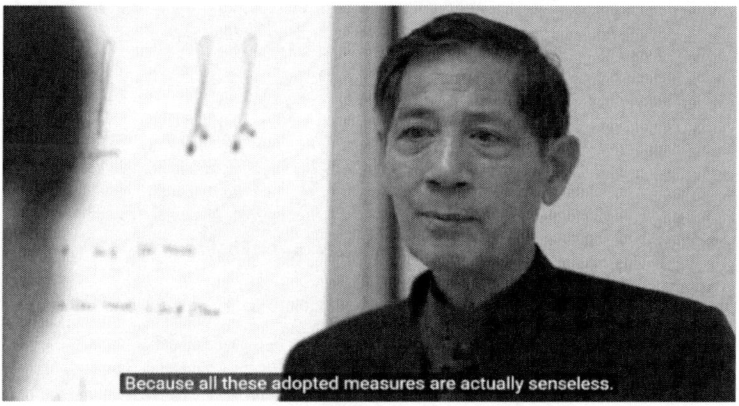
Because all these adopted measures are actually senseless.

Figure 4. Bhakti tells us that the adopted measure are “senseless”.

Bhakdi has recently published a series of open video-letters (see Figures 3-7), where he states that the Corona COVID-19 infection is just the common cold, which due to new test-methods and new ways of making statistics has come to look dangerous (9-15).

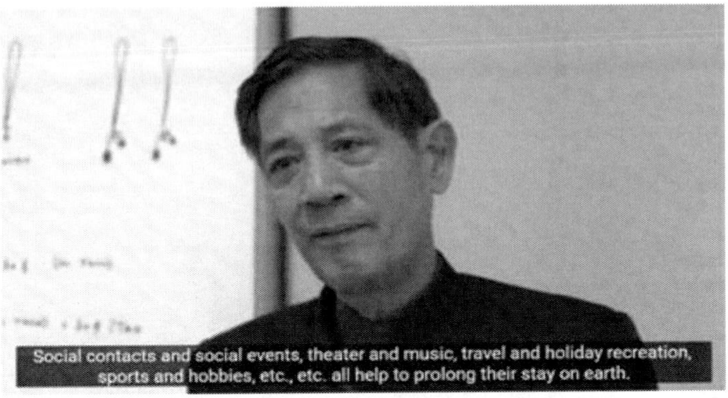
Social contacts and social events, theater and music, travel and holiday recreation, sports and hobbies, etc., etc. all help to prolong their stay on earth.

Figure 5. Bhakti tells us that the quarantine might shorten people's lives.

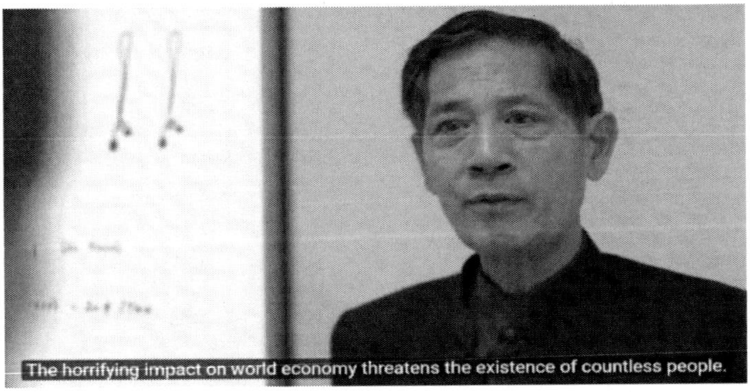
The horrifying impact on world economy threatens the existence of countless people.

Figure 6. Bhakti warns against the horrible consequences of damage on the world's economy.

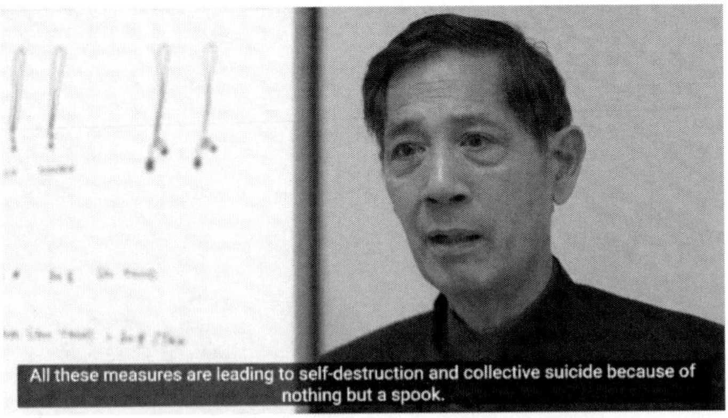

Figure 7. Bhakti calls the whole Corona pandemic hype a "spook".

BHAKDI'S ANALYSIS VIA AN INTERVIEW (10-15)

Interviewer: Professor Dr Sucharit Bhakdi, you are infectious disease specialist. You are one of the most highly cited medical research scientists of Germany. Today, we will talk about the Corona Virus. This virus spreads fear over the whole world. Also in Germany, a state of emergency imposes extreme restrictions. What are Corona viruses?

Bhakdi: These viruses co-exist with humans and animals around the globe. The viruses are the cause of very common, minor diseases of the respiratory tract. Very often, infections remain subclinical without symptoms. Severe courses occur almost exclusively in elderly patients with other underlying illnesses, in particular of lung and heart. Now, however, a new member is on stage spreading fear around the world.

Why? The new COVID-19 originated in China and spread rapidly. It appeared to be accompanied by an unexpectedly high number of deaths. Alarming reports followed from Northern Italy that concurred with the Chinese experience. It must, however, be pointed out that the large majority of other outbreaks in other parts of the world appeared to display lower apparent mortality rates and such high numbers of 4, 5 or 6% were not reached.

For example in South Korea the apparent mortality rate was 1%. Why "APPARENT" mortality rate? When patients concurrently have other illnesses, an infectious agent must not be held solely responsible for a lethal outcome. This happens for COVID-19, but such a conclusion is false and gives rise to the danger that other important factors are overlooked.

Different mortality rates may well be due to different local situations. For example, what does Northern Italy have in common with China? Answer: Horrific air pollution. The highest in the world. Northern Italy is the China of Europe. The lungs of inhabitants there have been chronically injured over decades and for this simple reason the situation may not be comparable to elsewhere.

What about Germany – the virus has also spread to us? Yes. It is spreading in Germany. One most important consequence being that we now have sufficient data to gauge the true danger of the virus in our country. Which is what the German experts and politicians have done. The highest alert level has been proclaimed and extreme preventive measures have been installed in the desperate attempt to retard spread of the virus.

Yes, and this is the incredible tragedy. Because all these adopted measures are actually senseless. Namely, the pressing questions are answered.

The first one: Does the virus generally cause more serious illness also in young people and kill patients who have no concurring illness? This would make them different from other everyday Corona viruses of the world. The answer is clearly: NO!

We have 10,000 infections reported (18 March 2020). 99.5% have no or only mild symptoms. Here, we already see that it is false and dangerous to talk about of 10,000 "patients"! They are not seriously ill. "Infection" is not identical with "disease". Of 10,000 infected people only 50-60 were severely ill. And 30 died to the present day. In 30 days.

So we have an apparent mortality rate of one COVID-19 positive case per day. Up to now. The looming worst case scenario that must be prevented according to the authorities: Then we would have 1,000,000 cases and maybe 3,000 death in 100 days.

This would mean 30 deaths a day. The aim is to prevent this "worst case scenario". All current emergency measures aim to slow down virus spread to save lives. Yes. But, we are looking already at the worst case scenario - with 30 deaths a day. 30 deaths a day may sound like very much. Keep in mind that every day, 2,200 over 65-year old depart from us, here in Germany. Keep in mind that many of these carry common Corona viruses. How many are not known, so let us just assume 1% (which is surely too low). This would translate to 22 a day. And these die every day.

The only difference is that we do not talk about "Corona-deaths". Because we know that these viruses are normally not the major cause of death. So, what we are doing in the moment is to prevent that these 22 are replaced by 30 COVID-19 positive patients. This is what is happening.

We are afraid, that 1,000,000 infections with the new virus will lead to 30 deaths a day over the next 100 days. But we do not realize that 20 or 30 or 40 or 100 patients positive for normal Corona viruses are already dying every day. To avoid that COVID-19 enters the scene instead of the other Corona viruses, extreme measures are installed.

Interviewer: So, what do you think about all these measures?

Bhakdi: They are grotesque, absurd and very dangerous. Our elderly citizens have every right to make efforts not to belong to the 2,200 that daily embark on their last journey. Social contacts and social events, theatre and music, travel and holiday recreation, sports and hobbies, etc., etc. all help to prolong their stay on earth. The life expectancy of millions is being shortened. The horrifying impact on world economy threatens the existence of countless people.

The consequences on medical care are profound. Already, services to patients who are in need are reduced, operations cancelled, practices empty, hospital personnel dwindling. All this will impact profoundly on our whole society.

I can only say: All these measures are leading to self-destruction and collective suicide because of nothing but a spook.

In a series of video-presentations Bhakdi elaborates on his viewpoints and bring further arguments (10-15).

JOHN PA IOANNIDIS (16)

John PA Ioannidis is professor of medicine and professor of epidemiology and population health, as well as professor by courtesy of biomedical data science at Stanford University School of Medicine, professor by courtesy of statistics at Stanford University School of Humanities and Sciences, and co-director of the Meta-Research Innovation Center at Stanford (METRICS) at Stanford University (see figure 8).

Born in New York City in 1965. He graduated in the top rank of his class at the University of Athens Medical School, then attended Harvard University for his medical residency in internal medicine. He did a fellowship at Tufts University for infectious disease. He was chairman at the Department of Hygiene and Epidemiology, University of Ioannina School of Medicine and adjunct professor at Tufts University School of

Medicine. He has also been President of the Society for Research Synthesis Methodology, and is one of the most-cited medical researchers.

Since 2010 Ioannidis is a Professor of Medicine, Health Research, Policy and Biomedical Data Science, at Stanford University School of Medicine and a Professor of Statistics at Stanford University School of Humanities and Sciences. He is director of the Stanford Prevention Research Center, and co-director, along with Steven N Goodman, of the Meta-Research Innovation Center at Stanford (METRICS). He is the editor-in-chief of the European Journal of Clinical Investigation. Ioannidis has received numerous awards and honorary titles and he is a member of the US National Academy of Medicine, of the European Academy of Sciences and Arts and an Einstein Fellow.

IOANNIDIS' VIDEOS AND WRITINGS (17-20)

We quote (17) in extenso: "The current coronavirus disease, Covid-19, has been called a once-in-a-century pandemic. But it may also be a once-in-a-century evidence fiasco.

At a time when everyone needs better information, from disease modellers and governments to people quarantined or just social distancing, we lack reliable evidence on how many people have been infected with SARS-CoV-2 or who continue to become infected. Better information is needed to guide decisions and actions of monumental significance and to monitor their impact.

Draconian countermeasures have been adopted in many countries. If the pandemic dissipates — either on its own or because of these measures — short-term extreme social distancing and lockdowns may be bearable. How long, though, should measures like these be continued if the pandemic churns across the globe unabated? How can policymakers tell if they are doing more good than harm?

The data collected so far on how many people are infected and how the epidemic is evolving are utterly unreliable. Given the limited testing to date, some deaths and probably the vast majority of infections due to SARS-CoV-2 are being missed. We do not know if we are failing to capture infections by a factor of three or 300. Three months after the outbreak emerged, most countries, including the US lack the ability to test a large number of people and no countries have reliable data on the prevalence of the virus in a representative random sample of the general population.

This evidence fiasco creates tremendous uncertainty about the risk of dying from Covid-19. Reported case fatality rates, like the official 3.4% rate from the World Health Organization, cause horror — and are meaningless. Patients who have been tested for SARS-CoV-2 are disproportionately those with severe symptoms and bad outcomes. As most health systems have limited testing capacity, selection bias may even worsen in the near future. Adding these extra sources of uncertainty, reasonable estimates for the case fatality ratio in the general US population vary from 0.05% to 1%.

That huge range markedly affects how severe the pandemic is and what should be done. A population-wide case fatality rate of 0.05% is lower than seasonal influenza. If that is the true rate, locking down the world with potentially tremendous social and financial consequences may be totally irrational. It's like an elephant being attacked by a house cat. Frustrated and trying to avoid the cat, the elephant accidentally jumps off a cliff and dies.

Could the Covid-19 case fatality rate be that low? No, some say, pointing to the high rate in elderly people. However, even some so-called mild or common-cold-type coronaviruses that have been known for decades can have case fatality rates as high as 8% when they infect elderly people in nursing homes. In fact, such "mild" coronaviruses infect tens of millions of people every year, and account for 3% to 11% of those hospitalized in the US with lower respiratory infections each winter.

These "mild" coronaviruses may be implicated in several thousands of deaths every year worldwide, though the vast majority of them are not documented with precise testing. Instead, they are lost as noise among 60 million deaths from various causes every year. Although successful surveillance systems have long existed for influenza, the disease is confirmed by a laboratory in a tiny minority of cases. In the US, for example, so far this season 1,073,976 specimens have been tested and 222,552 (20.7%) have tested positive for influenza. In the same period, the estimated number of influenza-like illnesses is between 36,000,000 and 51,000,000, with an estimated 22,000 to 55,000 flu deaths.

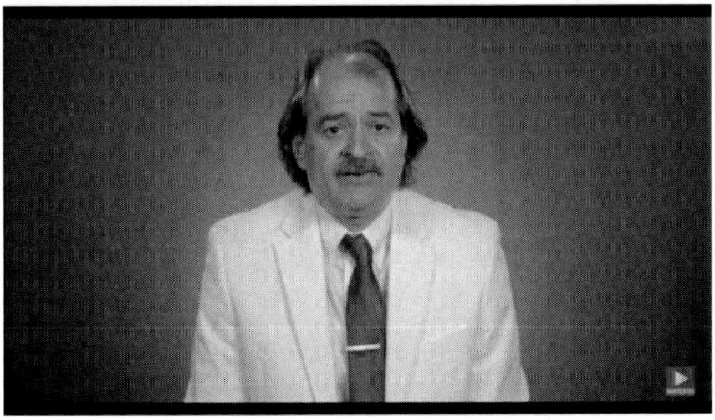

Figure 8. Professor Ioannidis from Stanford University speaks on the uncertainty around corona and the situation in Italy (19).

Note the uncertainty about influenza-like illness deaths: a 2.5-fold range, corresponding to tens of thousands of deaths. Every year, some of these deaths are due to influenza and some to other viruses, like common-cold coronaviruses.

In an autopsy series that tested for respiratory viruses in specimens from 57 elderly persons who died during the 2016 to 2017 influenza season, influenza viruses were detected in 18% of the specimens, while any kind of respiratory virus was found in 47%. In some people who die from viral respiratory pathogens, more than one virus is found upon autopsy and bacteria are often superimposed. A positive test for coronavirus does not mean necessarily that this virus is always primarily responsible for a patient's demise.

WHAT IS SCIENCE SAYING ABOUT CORONA COVID-19?

Coronaviruses are enveloped, positive single-stranded large RNA viruses that infect humans, but also a wide range of animals (79, 106). Coronaviruses were first described in 1966 by Tyrell and Bynoe, who cultivated the viruses from patients with common colds. Based on their morphology as spherical virions with a core shell and surface projections resembling a solar corona, they were termed coronaviruses (Latin: corona = crown). The genome size varies between 26 kb and 32 kb. The major four structural genes encode the nucleocapsid protein (N), the spike protein (S), a small membrane protein (SM) and the membrane glycoprotein (M) with an additional membrane glycoprotein (HE) occurring in the HCoV-OC43 and HKU1 beta-coronaviruses. SARS-CoV-2 is 96% identical at the whole-genome level to a bat coronavirus.

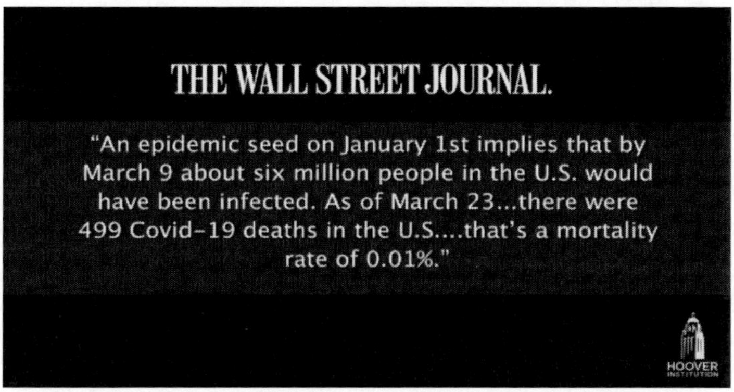

Figure 9. Slide from Professor of Medicine at Stanford University Jay Bhattacharya where he quotes his own article in the World Street Journal (22) presenting his conclusion that the Corona COVID-19 virus has a mortality rate of 0.01%.

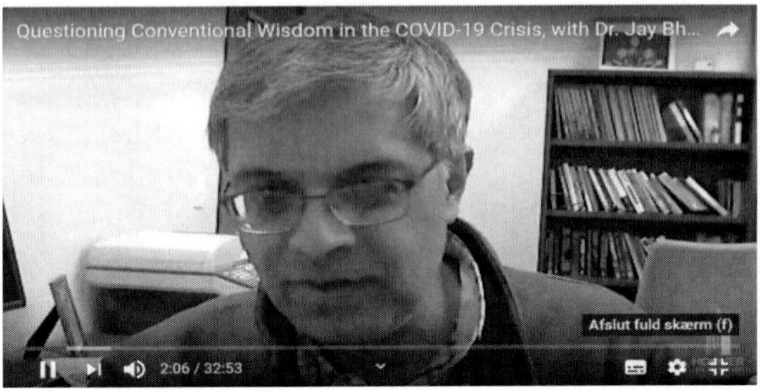

Figure 10. Professor of Medicine at Stanford University Jay Bhattacharya presents his conclusion that the Corona COVID-19 virus has a mortality rate of 0.01% (22).

We know from experience a lot about the danger and mortality of Corona virus, as it is one of the most common causes of the common cold. Very little is known on a scientific basis about the mortality of Corona virus, because no large-scale controlled studies have ever been made. A thorough review from 1974 by Monto (79) concludes that nobody ever died from a Corona virus infection. This is what every medical student in the world have learned until this day: The Corona virus is only dangerous for people with severely compromised immunity and a very poor health; and about 100 different, common viruses are dangerous for them.

A new study in the Lancet (80) concluded that Corona Covid-19 has a mortality of about 1%, but the study is model-based with a very low guess of the number of infected healthy people, and the number of dead patients are at the same time coming from the counting of already mortally ill patients, who also tested positive for Corona. So this study is suffering from exactly the same fundamental problems as Wodarg, Bhakdi and Ioannidis all are pointing out (1-22): it is based on statistics for the case mortality for Corona COVID-19 which is taken to be the mortality rate; how this article was published as a scientific study in the Lancet remains a deep mystery. When you look at the funding of this work, you see that WHO and Bill Gates Foundation are involved, raising the suspicion that this work is severely biased and not an objective scientific analysis of the Corona COVID-19 mortality. Unfortunately the publication of the study gives lay people reason to believe that Corona COVID-19 is dangerous, which add to the confusion.

New studies have showed us that at least 4 out of 5 Corona-infected people are asymptomatic (81), and that the asymptomatic carriers spread the Corona virus through micro-drops coming from normal breathing (82, 83).

PUBLIC DEBATE

Wolfgang Wodarg's position has been debated in Germany, i.e., in Der Spiegel (84), but here WHOs position and advices has just been repeated uncritically, while the documentation for the danger of the COVID-19 virus Wodarg has called for has not been provided - because it does not exist. Spiegel brought, instead of a serious debate about the important medical matters, an attack on Wodarg's person; he was indirectly associated with both Nazism and Satanism. We find no documented history of Wodarg being a believer of neither Nazism or Satan; how such strange accusations could appear in Der Spiegel remains a mystery, and this shows how emotional the debate is.

After Wodarg's whistleblowing, other experts in Germany and elsewhere have said the same. It is unknown if this is related to Wodarg's public appearance and the debate it has created. In Denmark, the former director of the National Board of Health Else Smith said to the newspaper Politiken: "There was and is no real health - professional basis for shutting down the entire country" (85).

Dr Else Smith is one of the leading experts on infectious diseases in Denmark and has worked with infectious medicine since the 1980s, preventing the spread of infectious diseases and managing epidemics, including at the National Serum Institute, where she worked with the HIV/AIDS epidemic. In 2009, she was in charge of managing the H1N1 Swine flu pandemic in Denmark. She is also an experienced leader in the health care sector with a good understanding of how things work. Smith stressed in Politiken March 15, 2020 that politics and not health-professional assessments closed Denmark down. In Politiken she explained it this way:

> Every two or three years, Denmark experiences a seasonal flu in which up to 1,500 people die. We accept that without much fuss and shutdowns, but it is precisely the same groups of people who are now at risk of infection and serious illness and death - the elderly, the debilitated, the chronically ill. The actions we take now, we could take every two to three years, which might protect many of these 1,500 citizens. But we don't," says Else Smith.
>
> For example, it is also voluntary if citizens of risk groups and health professionals can be vaccinated, she explains. After all, flu is just something you risk. Even though many weakened every year die.
>
> The National Board of Health has estimated that between 1,680 and 5,600 will die within the next 2-3 months of COVID-19. Depending on the spread of infection and the ability of hospitals to handle the most critically ill.
>
> Denmark shuts down in the biggest intervention ever in peacetime; people are fired, entire industries fear bankruptcy, the economy falters, so we come through a disease epidemic that at best kills as many particularly vulnerable citizens as it does with a generally more severe seasonal flu. At worst, three to four times as many.
>
> That's why I call it political. So there are also one, two, three ministers for each press conference. If it is purely health-related, you can ask what are they doing there?" she says.
>
> The spread of the infection is after the book…
>
> The question is whether this violent intervention in our society that can destroy our economy helps. After all, it's a virus that needs to strike a balance with us humans, and will probably end up as a seasonal virus of which we already have so many others," says Else Smith.

14 days after her public critique of the government's handling of the COVID-19 pandemics, she was forced to leave her job as vice director of the large Hvidovre Hospital (86), proving her point: The handling of the Corona pandemic is truly political. If you speak your opinion against the authorities in Denmark, where we have a public health care system and

where almost all doctors therefore are directly employed by the state, it has dire consequences.

This might be the reason for very few doctors engaging in the public debate in Denmark and other countries with nationalized health service. In spite of often sharing the opinion privately, that the political handling of the Corona COVID-19 pandemic is irrational because we are dealing with a Corona virus, which after all we know, is the same as the common cold, and therefore less dangerous than influenza, they chose to remain silent publicly (44).

QUESTIONS RAISED BY THE ANALYSES OF WODARG, BHAKDI AND IOANNIDIS OF THE CORONA COVID-19 PANDEMIC

The questions come in four series; the first is about the danger of the novel Corona COVID-19; the second series is about the psychosomatic nature of COVID-19 given the special social and psychological circumstances; the third is about the political actions taken during the pandemic; and the fourth series is about the political and economic interests, that could influence the circumstances around the Corona pandemic.

It might also be important to stress that the word “pandemic” in itself is not saying anything about the danger of the disease, only about the area it spreads in, namely a whole country or in the case of the Corona virus, the whole world. “Pandemic” which has become a negatively charged word in the public space does therefore not mean something bad; the word is frequently used about the common cold. The questions are meant to raise debate and encourage further investigation and analysis; we are in many cases not able to give final answers to the many questions.

Could it be that the new Corona Virus COVID-19 is just another common cold and not dangerous at all?

a. Is the Corona virus COVID-19 very dangerous, as the WHO says, or just another common cold, and not dangerous at all?
b. Is the Corona COVID-19 test valid, i.e., specific and precise? Has it been scientifically validated before use?
c. If the Corona COVID-19 statistics are made scientifically, and after the same formula, why are they so different from country to country? How are the new Corona statistics compared to the normal national monitoring of flu and common colds? How are they compared to the normal mortality statistics, are more people dying now that usually?
d. Can we trust the statistics on the Corona COVID-19 mortality? Who is counted as dead by Corona, and do we know the total number of infected people? Are we taking the *measured case fatality rate* to be the *Corona COVID-19 mortality rate*? If we do, why do we do so, when it is scientifically incorrect?
e. Do we stop thinking ourselves when we face the power of media and/or authorities? Or have we become weak, so we follow authority even when we know it is wrong?
f. If Corona COVID-19 is just the common cold, why are so few scientists and doctors saying this publicly?
g. Conclusion: Is the Corona COVID-19 infection more dangerous than a normal, harmless common cold?

Are we dealing with a brand new, unique and more dangerous Corona virus, or are the new clinical pictures we see everywhere a product of the rare and special circumstances where patients believe a common cold is a deadly new disease, and the whole society is panicking?

a. Is there a simple psychosomatic explanation for the unusual clinical picture sometimes with massive neurological symptoms, we see in some patients with Corona COVID-19 infection?

Could the actions taken to limit the spread of the infection in themselves be more harmful than the disease and even increase the Corona mortality?

a. Is it possible to prevent the spread of Corona virus, and is it desirable?
b. Do we need Corona infections to stay resistant to Corona virus?
c. What happens if people who do not need it go to the hospital? What happen with the patients who are not accepted to hospitals because the beds are reserved for Corona patients?
d. Is the media misleading us to believe that Corona is dangerous, thus creating strong fear in people of Corona COVID-19?
e. Are the political actions regarding the Corona COVID-19 pandemic taken on a scientific basis?
f. Could it be that the politicians enjoy their power too much, and like to play the role of the hero saving the voters, to an extent where the basic principles of freedom in our democracy are suspended?
g. If we harm the economy, how can we afford better health care?
h. How can we take care of the environment if we use all our resources to prevent that the very old and sick are dying?
i. Are the politicians making the wrong decisions when they are closing down our societies to prevent spread of the Corona COVID-19 infection?

Could it be that the Corona COVID-19 pandemic has been formed also by interests that potentially could benefit from the Corona COVID-19 virus being perceived as more harmful than it is?

a. Who has interests in "hyping" the Corona COVID-19 pandemic, and making it more dangerous than it is?
b. The pharmaceutical industry obviously benefit from the panic over the COVID-19 pandemic. Could it be that the pharmaceutical

companies have influenced how the mortality is measured and how the statistics are interpreted?

c. The World Health Organization (WHO) is guiding the world through the Corona COVID-19 pandemic but is WHO objective, neutral, and scientific, so we can trust the WHOs guidance?
d. We saw a misguidance in 2009 with the Swine Flu scandal where hundred countries were tricked to buy useless and unnecessary vaccines against a very mild influenza. Could the Corona COVID-19 alarm be just another Swine flu scandal?
e. The WHO has opened up to private companies for cooperation, and Linda and Bill Gates Foundation has invested billions of dollars in the WHO; can this affect how the WHO has been advising the world during the COVID-19 pandemic?
f. Do we have a New World Order, where the private companies have become so powerful that they have taken the lead in the world, and by that in practice ended the sovereignty of the national states, and thus democracy, as we know it?

Let us now take a close look at the questions that follows from the Whistle-blowers analyses. Could it be that the new Corona Virus COVID-19 is just another common cold, and not dangerous at all?

Is the Corona Virus COVID-19 very dangerous, as the WHO says, or just another common cold, and not dangerous at all? This is the most important question these days. We have looked into the background for the questions asked by Dr Wolfgang Wodarg (8): “How have you found out that the virus is dangerous?” (see figure 11) and we find it to be a relevant and valid question, justified by existing knowledge and science.

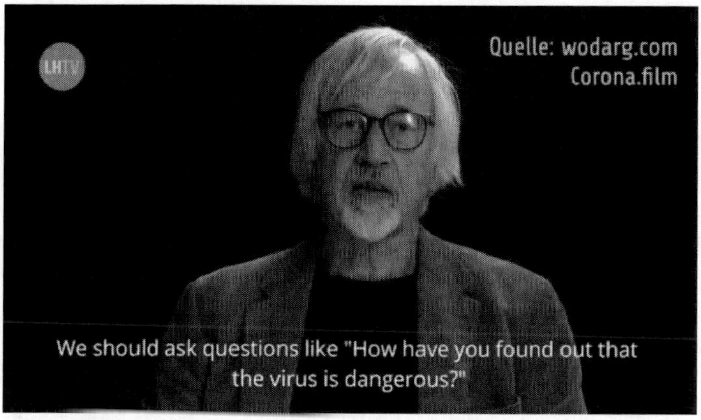
LHTV
Quelle: wodarg.com
Corona.film
We should ask questions like "How have you found out that the virus is dangerous?"

Figure 11. Wodarg asks the most fundamental question: How do we know that COVID-19 is dangerous? (8).

CORONA IS NOT NEW

The first thing Dr Wolfgang Wodarg emphasizes is that Corona viruses have been with us forever – it is one of the most common class of viruses causing the common cold - and it has been mutating and causing epidemics and pandemics every single year since the beginning of times. For the last 100 million years or so we must have had such viruses, which is why our mammal immune system has evolved; today all mammals are therefore able to tackle viruses like Corona viruses.

The coevolution of virus and immunological defence of the vulnerable mammal lung tissue has made viruses harmless to us if we are normally healthy; therefore, a common cold today is most often subclinical, i.e., not even experienced by the infected host of the virus. Many people do not even experience one cold or flu a year, in spite of getting and fighting infections by about 100 different viruses yearly.

In his presentation Wodarg shows the statistics from measurements in Glasgow (United Kingdom) where researchers yearly monitors the forest of about 100 different viruses that continuously mutates and infects us again and again, mostly without giving clinical symptoms. In his diagram (see figure 12) Corona viruses are marked with green; we see that a substantial part of the viruses that comes epidemically and pandemically every single year are Corona viruses.

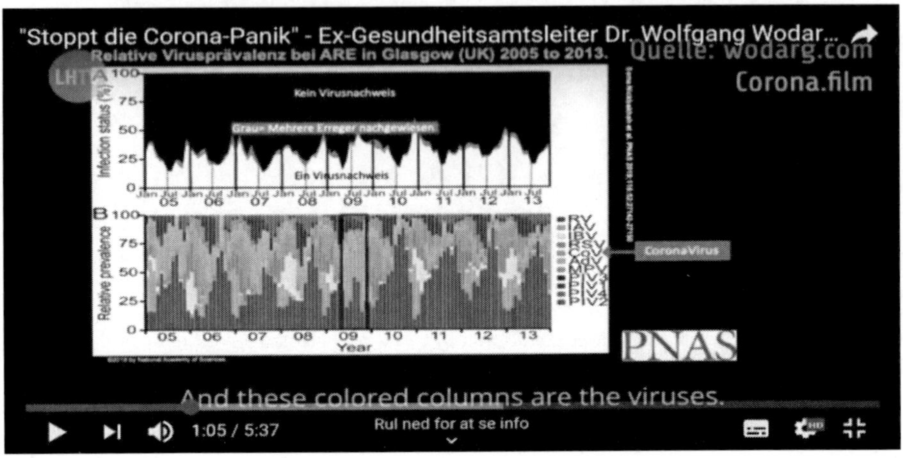

Figure 12. Every year we have a number of pandemics with Corona viruses (green); about 15% of all common colds are caused by Corona viruses (from Wodarg's presentation) (1).

Wodarg also points out that what we look at in the Covid-19 pandemic is a new way of measuring and following of the virus using a new kind of Corona test; we still also have all the normal indicators for colds and flues, including very reliable mortality statistics for the population.

While the statistics of the case mortality shows many people dying with Corona COVID-19 it is remarkable that the classical indicators DO NOT show any abnormal situation at all. Of course, you should look at these well-known indicators, which have been used for a long time, to estimate the true situation, because you here have the history, so you are able to tell what is actually happening. If you use a new and untested method, you do not know what is normal, so you are not able to interpret what you see, and this can easily lead to misinterpretation, overestimation of the danger, and unjustified panic. Also, the case mortality is not the Corona mortality, but only the mortality amongst the tested people who were already sick; and the count of people who died WITH Corona virus in their body is not the count of the people who died BY Corona virus infection, which is known from experience with Corona virus infection – the common cold - to be extremely rare. You simply do not die from a cold.

So when Dr Wolfgang Wodarg asks. "How have you find out that the Corona virus is dangerous?" This is a very good question. Because it should not be dangerous, after all we know about it, and after all we know about the pandemic.

Classical reviews on Corona virus also tell us that there never has been a single death from Corona virus (79), this is how harmless the common cold is normally considered to be. It must take some quite massive arguments to prove that there now exist a very harmful version of the Corona virus (87).

Of course, we need statistics on the mortality to prove it. However, the statistics we get these days are not designed to answer this question, according to Wodarg, Bhakdi and Ioannidis.

Is the Corona COVID-19 test valid? Specific and precise? Has it been scientifically validated before use?

What is new, according to Wodarg, is our ability to test for the Corona COVID-19 virus, thus making something that never has caught our attention before visible. The new Corona virus test has not been scientifically validated, and according to Wodarg there are big problems with the Corona test; many tested patients come out false-positive (they do not have it, but the test says they have), or false-negative (they have it but the test says they do not).

Up to 50% of everybody tested comes out as a false positive, says Wodarg. If this is true it means, that if you test the normal population, half would test positive even without having Corona COVID-19. This might be the reason for the WHO advice of only testing the very ill population. Furthermore, 15-50% of the tested people come out as false negative, depending of the test chosen (88). As the new Corona tests in use have not been scientifically validated, there are no good numbers for the errors of the tests yet (8).

It is likely that most of the Corona tests on the market react if you at some point had an infection with any of the Corona-virus in the sub-class of virus tested for. This means that the tests does not even test for the COVID-19 specifically; even with a positive test you could have one of the many other Corona viruses.

An educational case is the Cruise ship Diamond Princess, where 3,711 passengers were quarantined (mean age about 55 years) (18-21, 89). Between February 13-20, 2020, a total of 2,571 of those on board were tested, of which 460 were tested positive for coronavirus, but as many as 320 had no symptoms at all when the test was conducted. Ten of the passengers died. This happened in a closed environment where isolation of the sick passengers was impossible, because the staff visited everybody in their rooms and thus functioned as healthy virus-spreaders; at the same time a lot of tested infected, but false negative, people continued to spread the infection. In this situation it is not possible that only 460 became infected; most likely everybody on board got active Corona virus into their lungs from breathing small particles with Corona from the many healthy, but infected people. Everybody lived closely together and was breathing the same air for many weeks.

What we see here is, that the un-specific immune system (the line of immune cells like macrophages and Kupfer cells that does not need a molecular cue for acting) takes care of the micro-infection in most people (81, 82), so they do not become ill at all. These people had a Corona infection, but they did not have any symptoms, and they will not test positive on any known test, as they did not use antibodies, but cells to fight the disease. But they will most likely still acquire reinforced immunity to the Corona virus, as the information about the new virus is taken into the immune system for immunological learning, because the unspecific immune cells are presenting it for the immune system (90-93).

It is therefore very likely that the test has en additional error of 80% false negative, and that the true mortality for Corona COVID in the elderly population on Diamond Princess was 10/3711 = 0.27%, which is a much less than we see in a normal influenza.

If the Corona COVID-19 statistics are made scientifically, and after the same formula, why are they so different from country to country? Why are the new statistics on the Corona mortality so different from the normal national statistics monitoring of flues and colds? How are they compared to the normal mortality statistics - are more people dying now than usually?

In Italy, the statistics says that 7% of the Corona COVID-19 infected dies; in Germany, the statistics says that it is 0.3% of the infected that dies (26). Even the lowest number from Germany on 0.3% is many times the normal mortality for the common cold. So according to these statistics, we are haunted by the new Corona virus.

Here comes the next problem as Wodarg, Bhakdi, and Ioannidis all point out: If we only test the very sick and dying, and count every dead person with corona in his or her body as dead BY Corona COVID-19 virus and not WITH Corona virus, we artificially create a statistics that document the virus to be very dangerous and deadly. This is obviously what is happening all over the world, and this has been criticized by a series of leading researchers (20-22), also our three whistle blowers (1-19).

That these national statistics are very unreliable is easy to see from the differences in mortality in Italy and Germany – 7% of the Corona COVID-19 infected die in Italy, but only 0.3% of the infected dies in Germany. Of course, the same virus cannot be 20 times more dangerous in Italy than in Germany. Something is wrong here.

For about 10,000 people infected with Corona virus 100 experience a bad common cold, 10 go to the doctor or hospital with severe symptoms of infection. Of these 10, one dies. That is the normal statistic for the common cold. We do not have these numbers for COVID-19, but we have to assume that it is the case for this virus also, as this is the case for almost all Corona viruses. The people who cannot survive a common cold, or a flu which is much worse, are the very old, sick and therefore very weak people. Even in Italy the average age for the dead patients tested positive for Corona was 81 years old (8, 19).

Wodarg has compared the new WHO-guided COVID-19 statistics with the normal statistics for flu and common colds and found that the latter is showing a completely normal picture, while the WHO-guided statistics shows alarming figures (26). It is remarkable that nobody uses the classical measures, in a time, where we are desperate for good and reliable statistics.

We also have the normal death statistics and Wodarg has also here shown that the number of dead people are normal, not alarming in any way (2-8). Again, why is this important information not shared in the media, and used by the politicians in their decision-making - but only the alarming numbers from the WHO-guided, misinforming statistics. We refer to Wodarg's homepage (2) and to the videos of Bhakdi (10-15), and Ioannidis (18-20) for further documentation.

Can we trust the statistics on the Corona COVID-19 mortality? Who is counted as dead by Corona, and do we know the total number of infected people? Are we taking the measured case fatality rate to be the Corona COVID-19 mortality rate? If we do, why do we do so, when it is scientifically incorrect?

Professor Ioannidis from Stanford is one of the leading critiques of the way the statistic is made; according to him it is of vital importance to discriminate between patients dying WITH Corona virus, and patients dying BY Corona virus. As Corona virus is everywhere and in almost everybody, most people dies with Corona virus; but as Corona virus is known to be harmless, nobody really dies BY Corona virus.

If you test all dying or dead people, most deaths are not even closely related to a viral infection, i.e., Corona infection. In Denmark three deaths were counted as "Corona deaths" in the national statistics, but on scrutiny only one death had any relation to Corona at all (94). At the same time, we do not know the dark numbers, which might be very high, as Corona virus spreads very quickly in a population (83). The dark number is likely to be 10-100 times bigger than the number that comes from the sick and tested patients.

So to come from the official death numbers to relevant numbers for calculating mortality it is very likely that we must divide the number of deaths with 10. At the same time, and we must multiply the numbers of infected by a factor 10-100, to find the real number for the Corona COVID-19 mortality, as only the very sick are tested.

This gives an error of a factor 100 or more in the statistics the public is presented for every day in the media. Instead of a Corona mortality of 1% as the US government says, or 3.4% as the WHO says, the real mortality rate is probably 0.01% (1-22). The Corona COVID-19 virus is thus just another harmless virus out of about different 100 viruses that attack us in pandemics every single year.

Most of the countries follow the WHO's instructions for dealing with the Corona situation (95-97). The strategy where only the very sick are tested and all dead with corona infection are counted as "dead by Corona". Now we start to understand why we are getting these horrible statistics from almost all countries. When the mortality numbers are brought to the media without any critique, as the naked truth, people become terribly misinformed; and it is only natural that they get very scared. It seems to be a fatal error to publish these misleading statistics (1-12), and it creates the panic we see (see Figure 13) (98).

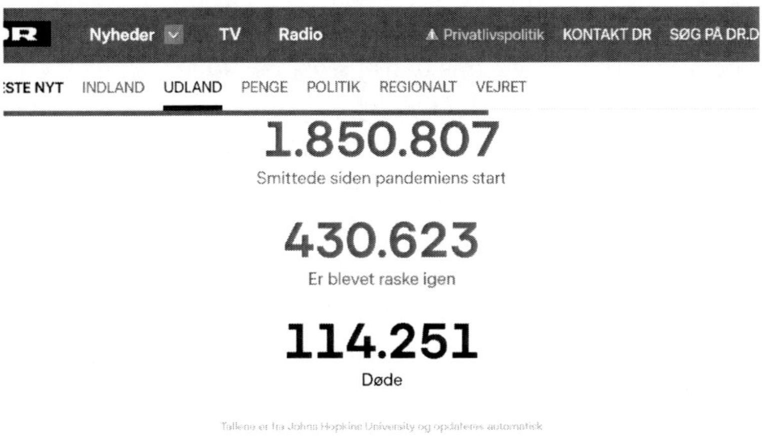

Figure 13. From the official webpage of the national Danish television (DR) April 15 2020. Obviously 6.17% of the COVID-19 infected are already dead and only 23% has recovered (13 April 2020). In truth, the number of people who has been infected in the world today is more likely several billions, and the number of patients dying BY Corona COVID-19, and not WITH Corona, is insignificantly small. Instead of bringing objective information, DR is misinforming the nation, creating panic overall. We see the media behaving this uncritical, irresponsible and senseless way in all European countries (98).

Do we stop thinking ourselves when we face the power of media and/or authorities? Or have we become weak, so we follow authority even when we know it is wrong?

The same desperate message is coming from everywhere – all media, every politician, every doctor, every single authority, even recently from the Danish Queen (99) blaming young people that they still meet and party, instead of sitting home alone.

Hippocrates said: "If you are not your own doctor you are a fool" (100). Because of our modern culture where we relay strongly on experts and outer authorities like doctors and little on ourselves, we have become easy victims of misinformation.

We also in Europe live in social democracies with a high degree of support and care for the individual citizens, and out of this comes naturally a strong faith in our politicians. We transfer much of the trust we have to our parents as small children to our politicians when we grow up. The media is often also seen as bringing the truth; both the reported data, which is often incorrect, and the conclusions, which often misfit the data, are taken to be true. The massive misinformation about the Corona COVID-19 coming from all the major media every single day, and at the same time from the politicians and national authorities, like the health system employees, the Police, and even the shop owners, creates a strong and reinforced belief that the Corona pandemic is mortally dangerous.

You can say that we are raised to trust, not to be critical. When we finally need to be critical, as in the case of COVID-19, we just follow and suspend our own rational judgment. Therefore, what is just a common cold, becomes the worst pandemic the world has ever seen. Remember that in 1920 with the Spanish flu, 1% died. When WHO says that the mortality of Corona COVID-19 is 3.4% (24), this is the worst pandemic the world has ever seen. How can we collectively just believe in such a thing?

We accept to close our societies down and give up on all civil rights. In most countries, there is almost no resistance to this madness, which comes with an enormous bill to us all, as pointed out by out three Whistle-Blowers (1-22). We have collectively become either pretty naïve so we have given up on knowing things and follow authorities blindly, or we have become so weak, that we follow outer authority in spite of knowing in ourselves what is right and rational. It is interesting that we blame people who blindly or out of fear follows outer authority when we are thinking of war-crimes, gang-crimes etc. Should we then not be eager to remove such weakness which is the root of these horrible things from our own culture?

If Corona COVID-19 is just the common cold, why are so few scientists and doctors saying this publicly?

The truth is that anybody with a scientific training knows that the statistics of mortality are made wrongly if you base it on case mortality; everybody trained in health sciences knows also that the Corona viruses are amongst the most common viruses giving us the common cold and that they are harmless. Nevertheless, few people with this background dare to speak openly about it; there is a strong resistance to speak against the public opinion, created by the scandal hungry media and the sadly misinformed politicians in cooperation.

Nevertheless, some people have the guts. March 15, 2020, as mentioned above, the former director of the Danish National Board of Health Else Smith said publicly, that "There was and is no real health - professional basis for shutting down the entire country" (85). March 29 she had to leave her job as hospital director for one of the biggest hospitals in the Copenhagen area (86). This shows the problem of free speech in Denmark, believed by many to be a well-functioning democracy. There is obviously no free speech for people employed in the public health care system during a pandemic; on the contrary, there is massive fear amongst the doctors – not for the Corona viruses - but for losing your job or other dire consequences if you speak you heart about what you know.

In Denmark Vibeke Manniche, MD, PhD has made a homepage under the headline "Hurrah – no signs of any dangerous Corona epidemic" (87), where she is questioning the statistics of the Corona COVID-19 mortality. She has suffered public humiliation for this in the national Danish TV (DR), because of a small calculation error she made, while nobody has acknowledged her brave contribution to the truth about Corona COVID-19 (101). Manniche reports (100) that many doctors write to her privately, that they believe that what is happening during the Corona pandemic is wrong. Hospital doctors complain that all the normal functions of the hospitals have been suspended, and all the beds are reserved for the Corona patients expected to come – except nobody is coming. The hospitals are empty, all functions have stopped; while the acute patients are suffering, maybe even dying, in their own homes.

Is the Corona COVID-19 infection more dangerous than a normal, harmless common cold?

In conclusion, the Corona COVID-19 virus is most likely less dangerous than a common influenza; Wodarg, Bhakdi and Ioannidis point at a mortality rate of 0.01% estimated from the data they have (1-22). We have no scientific reason to believe that Corona COVID-19 is dangerous at all; it is just the common cold made into a scary monster. All scientific knowledge seems to support the Whistle-Blowers common conclusion.

While Wodarg, Bhakdi and Ioannidis seems to be right, more and more experts line up with them, like Professor of Medicine at Stanford University Jay Bhattacharya who has engaged in the battle to make the world understand the simple, but fatal error that comes from *taking the measured case fatality rate to be identical with the corona mortality rate* (20-22) (see figures 9, 10). All these experts seems to agree that Corona COVID-19 is not dangerous; it is simply not a virus you can die from, if you are not very old and very sick or for other reasons having a severely compromised immunological function already.

If we look at the mortality rate around 0.01% this is 340 times less that WHOs estimate of 3.4% (24), and 100 times less than the 1% estimate of Anthony Fauci, the director of the US National Institute of Allergy and Infectious Diseases since 1984 (102).

A error of a factor 100 – two orders of magnitude - or even more is such a big error that it makes all the difference between a harmless common cold and a new fatal mutation that has come to wipe mankind off the planet. All our global troubles coming from the Corona COVID-19 pandemic, where more than three billion people have been quarantined or harmed in other ways, seem to come from the fact that neither politicians nor journalists have been able to understand this simple thing.

Are we dealing with a brand new, unique and more dangerous Corona COVID-19 virus?

We have created a world where many people in health matters are relying solely on medical experts, not on their own common sense and intuition; in this situation where the world is melting down in irrational fear of the global COVID-19 pandemic; we see the sad consequence of this development.

Could it be that all the trouble we these days face all over the world, with hundreds of thousands of people panicking and seeking doctors and hospital for their Corona infection, is actually caused by the conviction that they have a mortal viral infection? Can fear make you sick? Can social isolation weaken your immune system?

COVID-19 looks clinically like a brand new disease, a kind of virus we never have had before, attacking both body and brain at the same time. A general pattern in the new COVID-19 disease is according to these clinicians that the patients can feel very bad indeed; in some cases, COVID-19 may present as malaise, disorientation, or exhaustion (73, 74). They are also often difficult to get out of the ventilator. At the same time, the younger COVID-19 patients are known for using texts from the ventilators, something that the really sick patients never do. This brings us to our next question:

Is there a simple psychosomatic explanation for the unusual clinical picture sometimes with massive neurological symptoms, we see in some patients with Corona COVID-19 infection?

Imagine that you have a common cold, and that you know it is just a cold. What do you do? You stay home from work, seek a bed and find yourself a nice cup of chamomile tea and maybe a good book. You family will look after you, and you will be quite happy for a break in your busy life, to heal and get back to full health. Sometimes there is a cough, a running nose, fewer etc., which are annoying symptoms, but you have this coming every year, more or less, so you know the routine, and it is has never been a problem.

Now, image that you have the common cold, but *believe* that it is a new mutated, extremely dangerous virus with a mortality of 3.4%; and also imagine that you already from the media know all the bad symptoms of this new disease. Would you panic? Would you let your family take care of you? Would you seek a doctor? Would you be most happy to go to a hospital? Would you even experience all the symptoms you know this disease gives?

Of course, our perception of a disease - out experience of having a disease - is largely a product of what we know about the disease – of our *consciousness*. If we believe that it is a very dangerous new disease we have attracted, we behave very differently, and we experience the infection very differently. The common belief that COVID-19 is very dangerous makes people panic and seek medical attention. If the doctors also believe the new Corona virus is dangerous, they do a lot of testing, and isolates the patients, just to further increase the panic.

Everybody living in a city is every single day during the Corona COVID-19 pandemic massively hit by the (mis-)information that we face a life-threatening new virus; hundreds of times every day you are reminded of it. As we are psychophysical beings, there is a well-known psychosomatic component in all diseases. Can it enhance your symptoms and maybe even be dangerous to believe, that you have a deadly viral infection, while you only have the common cold? Yes it can (103-106).

Social isolation combined with fear of death is not healthy; we are socio-psycho-biological beings and therefore we have strong psychosomatic reactions. It must be expected, that there is a substantial contingency to the effect of the disease from the negative beliefs everybody shares about the COVID-19 virus. Psychosomatics could easily explain the damage we see, when the medical clinics and the hospitals are overflowed with sick patients. The instructions to the country's doctors that all COVID-19 patients should be carefully examined and treated thoroughly naturally also contributes to this. Psychosomatics could also explain the stronger symptoms we sometimes see in Corona COVID-19 than in the common cold: Many clinicians report that COVID-19 looks like a new disease. Anybody who has studied the emerging science of psycho-immunology/psychoneuroimmunology (107-112) will know that an innocent infection can manifest as a serious disease, if it is enhanced by strong fears and other negative emotions and beliefs.

In infection biology there are two known ways the psychosomatic impact can manifest; one way is that the experienced symptoms are enhanced (you could call it hysterical amplification); another way which might lead to increased mortality is that the immunological resistances is actually reduced, so an infection makes much more damage to the body. The weakening of the immune system has been found to correlate with stress (113).

Going to a hospital with a mortal disease can be compared to "detention in jail or other institution" and is given 63 point out of 100 possible on the Holmes-Rahe Life Stress Inventory (114). The impact is comparable to "divorce" (74 points), and "marital separation from mate" (65 points), and major personal injury or illness (53 points). Acute hospitalization for a patient, who believes COVID-19 is a mortal disease, is thus one of the most stressful events in life. In the inventory, you add your stressors to get your total stress-number. If you do that a Corona hospitalization with isolation from family and friends, this can add up to over 150. In the system, you then have 50% of risk for a major health breakdown with this level of stress (114).

The case of Prime Minister Boris Johnson of Great Britain is such a case where a common cold becomes a hospitalization (115). Johnson is send to the hospital by his own doctor, at a time where he is badly needed, and the hospital is taking him to the intensive care unit, because he is the prime minister, and because he feels bad. Here he gets oxygen. The news goes all around the world, that a healthy Boris Johnson got Corona, which sends him into intensive care. What actually happened? Nobody, especially not his own doctor, wanted to take responsibility, so Johnson was hospitalized - totally without reason. It was not an emergency hospitalization, but Johnson's doctor who thought it was best that he was admitted to take more tests. At the hospital you will be treated, especially if you feel bad. How could you not feel bad, if you are going to hospital with a viral infection, which you believe has a mortality of several percent?

The nocebo effect – the harmful effects of negative belief – is as well-known as the placebo effect in medicine. If you take an inert pill, but believe that it is a harmful drug, you will suffer the adverse effects you believe the drug has. Eight out of twenty had this reaction, and one out of twenty had it to such an extent that the patient in the experiment had to stop taking the chalk pill he was offered (116). Some people are more susceptible for self-suggestion, and they react more to nocebo. One out of 100 will have an extreme reaction. One out of 1,000 or 10,000 might even die. Do not underestimate nocebo, say the researchers working with it.

If you believe that you have a deadly virus, you will naturally panic and pay extreme attention to the symptoms, which enhance them maybe 2, 10 or 100 times, dependent on your personal tendency. Moreover, strong fear and strong symptoms of disease will force you to seek a doctor, and when the doctor is also scared believing in the mortality statistics, your fear is again boosted and the symptoms worsen; then you go to hospital. In the hospital you are treated as a person with a mortal infection and people are isolating you and looking after you dressed in space suits, scaring you even more, enhancing your symptoms even more, and by all that fear weakening you even more, so you in the end you might really die of what is truly a totally harmless virus. It is a kind of Voodoo. It really is. And yes, Voodoo also works, according to science (67).

The whole, modern area of psycho-immunology confirms the rationale behind psychosomatic medicine. It is well-known that fear, difficult emotions, and negative beliefs weakens our immune system and deteriorate our health (103-115), and the harmful effect of a negative psyche is much stronger that most people expect.

So yes, with the Corona COVID-19 panic, Corona has become a new disease with a new clinical picture, coloured strongly with neurological elements like confusion, fear and panic, disorientation, exhaustion and all kind of emotional reactions. It is still just the normal common cold, and virologically it is not more dangerous that normally; but a strong fear of death, the conviction that the end is near because you have attracted the most deadly virus ever seen in your country, provoked by social isolation, massive miss-information, and mass hysteria has turned it into a completely new experience. And knowing psycho-immunology, you might even be really sick from the Corona infection now. That is the biggest irony of it all.

Could the actions taken to limit the spread of the infection in themselves be more harmful than the disease and even increase the Corona mortality?

Extreme precautions like quarantines and lockdowns, the closure of airports and national borders, abandoning of work places, bans of public meetings, combined with strict emergency rules, precautions regarding the spread of infection, disinfection in shops and streets, etc. have severely compromised the quality of life of three billion people around the world.

Let's again consult Bhakdi's alarming (10-15):

> They [the measures taken] are grotesque, absurd and very dangerous. Our elderly citizens have every right to make efforts not to belong to the 2,200 that daily embark on their last journey. Social contacts and social events, theatre and music, travel and holiday recreation, sports and hobbies, etc., etc. all help to prolong their stay on earth. The life expectancy of millions is being shortened. The horrifying impact on world economy threatens the existence of countless people. The consequences on medical care are profound. Already, services to patients who are in need are reduced, operations cancelled, practices empty, hospital personnel dwindling. All this will impact profoundly on our whole society.

The actions and precautions taken worldwide these days have an impact on almost all parts of our society. Social interactions have been limited. In countries like Denmark public meetings in groups of more than 10 people have been forbidden; even the Danish Queen has asked people to stay at home (99). In many countries like the Czech Republic it is forbidden to leave your home without a good reason, and without a facemask. Similar emergency rules have only been seen in times of war.

The impact on the world's political systems, the global economy, the world's health, and the global environment is difficult to estimate, but experts from Financial Times and similar media believe it is enormous and devastating (118, 119). Let us have a look at the political actions and their consequences to find out if such political actions are justified, and what harm they might cause, justified or not.

Is it possible to prevent the spread of Corona virus and is it desirable?

A major reason for closing down countries, for closing borders and lockdowns, has been to avoid the impact of the COVID-19 virus by stopping the spread of the virus. More recently, in the realization of this being impossible, the intention has been to spread the mortal impact of the virus over time ("flatten the curve"), so the health systems at least could deal with the hundreds of thousands of dying people, the mortal Corona is predicted to cause. The whole political scenario builds on trust in the WHO´s prediction of 3.4% mortality for the Corona COVID-19.

But can you prevent Corona virus to spread? Clearly, you cannot. The small particles of 1 μm or less that come from normal breathing (82, 120) can infect you, so the safety distance is not the 1 or 2 meters, which go for infections carried by big droplets of 10-100 μm, but rather 10-100 meters. You cannot keep such distance in a city. Many people are wearing facemasks, but the question is if so small particles can be caught by a normal medical facemask; or if you need a military gasmask for that?

We have not been able to find scientific studies that prove that facemasks work on Corona virus spread. It is known from the 2002 and 2003 pandemics that health professionals who used the best medical masks on the market to protect themselves from SARS, got infected anyway (121), presumably because the masks cannot remove the infections micro-particles from the air. It does not help that it in practice is impossible to fit a facemask perfectly to the face; some percent of the air always go unfiltered into your lungs. You need a tight rubber fitting to avoid infection with Corona, like the ones used in military gasmasks.

If you look at the pores of the paper or fabric of a facemask, these are always much bigger (the best papers can filter down to 1-2 μm) than the very small micro-particles they are supposed to filter (0.01-4 μm particles coming from the opening and closing of the lung's alveoli) (120). A facemask filters well for bigger particles (98% of particles are removed for the air that goes through the mask), but only a few percent of the smaller particles are removed when particle size start to match the pore size of the paper or fabric.

Many countries have now laws that make it obligatory to wear facemasks outdoors; this effort seems judged on the data above to be without much effect. By far most of the people infecting us are healthy, infected people, who have no symptoms at all (79) - people who do not even notice that they are sick. This also means that the advice "Stay home if you are sick so you don't infect others" has little meaning. Based on these data we find it unlikely that it is possible to prevent a Corona virus from infecting every single person that lives in a city, where the Corona virus is flourishing.

There are about 100 known viruses that perform this pattern of infection and disease. To try to insulate us from getting them is simply impossible. Our immune system handle them well if we are normal and healthy persons, also if we are small children or old people; we even need these small and safe infections constantly to keep our immune system in good shape, as we will see below. Luckily, Corona is not, at least according to our Whistle-blowers, dangerous at all, so there is no reason to try to prevent anybody in getting the infection.

Do we need Corona infections to stay resistant to Corona virus?

It is believed amongst scientists in immunology, that we need regular infections with corona viruses to maintain your Corona-immunity, so infections stay subclinical (90-93). Becoming infected with Corona viruses is therefore healthy for us and not bad at all. It does not matter if you are one year old or 80 years old, you still need the infections to stay immune.

If you have serious diseases, like terminal cancer or acute coronary stenosis, a cold or a flu might be the cause that sends you to the other side. But then again, maybe this is for the best, because this is how Nature works (122). Known as "the father of modern medicine", Sir William Osler (1849-1919) appreciated the death caused by pneumonia and described it as "the old man's best friend" as death often occurs quickly and painlessly (123). Many old people wish to go, because their life has turned into suffering. Living does not make much sense anymore. The quality of life has gone low. In this case, it might be wise not to go against Nature.

What happens if people who do not need it go to the hospital? What happens to the patients who are not accepted to hospitals, because the beds are reserved for Corona patients?

The answer to the first question is a well-known. It is very dangerous to go to a hospital. The hospital infection you can get is often an infection with resistant bacteria, which is hard to treat, and the drugs you are likely to get have side effects, which can be serious; they can even increase mortality. 10-15% of all hospitalized people are getting an infection in the hospital, and the bacteria in hospitals are often resistant to antibiotics (124). Especially in Italy, Spain and the other countries where there have been big problems with the Corona COVID-19 virus, the hospital infections are frequent and often multi-resistant and therefore very dangerous (1-22). The treatment is broad-working antibiotics, which are known to be much more toxic that simple penicillin.

It is also very stressful to go to a hospital, and stress is known to weaken your immune system, making the infection you have more serious, see the discussion above. Fear is also not good for your health. So yes, it is very likely that massive hospitalization of the population with COVID-19 is increasing both morbidity and mortality. Everybody familiar with Ivan Illichs book "Medical nemesis" will smile when they read this. Because this is exactly Illichs point (77).

Is the media misleading us to believe that Corona is dangerous, thus creating strong fear in people of Corona COVID-19?

The media love scandals and sensations, and they have had a feast with the Corona COVID-19 pandemic. Instead of being cool and critical they have competed to bring the most bloody and terrible stories; they have not hesitate to communicate politicians warnings to the population about the mortal COVID-19 with 3.4% mortality rate, and have infused fear in their populations to such an extent that people with a common cold now want to see a doctor, and even want go to a hospital to feel safe.

Social phobia has exploded, and psychosomatic symptoms blossom. If you count the hours in the news and informative TV-programs on National TV in the European countries, you will find that few subject ever got so much – always negative - attention as the COVID-19 pandemic. Especially noteworthy is the media's agreement to deliver personal attacks on people like Wolfgang Wodarg who publicly have disagreed with the politicians and the WHO. Many people report censorship - it has been impossible to get through to the media with remarks that talked about being sensible, cool, and conservative. What happened to objectivity? What happened to independent thought and analysis?

Are the political actions regarding Corona taken on a scientific basis?

Wodarg, Bhakdi and Ioannidis are all very clear in their position here, and they share their viewpoint with many other researchers like Professor of Medicine at Stanford University Jay Bhattacharya: What is happening is irrational, it is political, it is definitely not based on science, as there is no reliable data to guide us. Actions not based on reason or common sense are irrational, and as such most likely harmful. When it comes to the question: "Is Corona COVID-19 dangerous?" there is no objective and scientific data to help us answer this question, as discussed above.

Now you could argue, that in that case it is better to be safe than sorry. But you can say that about all the 100 viruses that hits us all the time. You can say that about all new mutations of viruses.

There is a simple principle that rules both in science and in philosophy, Occam's razor (23): Suppose there are two explanations for an occurrence. In this case, the one that requires the smallest number of assumptions is usually correct. Another way of saying it is that the more assumptions you have to make, the more unlikely an explanation. In the case of the Corona danger, using Occam´s razor means that you need a good reason to believe that the new Corona COVID-19 is not just another common cold. If there is no such a reason, it is just the common cold.

Could it be that the politicians enjoy their power too much, and like to play the role of the hero saving the voters, to an extent where the basic principles of freedom in our democracy are suspended?

There is no doubt that many politicians enjoy their appearance in the media and especially the opportunity to appear as strong players saving the population from mortal danger. The politicians often have limited knowledge of science and biology, and therefore they are dependent on information they are getting from authorities in the field.

> Forcing millions of people to stay at home under pain of punishment is the road to Big Brother dominion. It's no accident that power-hungry Eurocrats were quick to follow the example set by China. And who drives panic more than the transnational World Health Organisation. If the H stood for Hysteria the shoe would fit equally well (119).

The WHO is often seen as the highest authority in health matters, in spite of the well-known fact that the WHO earlier has been unreliable, i.e., during the Swine Flu pandemic in 2009, and frequently has been criticized for corruption (27-70). Still, there is a feeling amongst politicians that if you refer to the WHO, nobody can really criticize you for it; you did what you should and could. If you rely on the WHO and believe in the dramatic statistics the WHO provides, showing a mortality rate of 3.4% for Corona COVID-19, then you better hurry to protect your nation!

The economy of our country, or the convenience and happiness of our people, cannot be more important than our people's lives. Everyone can understand that. So there they go, all the politicians act, and they also affirm each other in the position that these dramatic actions are the right thing to do. They even criticize countries like Sweden, which for a long time were not panicking and still keeps its borders open.

Can democracy survive massive abuse and political miss-guidance?

If it is true what Wodarg Bhakdi and Ioannidis say, that the politicians are making the failure of our life-time (17), will the truth, when it is finally realized by the people, weaken our trust in politicians to such a degree, that our democratic systems are falling apart (125-127)?

Can democracy survive dictatorial behaviour of governments that are not based in reason? Isn't there a fundamental conflict between democracy and top-ruling the way we see it these days all over the world, including in almost all European Countries? Isn't it too tempting for dictatorial tendencies in our politicians to use the argument of "public health" to control and regulate everybody's behaviour?

We are trying to prolong very old and very sick people's life a bit by preventing infections and making sure that there is space so they can be treated in a hospital - that is really what the whole thing is about now. Even if you believe that the Corona virus is dangerous for the elderly and the weak, is this worth losing our democracy for? Is it not too big prize to pay for the loss of personal freedom, the right to go to work and sustain our family, make meetings, and other democratic rights (125-127)?

Do we do serious harm to the economy?

Nearly three billion people around the globe under COVID-19 lockdowns as of March 26, 2020 (128). Analysts in Financial Times and similar places have warned against the severe negative impact of the political interventions following the Corona COVID-19 panic as the world's stock markets have reacted with a 20-25% drop (see figure 14) (118).

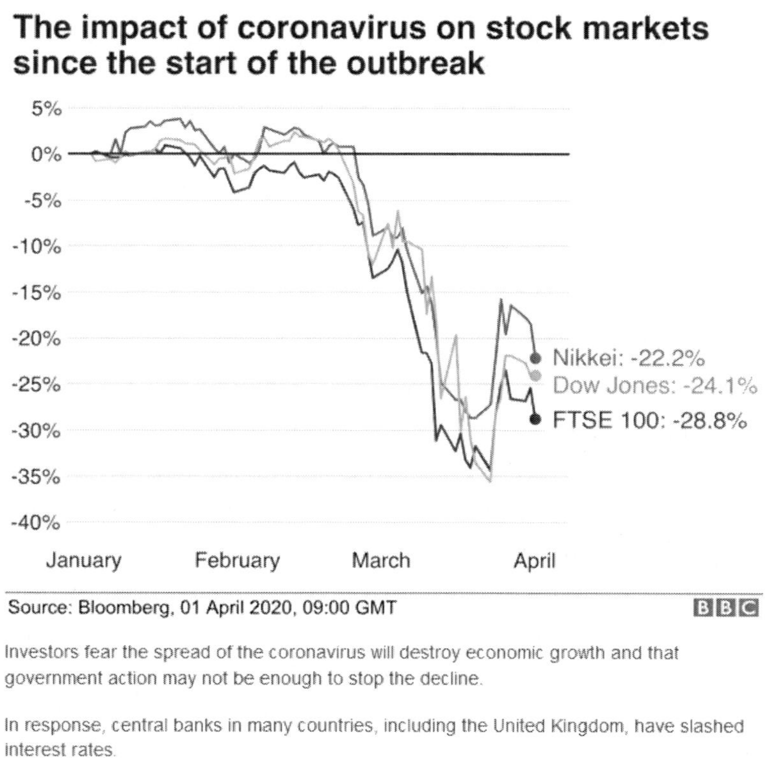

Figure 14. The international stock markets have reacted strongly to the COVID-19 pandemic (118).

The drastic measures used to prevent the WHO-predicted disaster of un-supported mass-death have called for massive critique by economists:

> "Policy makers and advisors have taken leave of their senses by forgetting that two elements make up the equation to understand the full impact of COVID-19. One element is the impact of the virus, the other, infinitely bigger, is the impact of the economic meltdown" (119)

If we need resources to take care of people, is it then wise to destroy the whole economy? If the Corona whistle-blowers are correct, all this is sadly unsubstantiated. The politicians of the world are committing the mistake of their lifetime. The blind – WHO – is leading the blind – our politicians.

How can we take care of the environment if we use all our resources to prevent that the very old and sick are dying?

During the last decades, we have seen a growing awareness of our fragile planet's need for care and support. Much attention has been given questions of sustainability, global warming etc. How can we take care of the global environment if we are investing this extreme amount of economic and social resources in protecting the oldest and weakest of our population?

It is also well-known that the chemical industries, amongst which the pharmaceutical industry is far the most powerful, are amongst the industries putting the biggest load on the environment (129). The willingness to put all our societies' resources into pharmaceutical medicine, as we see these days on a global level, are therefore a highly un-sustainable and regretful development.

Protecting the oldest and already mortally ill people from dying is the essence of what we are talking about in the Corona COVID-19 pandemic, as it is well-known that only this fraction of the population are troubled by Corona viruses. Again keep in mind that even in Italy, the most troubled by Corona COVID-19 of all nations, the average age of the dead with corona is still 81 years.

The willingness to sacrifice even the quality of life of people, personal freedom and democratic rights, just to prolong the life of the very sick, very old people a tiny bit, and the unwillingness to sacrifice even very little to save the planet's eco-system from future destruction and melt-down, is worth a deep thought. Why is the death of old, sick people a big problem to all politicians in the world, while the destruction of the whole humankind in a near future is not?

Our willingness to act with full throttle on a common cold, and our unwillingness to act on the obvious global climate- and nature problems are incomprehensible disproportional. Are the politicians making the wrong decisions when they are closing down our societies to prevent spread of the Corona COVID-19 infection?

In conclusion, what we face here is a global disaster, purely made by politicians, as pointed out by Wodarg, Bhakdi and Ioannidis. Based on no objective data, but mere rumours provided by the WHO, our politicians are sacrificing our whole culture, our democratic freedom, our economy, and thereby our ability to do something serious about the real problems of the world we collectively are facing.

Could it be that the Corona COVID-19 pandemic has been formed also by interests that potentially could benefit from the Corona COVID-19 virus being perceived as more harmful than it is?

This brings us to the final questions of why the Corona panic is happening. Facing a crisis on this global level naturally comes with many influential players and interests. Decisions these days do not only have local impact on single countries or communities, but can potentially impact a huge part of the world's population. Who are the players, global and local, that potentially could benefit from such a global crisis? Who has interests in "hyping" the Corona COVID-19 pandemic, and making it more dangerous than it is? This seems to be the most important question of all the questions, next to the question about the danger of COVID-19.

It is not an easy question to answer. The more you think about it, the harder it becomes. If you brainstorm, a number of people and organizations, states and companies, national and international, have interests. The simple answer, that the biggest interest lies with the most influential player in the Corona crisis, namely the WHO, is not necessarily true. Many interests may be bigger and more influential than the WHOs.

Governments and politicians could seek power; pharmaceutical industry and single players like Bill Gates could play a crucial rule. Even common people who would like to help, who would like to decide, lead and command, or who would like to escape reality and disappear into their own world, might find the pandemic a fine opportunity to realize their hidden dreams of a better live, by making a career out of the global tragedy.

It is still a good question, if the whistle-blowers are right, and COVID-19 actually is not more harmful than any other common cold, why would the WHO treat it like a dangerous pandemic with a mortal new virus? Could it be that the WHO has been misled by scientists who want to be important and get their research funded, as Wodarg supposes (8)? Or does the problem go deeper, so the WHO has its own interests in declaring such a disaster, as a privately funded organization with well-known strong bonds to the pharmaceutical industry that produces vaccines, tests, and medicine? Or is it true, what the most radical critiques have said for years: That the WHO is really run by the pharmaceutical companies, so the WHO functions like a giant marketing platform for the pharmaceutical industry?

The media also carries a big responsibility. In the competition for attention, scandals, catastrophes and emergencies are always welcome. Almost all big media have been playing along, creating a massive fear in the world's population. Small insignificant stories like a morgue in the Italian mountains running out of space, as it presumably does every other year due to the well-known under-capacity of the Italian public systems, has been the final proof for the world that we are facing a disaster worse than a nuclear war. The problem is that people through such small stories they can relate to are buying into the illusion that Corona COVID-19 is dangerous.

The most overlooked of all these factors seems to be *people's psychological needs* as mentioned above. About half the population suffers to some degrees from irrational fears and neurotic anxiety (130, 131). Our societies have never been safer for people; water has never been cleaner, food never better. Housing is great; work is safe, leisure activities plenty. So the fear and anxiety people feel are missing a reason. The "dangerous" Corona virus is giving people a reason to be as scared as they psychologically and existentially are.

Another psychological need is the need to help others and be of value. So many people have been helpful during the Corona pandemic; employees has taking care of the spacing between customers in lines in the shops, everybody has been responsible and avoided to infect each other by the use of hand-disinfections and facemasks etc. People have even been sewing facemasks to each other, when they were sold out in shops. In so many other ways, people have been considerate and helpful to each other, i.e., by not visiting the weak, sick, and elderly people. You can talk about the helper-egos of half the population being polished, and boosted by the Corona hype. Even people with a psychological need of being angry, has found something to be justified angry about. People with neurotic tendencies to isolate themselves, to be sad, to be disappointed, have found a good reason for doing so.

So the Corona pandemic has worldwide supported the egos of people and on an experiential level helped them out of difficult emotional and psychological problems. Of cause, the lock-down has also caused problems; countless families have been broken, and countless wife's and children battered; countless people have killed each other and even more have committed suicide, because of for example bankruptcies. Countless people have lost their jobs or at least a part of their income.

If you look at it with the understanding that Corona COVID-19 is just another common cold, you see the power of the social theatre, and understand the joy so many people feel by participating in it. Many people have built a completely new ego around the Corona pandemic. These people are the people that get angry if you tell them the wonderful news: that Corona COVID-19 is really harmless and just another common cold, and that our bodies have no problem at all handling it – unless we are 81 years old, and already dying from some serious disease.

Big Pharma

The pharmaceutical industry obviously benefit from the panic over the COVID-19 pandemic. Could it be that the pharmaceutical companies have influenced how the mortality is measured and how the statistics are interpreted? Could commercial interests from the pharmaceutical companies producing vaccines to the world influence the way the World Health Organization (WHO) operates, and the information, advises, and guidance the WHO gives to the world? Yes, it is possible, and it could explain how this whole Corona alarm and panic started.

The Cochrane movement, where thousands of doctors and researchers began to make new statistics of the good and bad effects of drugs, came from the understanding that interests make medical statistics unreliable (132-137). The stronger the interest, the less you can trust the data.

If there is money involved, you need to be especially sceptical. A medical statistic made by a provider or manufacturer of a drug or a vaccine is normally flawed and manipulated to such an extent that you cannot believe in the statistics (132-137). To answer this question about how big the influence of the pharma industry might be we need a deep exploration of the WHO, its peoples, the communication between internal organizations in the WHO, and with the industry and people related to the pharmaceutical industry. We need total transparency and full access to all communication in and with the WHO. The lack of openness has earlier made it difficult to investigate the WHO's processes (27-70).

The World Health Organization

The World Health Organization (WHO) is guiding the world through the Corona COVID-19 pandemic, but is WHO objective, neutral, and scientific, so we can trust the WHOs guidance? How come WHO is declaring a world catastrophe without having meaningful data to base such a declaration on? WHO is truly running with a rumour. It is just a make-up. It is pure abuse of authority.

We saw during the Swine flu pandemic in 2009 a very close bond between the WHO and the pharmaceutical companies; especially the companies producing vaccines (27-70). With such a bond, we need to be very careful when we need to interpret the information given to us by the WHO. We need to be sceptical and reluctant to follow the instructions for making the national statistics, i.e., regarding the danger and mortality of the Corona virus COVID-19. To judge the trustworthiness of the WHO we need to look carefully into WHOs earlier actions, especially in year 2009 during the Swine flu pandemic, and the changes in the WHO that has happened since then.

In 2010 a number of representatives from governments all over the world as well as a number of international organizations, i.e., the Council of Europe agreed that WHO had caused an international panic and disaster by declaring the mildest flu ever, the A/H1N1 "Swine flu" influenza, to be a pandemic threatening mankind. The Council of Europe pointed in a dire report to the problem of WHO going private as the true cause of all the trouble (28, 68). During 2010 the situation continued to develop and turned into a medical scandal of unknown proportions (27-70). Ineffective and dangerous medicines worth billions of dollars were sent for destruction. Close and secret links between the WHO and the pharmaceutical industry producing the vaccines was exposed. The Danish newspaper "Information" found that five researchers involving in advising WHO during the scandal had been paid around seven million EURO from the vaccine industry (27-70).

Unfortunately, it seems that the world's governments have forgotten what happened in 2009; there is little scepticism and often the results from the national statistics are presented as truth, both by the politicians and by the big media, who are loyal to the country, when intelligent criticism had been on its place. Why is WHO recommending the world to document the impact of Corona this way? Does the WHO want the Corona infection to look more dangerous and deadly than it is? The question is, could WHO have such an interest?

Again, knowing the close bond between the pharmaceutical industry and the WHO, it is easy to guess what is happening: A big scare of the world, to motivate every country in the world to by the pharmaceutical industries vaccines. So no, the WHO is not objective; its relations to the pharmaceutical industry and its sponsors has most likely biased it. We need a thorough investigation into this question to know what is happening.

We saw a misguidance in 2009 with the Swine flu scandal where many countries were tricked to buy useless and unnecessary vaccines against a very mild influenza. Could the Corona COVID-19 alarm is be just another Swine flu scandal? Many countries like Norway bought two portions per citizen. Nevertheless, these vaccines were never used and the government was fast to forget its mistake. For political reasons the WHO was not held responsible at that time. In addition, billions of dollars floated to the pharmaceutical industry.

Investigations in the years after 2009 into what then became known as the biggest WHO-scandal ever showed that the pharmaceutical industry was deeply involved in the WHO, and in so many ways had influenced WHOs behaviour (27-70). Wodarg said then: "The WHO's "false pandemic" flu campaign is one of the greatest medicine scandals of the century," and "The definition of an alarming pandemic must not be under the influence of drug-sellers" (37).

If you see what WHO suggest, as in the communique form April 13th, 2020, it seems obvious that the agenda is to sell vaccines against the common cold: "Our global connectedness means the risk of re-introduction and resurgence of COVID-19 will continue," WHO Director-General Tedros Adhanom Ghebreyesus told a virtual briefing from Geneva, stressing that "ultimately, the development and delivery of a safe and effective vaccine will be needed to fully interrupt transmission" (138). From all we know this is unnecessary, meaningless and, as all chemical medicine, also vaccines, have side-effects, also harmful.

What we face today might be exactly the same as we saw in 2009, just on a much larger scale, and much better planned. Again, the matter calls for thorough investigation.

The WHO has opened up to private companies for cooperation, and Linda and Bill Gates Foundation has invested billions of dollars in the WHO; can this affect how the WHO has been advising the world during the COVID-19 pandemic? Bill Gates says in a recent TV-interview (75) that he has invested billions of dollars in the vaccine industry and we know that he has also donated a billion dollars to the WHO.

The question this raises is if Bill Gates in seeing the WHO as a marketing platform for his vaccines. It might also be the other way round; that people use the fact that Gates' main area of expertise is computers and not biology to trick him with stories about "the dangerous virus" to invest his money in their industries. We know little about the lobbyism of these companies towards the WHO, but it is well-known that the pharmaceutical industry has thousands of lobbyists, of which many focused on governments and super-national health organizations like the WHO.

Is Bill Gates guilty of manipulating the WHO into creating a panic that will sell his vaccines? Or is Bill Gates just naive, and in good faith and will to help, exploited by the pharmaceutical industry? Do we see common interest between Gates and the industry, both perusing a big plan for honour and wealth? We all know the old saying that "The road to hell is paved with good intentions."

In accordance with this, the COVID-19 pandemic is followed by fundraising from the WHO, here from the WHO-calendar: "13 March 2020 COVID-19 Solidarity Response Fund launched to receive donations from private individuals, corporations and institutions" (139). As mentioned above, it might also be that the WHO is acting in its own interest of fundraising.

A New World Order?

Do we have a New World Order, where the private companies have become so powerful that they have taken the lead in the world, and by that in practice ended the sovereignty of the national states, and thus democracy, as we know it? If Wodarg, Bhakdi and Ioannidis are right and the whole Corona COVID-19 is a "hype", planted in the international society through the WHO by people and organizations with interests.

A natural suspicion given the Swine flu scandal is that it is the enormously large and powerful pharmaceutical companies, together with other global players, that is taking control over the world and its nations (27-70). With companies growing still bigger and being multinational, there comes a point where the power tips from being in the hand of national politician to being in the hand of the leaders of the world's big companies. If Wodarg, Bhakdi, and Ioannidis are right, we could have this new world order here, today and this is extremely problematic.

A central critique raised by amongst others the Danish professor and former director of the Nordic Cochrane Institute Peter Gøtzsche (which he created before he was fired because he opened his mouth) is that the pharmaceutical industry takes care of its own economic interest in unethical ways, manipulating research data, and often disregarding people's needs, and good business customs, as well as national and international laws (134-136).

Can we stop this development into a New World Order where money, and not people, rules? Can we avoid the world becoming one unit to such an extent, that it can be controlled and taken over by single organizations and companies or industrial complexes (like the medico-industrial complex where all doctors and all the big pharmaceutical companies are lining up together, driven by the unfathomable incomes from the complex)? Can we stop the development towards a politically and economically amalgamated world, under the command of the big companies, which seems to be where the world is going? Many questions and few answers.

Discussion

It is time to examine what we know for sure, and also to thoroughly examine the sources from where we know it. In our culture, we share a lot of information that takes the form of *beliefs* (82). We think science is true, but the basis for science is also beliefs. Even the basis for mathematics is beliefs, callcd axioms. They are sometimes useful, but they are never absolutely true. We cannot substitute our common sense, our sense of rationality and truth, our cool minds and direct seeing of the world, with scientific book knowledge. Much less can we do so, if the people writing the books and articles we read are paid to do what they do, say what they say, and think what they think. Beliefs are what our common reality is based on, our society and our culture, but beliefs are not true, they are still just beliefs.

Something that is obvious for anybody who spent some time in medical research is that anywhere there is big economic interests, there is manipulation, distortion of information, and erroneous interpretations; because it is simply too tempting for us human beings to go for the money instead of the truth. Very few companies run the world today and they become more powerful every day (141-143). One of the biggest and wealthiest industries today is the much criticized pharmaceutical industry (27-70, 132-137, 143).

We learned sadly that the pharmaceutical industry has taken control over the World Health Organization (WHO) during the 2009 Swine flu pandemic (27-70,). Wodarg said then: "The WHO's "false pandemic" flu campaign is one of the greatest medicine scandals of the century." He spoke his heart courageously. The commercial interest in vaccines are so strong, and the bonds between this pharmaceutical industry and the WHO so strong, that you cannot any longer trust the information that comes from the WHO regarding pandemics. Unfortunately WHO has been able to controls both the way national statistics on Corona mortality are made, and the way they are interpreted, which have led to massive misinformation about the Corona COVID-19 mortality. The WHO has said it is 3.4% of the infected that dies by Corona; the truth according to Wodarg, Bhakdi, and Ioannidis is that it is 0.01% of the infected people that dies, and these people are in average over 80 years old, and has at least one severe disease already, often two or three.

But the fake news that the Corona COVID-19 has a mortality rate of 3.4% has been spread by authorities to almost every single human being on planet Earth. The false statistics gives the impression that we are facing a fatal, new virus, a type of virus we need to fear, which easily could be the end of our culture. But, on the other hand our three whistle-blowers Wodarg, Bhakdi and Ioannidis tells us, that there is simply no data to back such a statement up (1-22). There is no scientific reason at all to believe in that mortality rate. The statistics are made in such a way that the Corona virus looks dangerous; it is manipulation. And we are falling for it, because we are naïve, uncritical and scared. We really should stop following the WHO's advices blindly, in the understanding that they are not objective, which now even President Trump has realized.

The infection with Corona virus is the same as the common cold; Corona virus have mutated every single year and created epidemics for maybe a million years, without ever threatening our life or existence. The COVID-19 is not different. But of course the clinical picture of a Corona infection is brand new, because for the first time in history people *believe* that a common cold can kill you. They seek doctors and hospitals, find themselves surrounded by catastrophe procedures and medics and paramedics in space suits; they are isolated from their family and friends; they are treated as if they had a diseases worse than Ebola. Of course, they feel bad. Therefore, they get treatments, like oxygen, tranquillizers, sleeping pills etc. They also often get hospital infections, as anybody else going to a hospital, and then they often get side effects from the strong drugs they take. Again, people believe that what they feel comes from the deadly infection they have attracted.

Of course, the clinical picture of the common cold is different under such circumstances! We are psychophysical beings and we have strong psychosomatic reactions to fear and negative beliefs, as science has clearly showed us the last four decades.

Are people dying? Yes of course; weak and old people, who are very sick already, might die a few weeks earlier if they get the Corona virus, than if they did not catch the common cold. That is the danger we are talking about here. That is what we are putting the world on the other end to avoid. Mass hysteria, mass psychosis, mass psychogenic illness, call it what you like, but this is what we are dealing with here.

The question that comes to mind in this situation is: How could the world go so mad? How can so many people suddenly believe in such a lie, in such a construction that is obviously serving the interests of pharmaceutical industry? Is it because it is at the same time serving the interest of the researches and their organization that needs funding, of the politicians in their need for power, and the media in their need for good stories? Maybe even the people of the Earth need some novelty, some change, some variation in a life that has been too boring, too eventless, and too predictable?

In addition, how could the most important question of our time, namely the question of global sustainability, suddenly be forgotten from one day to the other, just because a common cold is spreading, as it have done every year for millennia? We need to understand that our modern culture has become a collective dream; the content of this dream is provided by authorities, who speak to us through the media. In a way, we are collectively repeating our childhood, where we allowed our parent so tell us the truth about the world, and create our idea of reality. We never woke up, we never grew up, and we never found our independent eyes on the world.

In our hunger for comfort and a pain free, easy living, we have completely forgotten our inner compass of wisdom; we have lost our common sense, our feeling of what is true and what is not. The Corona COVID-19 story has taught us, that we affirm each other in our collective beliefs, and when we collectively act on these believes, they become even more solid. When our authorities make everybody act on these beliefs, they become established as *the highest truth*. History repeats itself. Wodarg tells us: The Emperor is naked! You and the whole world have been fooled. And you have been easy pray for the illusion somebody has wanted to create, to milk you and your country, exactly like the dumb emperor in Hans Christian Andersen's (1805-1885) famous story (140):

> So off went the Emperor in procession under his splendid canopy. Everyone in the streets and the windows said, "Oh, how fine are the Emperor's new clothes! Don't they fit him to perfection? And see his

long train!" Nobody would confess that he couldn't see anything, for that would prove him either unfit for his position, or a fool. No costume the Emperor had worn before was ever such a complete success.

But he hasn't got anything on," a little child said.

Did you ever hear such innocent prattle?" said its father. And one person whispered to another what the child had said, "He hasn't anything on. A child says he hasn't anything on."

"But he hasn't got anything on!" the whole town cried out at last.

The Emperor shivered, for he suspected they were right. But he thought, "This procession has got to go on." So he walked more proudly than ever, as his noblemen held high the train that wasn't there at all."

Information is always impure when there is interest. The stronger the interest, the bigger the impurity. Explore this old truth for yourself. Do not let the pharmaceutical industry, the WHO, and the politicians create a new world order together, based alone on your fear.

We just broke free of 1,000 years of slavery from the church and the feudal kings. Humankind stands today on the edge of a wonderful new time with democracy and spiritual freedom. Let us not again fall into slavery of ignorance and outer authority. The bill for the illusion we now share collectively is already immense; and if we do not break the spell, we will all be paying for the new world order for a long time to come.

CONCLUSION

"Forcing millions of people to stay at home under pain of punishment is the road to Big Brother dominion. It's no accident that power-hungry Eurocrats were quick to follow the example set by China. And who drives panic more than the transnational World Health Organisation. If the H stood for Hysteria the shoe would fit equally well." Apfel 2020 (119)

An important player in the COVID-19 pandemic is Bill Gates, who in a TED talk in 2015 (76) said: "When we were kids, the disaster we worried about most was a nuclear war. That's why we had a barrel down in our basement, filled with cans of food and water. When the nuclear attack came, we were supposed to go downstairs, hunker down, and eat out of that barrel. Today the greatest risk of global catastrophe doesn't look like this" (see Figure 15). "Instead, it looks like this something else" (as shown in figure 16). "If anything kills over 10 million people in the next few decades, it is most likely to be a highly infectious virus rather than a war. Not missiles, but microbes". Bill Gates has since invested billions of dollars in the vaccine industry, and at the same time supported the WHO with similar amounts (75).

We are during the Corona COVID-19 (SARS-CoV-2) pandemic facing a global disaster, which seemingly is caused by new deadly virus the whole world is trying to cope with after warning from the World Health Organization about a mortality of 3.4%. Three leading experts in infectious diseases, Wodarg, Bhakdi and Ioannidis are holding the position that we are misinterpreting the statistics and what we are facing is a misinformation campaign, not a dangerous new virus (1-22).

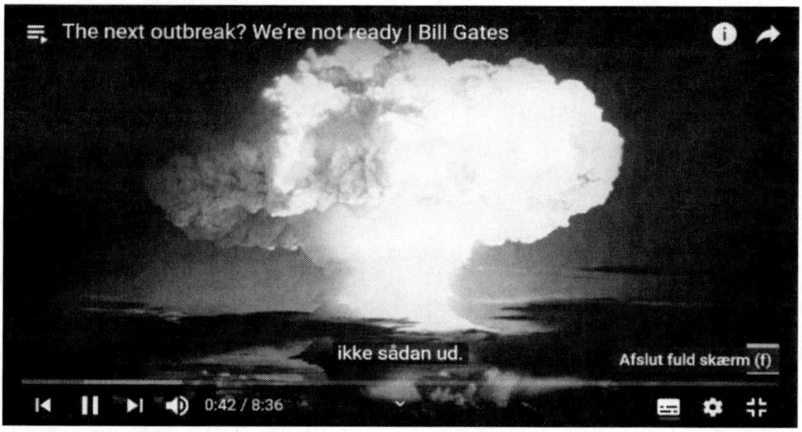

Figure 15. According to Bill Gates, this is no longer a serious threat to mankind: The Nuclear war.

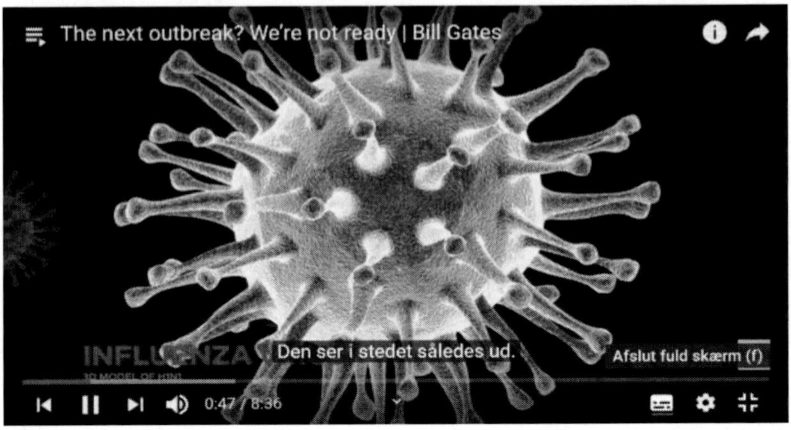

Figure 16. Instead, we must fear the Corona and the flu viruses… They are much more dangerous. However, this is not what scientists on the matter believe.

We have found the Whistle-Blowers statements to be true: The WHO is counting the death-by-Corona numbers wrongly using the *Corona case fatality rate* as the same as the *Corona mortality rate*; the WHO is counting "patients dead WITH Corona" for "patients dead BY Corona", and it is ignoring large dark numbers of COVID-19 infected people.

Furthermore, the WHO is ignoring all we already know about Corona viruses, and all the well-established traditional statistics on colds and flues, we have access to as well. The WHO is also ignoring the well-established and reliable statistics on mortality in the population, we also have access to, thus creating an image of a mortal pandemic, there according to science does not exist at all. *In short, the WHO is running with, or fabricating a rumour, a belief with no scientific basis.*

Unfortunately the politicians of the world has reacted to the WHO campaign as if it was true, creating massive fear in the population, that now has come to believe that we are facing a deathly new viral infection. Massive fear boosts the symptoms of Corona COVID-19 patients strongly in susceptible, suggestible individual, which happens for well-known psychosomatic reasons: If you believe you have a mortal infection, and everybody, including your own doctor and the hospital affirms you in this belief, it is only natural that you feel bad. If you feel bad at the hospital, you will get treated. Hospitalization, ventilators, and drugs give hospital infections, side effects, and increase mortality. In this way, the world has affirmed itself in the illusion of a mortal pandemic, which simply does not exist to begin with. The patients infected with Corona virus, who believe in the grim WHO mortality statistic, and therefore are convinced that they suffer from a mortal disease, present a clinical picture, not of a common cold, but of a new, much more serious disease.

If we take into account what we know scientifically about psychosomatics, there is little doubt that this new symptomatology is created by the panic of the society hitting the vulnerable patients hard; and not by the novel Corona COVID-19 (SARS-CoV-2) virus.

As there is no dangerous virus in the COVID-19 pandemic, we can all just go back to our normal way of living. The worldwide Corona mass-hysteria must end now. There is no reason to keep distance from anybody because of COVID-19 - it is not dangerous even for very old people, if they do not have a serious disease threatening their life already. There is no reason to avoid being infected. There is no way you can avoid getting the infection if you live in a city, but most likely you will not even notice it, as 99% or so of infections are subclinical. There is no reason for closed borders, and lock-downs, closed restaurants, workplaces, schools, etc. Getting the COVID-19 infection will strengthen your immune system, so you also will be immune to the next common cold you attract. Every healthy carrier spreads the harmless COVID-19 virus to countless other people through very small droplets (4-0.01m) we exhale. There is no reason for the use of facemasks, as a facemask cannot filter these small droplets. There is no way we can avoid getting the infection if we live in a city. There is therefore no reason for hygienic and antiseptic procedures to try to avoid COVID-19. There is no need for drugs or vaccines against COVID-19; a vaccine has adverse effects and a general, global vaccination program for the harmless COVID-19, which WHO has suggested, will not benefit but only harm countless people. The politicians and the media responsible for the unfortunate situation of the world must do their best to undo the damage they have caused, by uncritically believing in the World Health Organization (WHO) and following its advices. Common, immediate and strong efforts on a global scale must focus on avoiding lasting harm on the wellbeing of the people, the economy, and the culture of human relations.

Recommendations

The World Health Organizations (WHO) a decade ago opened up for private funding and sponsorships, which has made the cooperation between private companies and the WHO much closer. Unfortunately this has given us a WHO controlled by the wealthy and powerful players around WHO, as we have seen many examples of. One important example is the Swine flu scandal in 2009, another the fact that WHO during the last decade systematically has followed the industrial data for the drugs and vaccines in its recommendations, instead of independent studies of higher quality; now we see, at least according to our three whistle-blowers, another example of massive and systematic misinformation of the world on the Corona COVID-19 mortality rate, followed by recommendations of global vaccination for a totally harmless common cold.

We have seen a WHO that did not regret, or apologize, its actions after the corruption was documented in 2009 in the biggest scandal in WHOs history; neither saw we any change in WHOs behaviour or the way WHO was organized or structures as a consequence of the scandal. Most sadly, there has been little change in the level of secrecy WHO operates in, which makes it very difficult for the public, the media, and the member states to control WHO for corruption and other unethical and inappropriate behaviour, and most importantly, lack of scientific quality and scientific basis of actions and recommendations.

In the recommendation of pharmaceutical drugs, a scientific basis is especially important, as the patients will get the wrong pills; we have seen the WHO continue to recommend the use of many classes of drugs, which many Cochrane reviews have shown have no significant effect, but very significant and harmful side effect (137). Likewise, WHO's recommendation of Chloroquine and other drugs to treat and prevent

Corona COVID-19 is meaningless and dangerous, and without scientific foundation (2). According to Wodarg, the WHOs recommendation of the use of Chloroquine is likely to be followed in Africa, where it will cause massive harm to the population (2).

It seems to be a fact that the mortality rate of Corona virus COVID-19 (SARS-CoV-2) is not 3.4% as WHO has continued to say through the whole pandemic, but 0.01%, or a factor 340 less than the WHO says.

It is time to hold the WHO responsible for the global crisis its misinformation of the member states and the public has caused. There can be no doubt that WHO has out-played its role as a wise, global guide in health matters. President Trump has already seen the light and cancelled United States participation of the WHO budget.

We strongly recommend the member states to immediately close the World Health Organization (WHO), and make national advising boards in medicine with people well trained in scientific methodology, and strictly without any links to the pharmaceutical industry, and without any history of links to the pharmaceutical industry. When international efforts are needed in health areas, we recommend that ad-hoc committees are made with the leading scientists in the different fields; these committees should only exist until a problem is solved, and the issue for a committee should be narrow and well-defined. All communication should be public, and the economy of the project should be run by professionals with no interest in the matter at all, and with no connection to players with interest. Only in this way we can make sure that science and not money and politics rules.

It is important to stress that the role of the pharmaceutical companies in the Corona COVID-19 global crisis at this point is unknown. We recommend a thorough investigation into the WHO to see if we again have become victims to fraud and corruption by the pharmaceutical industry.

We furthermore suggest funding of psychosomatic and psycho-immunological research, as a better understanding of the connection between mind and body in infectious diseases would have made it easier to understand the nature of the global crisis at an earlier point in the Corona COVID-19 pandemic.

COVID-19 MORTALITY RATE BASED ON DATA FROM THE NORDIC COUNTRIES PER MARCH 15TH, 2020

The infection caused by the new Corona virus SARS-CoV-2 is the same as the common cold, and the mortality of COVID-19 is 0.01-0.03%, which is now known from Denmark, Sweden and Norway, where national statistics are reliable.

On March the 15th, 2020, we had enough data from Denmark, Norway and Sweden to make a significant and valid analysis of the mortality of the COVID-19, and we found the following for the Nordic Countries (see Table 1). There are 3,154 people who were tested and found positive for Corona; most of these people had severe symptoms and went therefore to a doctor or a hospital. From this we can estimate the real number of infected to 9,000-30,000. The official number of dead from the Corona virus in the three Nordic countries are nine, giving us a mortality of 0.03-0.01%. The average age of the dead was 82 years. We are facing the pattern of a common cold, and most common colds are actually corona viruses, so this fits.

But then there is the counting. We know from Denmark that out of the three dead, only one actually died where the corona virus could have been a co-factor; the other two died from unrelated courses (2). We suspect that they were included in the counting for political reasons. The same is most likely the case in Norway and Sweden, but we are unable to get the information about the dead people there. From what we do know, we suggest that the mortality is actually only 0.01-0.03%. We are thus talking about an infection that in the worst case course harm similar to a mild common cold. The calculations based on the given data gives us a final figure for COVID-19 mortality of 0.02-0.07%.

Table 1. The mortality of COVID-19 is 0.02-0.07% based on figures from the Nordic Countries (2)

Country	Number of infected, tested	Real number of infected (estimate)		Number of dead	Number of dead if you only include the people who actually died of corona infection	Average age, dead	Mortality as percent of infected	
	OBS: Only seriously ill are tested	Min	Max				% high	% low
Denmark	864	3000	10000	3	1*)	80,3	0,03	0,01
Sweden	1040	3000	10000	3	?	85 (?)	0,1	0,03
Norway	1250	3000	10000	3	?	80 (?)	0,1	0,03
The Nordic Countries	3154	9000	30000	9	?	81,77	0,077	0,023

However, as the data on the mortality is obviously not correct for Sweden and Norway, but likely to be at factor three too high the estimate for the mortality of Corona COVID-19 remains 0.01-0.03%.

The data from the Nordic countries shows that Corona Virus COVID-19 is not at all different from the seasonal common cold we have every year with a mortality of 0.01%-0.03% ($p = 0.05$), and is less dangerous than influenza. The Corona COVID-19 virus is just the common cold, and it is not more dangerous than it always has been.

The 18th of April 2020 we were able to check this result again using the national mortality statistics from Danmarks Statistik (Denmark's National Statistics), at a time where the national experts in Denmark agree that the pandemic is over and the country slowly is opening up again and ending its lock-down. The conclusion from the statisticians is that there is no over-death in Denmark for the first four month of 2020, where the pandemic spread in Denmark (71). This shows clearly that COVID-19 is a *common cold*, and not a mortally dangerous new virus, as the WHO for the last six month has insisted on, without having any scientific data to back this up. Now we have the data and now we know.

The precautions taken in Denmark have not been able to stop the spreading of the virus, and this was not the intention of the precautions; the predicted problems with a high number of people in respiratory problems overwhelming the hospitals never happened. There is therefore no possibility to explain the low mortality from the political actions taken regarding Corona; the reason nobody died from Corona is that it is not dangerous.

COVID-19 MORTALITY RATE BASED ON DATA FROM AUTOPSY STUDIES PER APRIL 28TH, 2020

Update 28-04-2020. Professor Klaus Püschel at the Universitätsklinikum Hamburger-Eppendorf has made autopsy on all corona positive patients dead in Hamburg, and found that not one single of these patients WITH COVID-19 died BY Corona COVID 19. From this, we can learn that the true mortality rate of Corona virus is less than one in 100,000, or ≤0.001%, which is even 10 times less than the whistle-blowers' estimate. The average age of the dead with Corona he did autopsy on were 80 years old, and they all had one or more severe diseases that could explain why they died. Therefore, it was not the Corona COVID-19 virus that killed them. Professor Püschel concludes that we have absolute no reason to fear that the virus will kill us (144). His findings are in accordance with a number of similar autopsy studies that now have come from many countries.

ACKNOWLEDGMENTS TO THE CORONA COVID-19 WHISTLE-BLOWERS

We want acknowledge the following 46 doctors and experts who during the 2019-2020 pandemic publicly have expressed, that they find the Corona COVID-19 mortality rate to be very low, around 0.01%, and much lower than the WHO's claimed mortality rate of 3.4%:

Dr. Bodo Schiffmann
Dr. David Katz
Dr. Else Smith
Dr. Gérard Krause

Dr. Heiko Schöning
Dr. Jaroslav Belsky
Dr. Jenö Ebert
Dr. Joel Kettner
Dr. Karl J Probs,
Dr. Leonard Coldwell
Dr. Mark Fiddike
Dr. med. Claus Köhnlein
Dr. Michael T Osterholm
Dr. MUDr. Martin Balík, Ph.D.
Dr. Peer Eifler
Dr. Shiva Ayyadurai
Dr. Vibeke Manniche
Dr. Wolfgang Wodarg
Dr. Yanis Roussel
MUDr. Jaroslav Svoboda
MUDr. Zdeněk Kalvach, CSc.
Prof. DDr. Martin Haditsch
Prof. Dr. Carsten Scheller
Prof. Dr. Jochen A Werner
Prof. Dr. John lonannidis
Prof. Dr. Matteo Bassetti
Prof. Dr. Pietro Vernazza
Prof. Dr. Stefan Hockertz
Prof. Dr. Sucharit Bhakdi
Prof. Dr. Yoram Lass
Prof. Erich Bendavid
Prof. Frank Ulrich Montgomery
Prof. Hendrik Streeck
Prof. Jay Bhattacharya
Prof. Karin Mölling
Prof. Klaus Püschel
Prof. Maria Rita Gismondo
Prof. MUDr. Cyril Höschl, DrSc.

Prof. MUDr. Jan Pirk, DrSc
Prof. MUDr. Jiří Neuwirth, CSc, MBA
Prof. MUDr. Jiřina Bartůňková, DrSc, MBA
Prof. MUDr. Julius Špičák, CSc
Prof. MUDr. Robert Lischke, PhD
Prof. MUDr. Tomáš Zima, DrSc, MBA
Prof. PaedDr. Pavel Kolář, PhD
Prof. Peter C Gøtzsche

This list of Corona Whistle-blowers is far from complete. We wish to express our deepest gratitude for their courage to speak openly against the authorities that have chosen to follow the WHO instead of the scientific experts, in a time where many who know do not dare to speak.

ACKNOWLEDGEMENTS

This chapter is an update of Ventegodt S, Merrick J. A tribute to the Corona virus COVID-19 (SARS-CoV-2) whistle-blowers. J Altern Med Res 2020;12(2), in print.

REFERENCES

[1] Wodarg W. Wikipedia. URL: https://en.wikipedia.org/wiki/Wolfgang_Wodarg.
[2] Wodarg W. Home page. URL: https://www.wodarg.com/.
[3] Frontal21 ZDF. [Lungenfacharzt Wolfgang Wodarg spricht jetzt LIVE über die Auswirkungen des Corona Virus]. Frontal21 2020 Mar 10. URL: https://www.youtube.com/watch?v=hW4qzAPP5pU. [German] [Pulmonologist Wolfgang Wodarg now speaks LIVE about the effects of the corona virus]
[4] Frontal21 ZDF. [Coronavirus - nicht schlimmer als eine "schwere Grippewelle"?] 2020 Mar 10. URL: https://www.youtube.com/watch?v=7_uKN9vdigE. [German] [Coronavirus - not worse than a "severe flu wave"?]

[5] Rubikon. [Dr. Wolfgang Wodarg zur Corona-Krise (Ostern 2020)] 2020 April 13. URL: https://www.youtube.com/watch?v=bZcG_7k4LaM. [German] [Dr. Wolfgang Wodarg on the corona crisis (Easter 2020)]
[6] Radio München. [Covid 19 - Test ist unspezifisch - Dr. Wolfgang Wodarg.] 2020 Mar 27. URL: https://soundcloud.com/radiomuenchen/covid-19-test-testet-alle-corona-viren-dr-wolfgang-wodarg. [German] [Covid 19 - test is unspecific - Dr. Wolfgang Wodarg]
[7] Frontal 21 ZDF. [Coronavirus - nicht schlimmer als eine "schwere Grippewelle – Faktencheck] 2020 Apr 09. URL: https://www.youtube.com/watch?v=cmoh BuUvsLE. [German] [Coronavirus - no worse than a "severe flu wave" fact check]
[8] LokalHeute TV. [Stoppt die Corona-Panik" - Ex-Gesundheitsamtsleiter Dr. Wolfgang Wodarg]. Interview, Dockumentation. 2020 Mar 17. URL: https://m youtube.com/watch?v=XnlT3rPNUp0. [German] [Stop the Corona Panic "- Ex-Health Director Dr. Wolfgang Wodarg]
[9] Wikipedia. Professor Dr Sucharit Bhakdi. URL: https://de.wikipedia.org/ wiki/Sucharit_Bhakdi.
[10] Bhakdi S. CV-9Teen. Open letter from Professor Sucharit Bhakdi to German Chancellor Angela Merkel 2020 Mar 29. URL: https://www.youtube.com/ watch?v=CGCJEBh80gg&app=desktop.
[11] Bhakdi S. Youtube channel. URL: https://www.youtube.com/channel/UCgjx QLDkeoa-uJu4sE0eNrg.
[12] Bhakdi S. [Corona-Krise: Offener Brief an die Bundeskanzlerin von Prof. Sucharit Bhakdi 2020 Mar 29]. URL: https://www.youtube.com/watch?v=LsEx PrHCHbw. [German] [Corona crisis: Open letter to the Federal Chancellor from Prof. Sucharit Bhakdi]
[13] Bhakdi S. [Corona-Krise: Professor Sucharit Bhakdi erklärt warum die Maßnahmen sinnlos und selbstzerstörerisch sind 2020 Mar 19]. URL: https://www.youtube.com/ watch?v=JBB9bA-gXL4. [German] [Corona crisis: Professor Sucharit Bhakdi explains why the measures are senseless and self-destructive 2020 Mar 19]
[14] Bhakdi S. [Sucharit Bhakdi - Corona-Nachtrag 1: Belastbarkeit des Gesundheitssystems 2020 Mar 22]. URL: https://www.youtube.com/watch?v= lJEJBKiBVlA. [German] [Sucharit Bhakdi - Corona addendum 1: Resilience of the health system]
[15] Bhakdi S. [Sucharit Bhakdi - Corona-Krise Nachtrag 2 - Schreckensszenario Italien 2020 Mar 22]. URL: https://www.youtube.com/watch?v=MARVdS-pHdQ. [German] [Sucharit Bhakdi - Corona Crisis Addendum 2 - Dread Scenario Italy]
[16] Wikipedia. John Ioannidis. URL: https://en. wikipedia.org/wiki/John_Ioannidis.
[17] Ioannidis JPA. A fiasco in the making? As the coronavirus pandemic takes hold, we are making decisions without reliable data, 2020 Mar 17. URL: https://www. statnews.com/2020/03/17/a-fiasco-in-the-making-as-the-coronavirus-pandemic-takes-hold-we-are-making-decisions-without-reliable-data/.

[18] Ioannidis JPA. Perspectives on the pandemic, Episode 1, 2020 Mar 26. URL: https://www.youtube. com/watch?v=d6MZy-2fcBw.

[19] Ovalmedia. Professor Ioannidis from Stanford University on the uncertainty around corona and the situation in Italy, 2020 Apr 03. URL: https://www.youtube. com/watch?v=NPtwcbWUg2I.

[20] Ioannidis J. Dr Ioannidis on why we don't have reliable data surrounding COVID-19, 2020 Apr 03. URL: https://www.youtube.com/watch?v=QUvWaxuurzQ.

[21] Hoover Institute. Questioning conventional wisdom in the COVID-19 crisis, with Dr. Jay Bhattacharya 2020 Mar 31. URL: https://www.youtube.com/watch?v=-UO3Wd5urg0.

[22] Bendavid E, Bhattacharya J. Is the Coronavirus as deadly as they say? Current estimates about the Covid-19 fatality rate may be too high by orders of magnitude. Wall Street Journal 2020 Mar 24. URL: https://www.wsj.com/articles/is-the-coronavirus-as-deadly-as-they-say-11585088464.

[23] Use Occam's razor to keep it simple. The English Farm 2019 Aug 10. URL: https://theenglishfarm.com/blog/use-occams-razor-keep-it-simple.

[24] Lovelae Jr B, Higgins-Dunn N. WHO says coronavirus death rate is 3.4% globally, higher than previously thought. CNBC 2020 Mar 03. URL: https://www.cnbc.com/ 2020/03/03/who-says-coronavirus-death-rate-is-3point4percent-globally-higher-than-previously-thought.html.

[25] Ducharme J, Wolfson E. The WHO estimated COVID-19 mortality at 3.4%. That doesn't tell the whole story. Time 2020 Mar 09. URL: https://time.com/ 5798168/coronavirus-mortality-rate/.

[26] The Editor. Overview - the days numbers and the most important news on the Corona virus. [lynoverblik-dagens-tal-og-vigtigste-nyheder-om-coronavirus]. Sundhedspolitisk Tidsskr 2020 Mar 15. URL: https://sundhedspolitisktidsskrift. dk/nyheder/3073-lynoverblik-dagens-tal-og-vigtigste-nyheder-om-coronavirus.html.

[27] Wodarg W, Baselga AF, Ayva L, Conde BA, Czinege IFP, Grozdanova D, et al. Faked pandemics - a threat for health (PDF). Parliamentary Assembly of the Council of Europe, 2009 Dec 18.

[28] Wodarg W. Faked pandemics, a threat to health. PACE Plenary session social affairs Council of Europe to investigate WHO. Council of Europe 2010 Jan 25-29.

[29] Stoer J. Stop funding WHO until it cleans up its act. Natl Rev 2017 Jun14. URL: https://www.nationalreview.com/2017/06/world-health-organization-corrupt-wasteful/.

[30] WHO swine flu experts 'linked' with drug companies. BBC 2010 Jun 04. URL: https://www.bbc.com/news/10235558.

[31] Bethge P, Elger K, Glüsing J, Grill M, Hachenbroch V, Puhl J, et al. Reconstruction of a mass hysteria: The Swine flu panic of 2009. Der Spiegel Part 1 2010.

[32] Bethge P, Elger K, Glüsing J, Grill M, Hachenbroch V, Puhl J, et al. Reconstruction of a mass hysteria: The Swine flu panic of 2009. Der Spiegel Part 2 2010.

[33] Ramesh R. Report condemns swine flu experts' ties to big pharma. The Guardian 2010.

[34] Ventegodt S. Why the Corruption of the World Health Organization (WHO) is the biggest threat to the World's public health of our time. J Integrative Med Ther 2015;2(1):5.

[35] Franck L. Trust WHO. Oval Media Film 2018.

[36] A message from Oval Media, producers of trust WHO: Trust WHO filmmakers respond to Vimeo censorship, 2020 Apr 17. URL: https://www.youtube.com/watch?v=VjQGyqVN5RM.

[37] Taylor L. EU to probe pharma over "false pandemic". PharmaTimes Online 2010 Jan 04. URL: http://www.pharmatimes.com/news/eu_to_probe_pharma_over_false_pandemic 982876.

[38] Braillon A. The World Health Organization: No game of thrones. BMJ 2014;348:g4265. URL: https://www. bmj.com/content/348/bmj.g4265/rr/703675.

[39] Cohen D, Carter P. Conflicts of interest- WHO and the pandemic flu "conspiracies". BMJ 2010;340:c2912. URL: https://www.bmj.com/content/340/bmj.c2912.

[40] Cohen D, Carter P. WHO and the pandemic flu "conspiracies". BMJ 2010;340:c2912.

[41] Doshi P, Jefferson T. WHO and pandemic flu. Another question for GSK. BMJ 2010;340:c3455. URL: https://www.bmj.com/content/340/bmj.c3455.full.

[42] Jefferson T, Doshi P. Multisystem failure: the story of anti-influenza drugs. Recenti Prog Med 2014;105:187-90.

[43] Jefferson T, Doshi P. WHO and pandemic flu. Time for change, WHO. BMJ 2010;340: c3461. URL: https://www.bmj.com/content/340/bmj.c3461.

[44] Law R. WHO and pandemic flu. There was also no new subtype. BMJ 2010;340:c3460. URL: https://www.bmj.com/content/340/bmj.c3460.long.

[45] Payne D. Tamiflu: The battle for secret drug data. BMJ 2012;345:e7303 URL: https://www.bmj.com/content/345/bmj.e7303.long.

[46] Watson R. WHO is accused of "crying wolf" over swine flu pandemic. BMJ 2010;340: c1904. URL: https://www.bmj.com/content/340/bmj.c1904.long.

[47] Zarocostas J. Swine flu pandemic review panel seeks access to confidential documents between WHO and drug companies. BMJ 2010;340: c2792. URL: https://www.bmj.com/content/340/bmj.c2792.long.

[48] Neale T. World Health Organization scientists linked to swine flu vaccine makers. ABC News 2010. URL: https://abcnews.go.com/Health/SwineFlu/swine-flu-pandemic-world-health-organization-scientists-linked/story?id=10829940.

[49] Way opened for Pandemrix swine flu jab compensation. BBC 2013. URL: https://www.bbc.com/news/health-24172715.

[50] Holder R, Loertscher S, Rohner D. Biased experts, costly lies, and binary decisions. SSRN 2010. URL: https://papers.ssrn.com/sol3/papers.cfm?abstract_id=1639351.

[51] Walsh F. WHO swine flu experts 'linked' with drug companies. BBC 2010. URL: https://www.bbc.com/news/10235558.

[52] Cohen D, Carter P. WHO and the pandemic flu "conspiracies". BMJ 2010;340:c2912. URL: https://www.researchgate.net/publication/232266547_WHO_and_the_pandemic_flu_conspiracies.

[53] MB. Australian journalist wins prestigious award for exposing flu vaccine scandal. The Refusers 2011. URL: http://nhne-pulse.org/australian-journalist-wins-prestigious-award-for-exposing-flu-vaccine-scandal/.

[54] Edwards T. Big pharma probed for 'false' swine flu pandemic 2010.

[55] Fletcher V. Swine flu scandal: Billions of pounds are wasted on vaccines. Express 2010. URL: https://www.express.co.uk/news/uk/156359/Swine-flu-scandal-Billions-of-pounds-are-wasted-on-vaccines.

[56] Galushko I. The reality behind the swine flu conspiracy. RT 2009. URL: https://www.rt.com/russia/reality-swine-flu-conspiracy/.

[57] Voller L. Can we trust WHO? [Tør vi stole på WHO?]. Information 2009. URL: https://www.information.dk/debat/leder/2009/12/toer-stole-paa-who.

[58] Mercola J. Major victory with swine flu scandal. Infowars 2009. Retrieved 2020-04-18 from https://www.infowars.com/major-victory-with-swine-flu-scandal/.

[59] Rappoport J. A new giant vaccine scandal exposes government lies and psyops. Jon Rappoport's Blog 2013. URL: http://flyingtigercomics.blogspot.com/2013/06/a-new-giant-vaccine-scandal-exposes.html.

[60] Ramesh R. Report condemns swine flu experts' ties to big pharma. The Guardian 2010. URL: https://www.theguardian.com/business/2010/jun/04/swine-flu-experts-big-pharmaceutical.

[61] Shanahan C. Law firm not expecting swine flu narcolepsy case in court before 2016. Irish Examiner 2014. URL: https://www.irishexaminer.com/ireland/law-firm-not-expecting-swine-flu-narcolepsy-case-in-court-before-2016-286331.html.

[62] Stein R. Reports accuse WHO of exaggerating H1N1 threat, possible ties to drug makers. Washington Post 2010 Jun 04. URL: http://commonamericanjournal.com/reports-accuse-who-of-exaggerating-h1n1-threat-possible-ties-to-drug-makers/.

[63] Special Court not competent in swine flu vaccine case. B92.net 2012 Jul 26. URL: https://www.b92.net/eng/news/crimes.php?yyyy=2012&mm=07&dd=26&nav_id=81470.

[64] Villesen K, Voller L. Secrete committee gives advices to WHO on Swine flu [Hemmeligkomitérådgiver WHO on svine influenza]. Information 2009. URL: https://www.information.dk/udland/2009/12/hemmelig-komite-raadgiver-who-svineinfluenza.

[65] Voller L, Villesen K. WHO-advisers hides million-euro contributions from the pharmaceutical industry [WHO-rådgiver skjuler millionbidrag fra medicinalindustrien]. Information 2009. URL: https://www.information.dk/indland/2009/12/who-raadgiver-skjuler-millionbidrag-medicinalindustrien,

[66] Wikipedia. 2009 flu pandemic by country. URL: https://en.wikipedia.org/wiki/2009_swine_flu_pandemic_by_country.

[67] William FE. Mega corruption at the WHO. Rense.com 2009.

[68] Flynn P. The handling of the H1N1 pandemic: More transparency needed. Council of Europe 2010. URL: https://assembly.coe.int/CommitteeDocs/2010/20100604_H1N1pandemic_e.pdf.

[69] Polish Health Ministry. Mrs Ewa Kopacz gives speech in Polish Parliament. Youtube 2009. URL: https://www.youtube.com/watch?v=RhZesZe33cw.

[70] Grolle J, Hackenbroch V. Interview with epidemiologist Tom Jefferson "A whole industry is waiting for a pandemic." Der Spiegel 2009. URL: https://www.spiegel.de/international/world/interview-with-epidemiologist-tom-jefferson-a-whole-industry-is-waiting-for-a-pandemic-a-637119.html.

[71] Ritzau Bureau. Ifølge Danmarks Statistik er der i år ikke nogen overdødelighed sammenlignet med tidligere år. Ritzau 2020 Apr 17. URL: https://nyheder.tv2.dk/2020-04-17-corona-ser-ikke-ud-til-at-give-flere-doedsfald-end-normalt. [Danish] [According to Statistics Denmark, there is no mortality this year compared to previous years.]

[72] Posch M, Bauer P, Posch A, König F. [Erste Analysen österreichischer Covid-19 Sterbezahlen nach Alter und Geschlecht 2020 Apr 10]. URL: https://cemsiis.meduniwien.ac.at/fileadmin/cemsiis/MS/data/2020_04_06_COVID_19_Analyse_Sterbezahlen.pdf. [German] [First analyzes of Austrian Covid-19 deaths by age and gender]

[73] Landsverk G. Some COVID-19 symptoms are turning out to be atypical. Here's what we know so far. Science Alert 2020 Apr 01. URL: https://www.sciencealert.com/10-coronavirus-symptoms-you-may-not-be-aware-of.

[74] Smith C. Doctors have discovered unusual new coronavirus symptoms. BGR 2020 Apr 02. URL: https://bgr.com/2020/04/02/coronavirus-symptoms-neurological-signs-point-to-covid-19-infection/

[75] CGTN. Bill Gates responds to vaccine conspiracy theories. CCTV 2020 Apr 10. URL: https://www.youtube.com/watch?v=nFUdX_0PpT0.

[76] Gates B. The next outbreak? We're not ready. Bill Gates – YouTube. TED Talkes 2015 Apr 03. URL: https://www.youtube.com/watch?v=6Af6b_wyiwI&list=PLh9VQRAGyrKMmFns4uG4vW9NyfTjHySeD.

[77] Illich II. Medical nemesis. London: Calder Boyars, 1974.

[78] Wikipedia. List of mass hysteria cases. URL: https://en.wikipedia.org/wiki/List_of_mass_hysteria_cases.

[79] Monto AS. Medical reviews. Coronaviruses. Yale J Biol Med 1974;47(4):234-51.

[80] Verity R, Okell LC, Dorigatti I, Winskill P, Whittaker C, Imai N, et al. Estimates of the severity of coronavirus disease 2019: a model-based analysis. Lancet Open 2020 Mar 30. doi: https://doin.org/10.1016/S1473-3099(20)30243-7.

[81] Day M. Covid-19: Four fifths of cases are asymptomatic, China figures indicate. BMJ 2020 Apr 02. URL: https://www.bmj.com/content/369/bmj.m1375.

[82] Service RF. You may be able to spread coronavirus just by breathing, new report finds. Science 2020 Apr 02. URL: https://www.sciencemag.org/news/2020/04/you-may-be-able-spread-coronavirus-just-breathing-new-report-finds.

[83] Stieb M. Oxford model: Coronavirus may have already infected half of UK population. Nymag 2020 Mar 24. URL: https://nymag.com/intelligencer/2020/03/oxford-study-coronavirus-may-have-infected-half-of-u-k.html.

[84] Merlot J. [Faktencheck. Die gefährlichen Falschinformationen des Wolfgang Wodarg]. Der Spiegel 2020 Mar 20. URL: https://www.spiegel.de/consent-a-?targetUrl=https%3 A%2F%2Fwww.spiegel.de%2Fwissenschaft%2Fmedizin%2Fcoronavirus-die-gefaehrlichen-falschinformationen-des-wolfgang-wodarg-a-f74bc73b-aac5-469e-a4e4-2ebe7aa6c270%3Ffbclid%3DIwAR3ckelFZIOynoQS3cXoJLDPnfKLjbYqMIWWmJwXK1eZRTh6Mm0DrGqCTY0&ref=https%3A%2F%2Fl.facebook.com%2F. [German] [Fact check. The dangerous false information of Wolfgang Wodarg]

[85] Rasmussen LI. Former Director of the Board of Health: There was and is no real health - professional basis for shutting down the entire country. Politics and not a purely health professional assessment closed large parts of Denmark on Wednesday, says the assessment from former director of the National Board of Health Else Smith. Politiken 2020 Mar 15. URL: https://politiken.dk/forbrugogliv/sundhedogmotion/art7703620/Der-var-og-er-intet-reelt-sundheds-fagligt-bel%C3%A6g-for-at-lukke-hele-landet-ned. [Danish]

[86] Döllner N. Else Smith: "Ja, jeg er jobsøgende" Vicedirektør på Hvidovre og Amager Hospital stopper med øjeblikkelig virkning. Dagens Medicin 2020 Mar 29. URL: https://dagensmedicin.dk/else-smith-ja-jeg-er-jobsoegende/. [Danish] ["Yes, I am a job seeker" Deputy Director at Hvidovre and Amager Hospital stops with immediate effect. Today's Medicine]

[87] Homepage. Vibeke Manniches. Hurra – intet tegn på faretruende corona-epidemi. URL: http://vibekemanniche.dk/. [Vibeke Manniches. Hurray - no sign of the endangered corona epidemic.]

[88] Weaver C. Questions about accuracy of Coronavirus tests sow worry. Wall Street Journal 2020 Apr 02. URL: https://www.wsj.com/articles/questions-about-accuracy-of-coronavirus-tests-sow-worry-11585836001.

[89] Møller P. Krydstogtskibet var forladt i 17 dage, men lægerne fandt stadig spor af virus. TV2 2020 Mar 28. URL: https://nyheder.tv2.dk/udland/2020-03-28-krydstogtskibet-var-forladt-i-17-dage-men-laegerne-fandt-stadig-spor-af-virus. [Danish] [The cruise ship was abandoned for 17 days, but doctors still found traces of viruses]

[90] Alberts B, Bray D, Raff JLM, Roberts K, Watson JD. The cell: Molecular biology of the cell. New York: Garland, 1983.

[91] Roitt I, Brostoff J, Male D. Immunology. London; Gower Medical, 1985.

[92] Klein, J. Natural history of the major histocompability complex. New York: John Wiley Sons, 1986.

[93] Klein J. The science of self - Nonself discrimination. New York: John Wiley Sons, 1982.

[94] Denmark Coronavirus. URL: https://sundheds politisktidsskrift.dk/nyheder/3073-lynoverblik-dagens-tal-og-vigtigste-nyheder-om-coronavirus.html. [Danish]

[95] World Health Organization. Homepage. URL: https://www.who.int.

[96] World Health Organization. Coronavirus. URL: https://www.who.int/emergencies/diseases/novel-coronavirus-2019.

[97] World Health Organization. Draft as of 12 February 2020. COVID-19 Strategic Preparedness and Response Plan. Operational Planning Guidelines. Geneva: WHO, 2020. URL: https://www.who.int/docs/default-source/coronaviruse/covid-19-sprp-unct-guidelines.pdf?sfvrsn=81ff43d8_4.

[98] Danish television DR. COVID data for the world presented 2020 Apr 13. URL: www.dr.dk. [Danish]

[99] Gøttler SØ. Opsang fra dronningen i historisk tale: Tankeløst og hensynsløst. Jyllands Posten 2020 Mar 17. URL: https://jyllands-posten.dk/indland/ECE12017622/opsang-fra-dronningen-i-historisk-tale-tankeloest-og-hensynsloest/. [Danish] [Songs from the Queen in Historical Speech: Thoughtless and Reckless. Jyllands]

[100] Jones WHS. Hippocrates, Vol. I–IV. London: William Heinemann, 1923-1931.

[101] Østergaard A. [Detektor: Lægen Vibeke Manniche vildleder med hjemmelavet corona-graf. Vibeke Manniche nedtoner igen og igen alvoren af corona-epidemi med en fejlagtig graf]. DR 2020 Mar 25. URL: https://www.dr.dk/nyheder/detektor/detektor-laegen-vibeke-manniche-vildleder-med-hjemmelavet-corona-graf. [Danish] [Detector: Doctor Vibeke Manniche misleads with homemade corona graph. Vibeke Manniche dims again and again the seriousness of the corona epidemic with a faulty graph]

[102] Bloomberg Market and Finance. Coronavirus is 10 times more lethal than seasonal flu, Fauci says. National Institute of Allergy and Infectious Diseases Director Anthony Fauci tells the House Oversight and Reform Committee that the novel coronavirus spreading across the globe is "10 times more lethal than the seasonal flu" 2020 Mar 11. URL: https://www.youtube.com/watch?v=2DekzGCJhJw

[103] Broadbent DE, Broadbent MHP, Phillpotts RJ, Wallace J. Some further studies on the prediction of experimental colds in volunteers by psychological factors. J Psychosom Res 1984;28(6):511-23.

[104] Clover RD, Abell T, Becker LA, Crawford S, Ramsey CN. Family functioning and stress as predictors of influenza B infection. J Fam Pract 1989;28:535-9.

[105] Cohen S, Tyrrell DA, Smith AP. Psychological stress and susceptibility to the common cold. N Engl J Med 1991;325(9):606–12. doi:10.1056/nejm199108293250903.

[106] Velavan TP, Meyer CG. Editorial. The COVID-19 epidemic. TMIH 2020 Febr 12. URL: https://doi.org/10.1111/tmi.13383.

[107] Irwin M, Vedhara K. Human psychoneuroimmunology. New York: Oxford University Press, 2005.

[108] Segerstrom SC, ed. The Oxford handbook of psychoneuroimmunology. New York: Oxford University Press, 2012.

[109] Sheridan JF Dobbs C, Brown D, Willing B. Psychoneuroimmunology: Stress effects on pathogenesis and immunity during infection. Clin Microbiol Rev 1994;7:200-12.

[110] Lloyd, R. Explorations in psychoneuroimmunology. Orlando, FL: Grune Stratton, 1987.

[111] Locke S, Ader R, Besedovsky H, Hal, N, Solomon G, Aron T. Foundations of psychoneuroimmunology. New York: Aldine, 1985.

[112] Ventegodt S, Flensborg-Madsen T, Andersen NJ, Nielsen M, Morad M, Merrick J. Global quality of life (QOL), health and ability are primarily determined by our consciousness. Research findings from Denmark 1991-2004. Soc Indicator Res 2005;71;87-122.

[113] Cohen S, Williamson GM. Stress and infectious disease in humans. Psychol Bull 1991;109(1):5–24.

[114] Holmes TH, Rahe RH. The Holmes-Rahe Life Stress Inventory. URL: https://www.stress.org/wp-content/uploads/2019/04/stress-inventory-1.pdf.

[115] The British Prime Minister Boris Johnson is out of intensive care. [Den britiske premierminister, Boris Johnson, er ude af intensiv.] DR 2020 Apr 09. URL: https://www.dr.dk/nyheder/udland/boris-johnson-er-ude-af-intensiv. [Danish]

[116] Mitsikostas DD. Nocebo in headache. Curr Opin Neurol. 2016;29(3):331-6. doi: 10.1097/WCO.0000000000000313.

[117] Lester D. Voodoo death. Omega (Westport) 2009;59(1):1-18.

[118] Jones L, Brown D, Palumbo D. Coronavirus: A visual guide to the economic impact. BBC News 2020 Apr 03. URL: https://www.bbc.com/news/business-5170 6225.

[119] Apfel S. Covid-19: The forgotten equation wreaks havoc. Doesn't anyone realize that shrinkage of the economy puts new demands on public health well out of reach? The economy has to be put into the equation. Israel National News 2020 Mar 29. URL http://www.israelnationalnews.com/Articles/Article.aspx/25455.

[120] Bake B, Larsson P, Ljungkvist G, Ljungstrom E, Olin A-C. Exhaled particles and small airways. Respir Res 2019;20:8. doi.org/10.1186/s12931-019-0970-9.

[121] Does facemasks protect against Corona viruses? [Beskytter ansigtsmasker mod coronavirus?] Illustreret Videnskab URL: https://illvid.dk/medicin/beskytter-ansigtsmasker-mod-coronavirus. [Danish]

[122] Poletti RA. Ethics of death and dying. Int J Nurs Stud 1985;22(4):329-34.

[123] WIKI. Pneumonia. URL: https://da.wikipedia.org/wiki/Lungebet%C3%A6ndelse.

[124] Ogwang M, Paramatti D, Molteni T, Ochola E, Okello TR, Ortiz Salgado JC, et al. Prevalence of hospital-associated infections can be decreased effectively in developing countries. J Hosp Infect 2013;84(2):138-42. doi: 10.1016/j.jhin. 2013.02.016.

[125] Herszenhorn DM. Democracy in critical care as coronavirus disrupts governments. Travel bans and social distancing prompt changes to politics as usual — and fears of executive overreach. Politico 2020 Apr 03. URL: https://www.politico.eu/article/ democracy-in-critical-care-as-coronavirus-disrupts-governments/.

[126] Wigura K, Kuisz J. Coronavirus is now contaminating Europe's democracy. The Guardian 2020 Apr 01. URL: https://www.theguardian.com/world/commentisfree/ 2020/apr/01/coronavirus-contaminating-europe-democracy-viktor-orban-seize-more-power.

[127] Szymanowski G. How coronavirus challenges open democracies. The corona pandemic is not just a health hazard. A permanent mode of crisis can also endanger open societies. In a state of emergency, the course is set for an uncertain post-corona world. DW 2020 Mar 25. URL: https://www.dw.com/en/how-coronavirus-challenges-open-democracies/a-52917307.

[128] Lacina L. Nearly 3 billion people around the globe under COVID-19 lockdowns - Today's coronavirus updates. World Economic Forum 2020 Mar 26. URL: https://www.weforum.org/agenda/2020/03/todays-coronavirus-updates/.

[129] Ventegodt S. A comparative analysis of the environmental consequences of the world's different types of medicine: Consciousness-based holistic medicine versus pharmaceutical medicine. J Altern Med Res 2019:11(1):67-78.

[130] Ventegodt S. [Livskvalitet i Danmark]. Quality of life in Denmark. Results from a population survey. Copenhagen: Forskningscentrets Forlag, 1995. [partly in Danish]

[131] Ventegodt S. [Livskvalitet hos 4500 31-33 årige]. The quality of life of 4500 31-33 year-olds. Result from a study of the Prospective Pediatric Cohort of persons born at the University Hospital in Copenhagen. Copenhagen: Forskningscentrets Forlag, 1996. [partly in Danish]

[132] Jefferson T, Zarra L. Bufala spotting, part one: assessing research papers. J Royal Soc Med 2007 Jan 1. URL: https://doi.org/10.1177/014107680710000114.

[133] Jefferson T, Zarra L. Bufale spotting, part two: assessing systematic reviews. J Royal Soc Med 2007 Apr 1. URL: https://doi.org/10.1177/014107680710 011413.

[134] Gøtzsche PC. Vaccines: Truth, lies and controversy. Copenhagen: Peoples Press, 2020.

[135] Gøtzsche PC. Deadly medicines and organised crime: How Big Pharma has corrupted healthcare". New York: Radcliffe, 2013.

[136] Gøtzsche PC. Deadly psychiatry and organised denial. Copenhagen: People Press, 2017.

[137] Ventegodt S. A review of World Health Organization's recommendations in "WHO's model list of essential medicines": Who provides the data for the drug register? Altern Med Res 2016;8(4):347-57.

[138] AFP - Agence France Presse. Vaccine needed to fully halt spread of COVID-19. URL: https://www. barrons.com/news/vaccine-needed-to-fully-halt-spread-of-covid-19-who-01586794505?refsec=afp-news.
[139] WHO Timeline. COVID-19. 2020 April 12. URL: https://www.who.int/news-room/detail/08-04-2020-who-timeline---covid-19.
[140] Hersholt J. The Emperor's new clothes. [En oversættelse af HC Andersens "Keiserens nye Klæder".] URL: https://andersen.sdu.dk/vaerk/hersholt/The EmperorsNewClothes.html.
[141] Who control the World? A surprisingly small number of corporations control massive global market shares. International Business Guide 2020. URL: https:// internationalbusinessguide.org/corporations.
[142] Taylor K. These 10 companies control everything you buy. Independent 2017 Apr 17. URL: https://www.independent.co.uk/life-style/companies-control-everything-you-buy-kelloggs-nestle-unilever-a7666731.html.
[143] Hagopian J. The evils of Big Pharma exposed. Global Research 2018 Jul 19. URL: https://www.globalresearch.ca/the-evils-of-big-pharma-exposed/5425382.
[144] Püschel C. Corona-Obduktionen: Von den Toten lernen. Hamburg Journal. NDR 28-04-2020. URL: https://www.ndr.de/fernsehen/sendungen/hamburg_journal/ Hamburg-Journal.sendung1020130.html. [German] [Corona autopsies: learning from the dead]

Chapter 3

THE MEDIA AND THE CORONA PANDEMIC

The media have brought so many stories that have convinced people that we are in the middle of a very dangerous viral pandemic; but the media have totally misinformed and mislead people. The media have explored the situation ruthlessly; they have had a feast, at the world's expense. Now that we know that the Corona COVID-19 virus is not dangerous at all, we have a big job to do explaining people how they were tricked to believe that the virus was dangerous. A big part of this is to teach people to be critical to the media, so they can be a little harder to manipulate next time the world go totally crazy. We also need to teach people to be critical to authorities, because the authorities are not always serving our best interest. Sometimes other interests, like big money, comes into the play, which makes things skew and irrational. As we have seen in the COVID-19 pandemic in 2020.

INTRODUCTION

It has been very interesting to watch how the interplay between the media and the population's understanding of Corona COVID-19 has been. Most people are unfamiliar with the mechanism and logic behind the production of stories to the media.

A good story is a story that fits well to our expectations; a story that runs on a theme we already are giving a lot of attention. It is a story that scares us, that raises emotions, and confirms us in what we believe, or take our doubt away.

The emotional angle sells papers, which is why the media are full of stories about murder, rape, disasters, abuse, fraud and more. In the Corona pandemic, the media have had a feast. Good stories have been provided from all over the world, and have filled the media every day, and one media has fed the next. The stories have been so good that the same story could go in all newspapers and all TV-news programs the same day.

Unfortunately, what really characterizes the good story is that it is sensational, un-usual, about something new and unseen. Every story is angled; every story is made in such a way that your attention and curiosity has been awakened. Very often, a simple reason for what we see, that takes the sensational out of the story, is omitted. Like in the stories about the overfilled morgues. Did we hear that the Italian authorities moved all the old, dying people from the elderly homes to the central hospitals, where the morgues therefore filled up? No, we did not. Why? Because if that part had been in the story, it would have been a story about bad management in the Italian health care system.

If you manage to see our Whistleblowers' many videos, you will hear severe critique of how the Corona pandemic was handled in Italy by the authorities, which was what created the problems you saw in the media. Of course, that would not have been a good story. People were waiting for the World Health Organisation (WHO) prediction about a COVID-19 killing millions of people, so when the stories came from Italy, the whole world learned that now the pandemic had started to create hell in Europe. You can say that hell came. Except it was not the virus that created this hell, it was the politicians following the irrational WHO instructions and believing in the WHOs number of 3.4% for the COVID-19 mortality rate.

Media stories

During the COVID-19 pandemic, the media have been filled with the most incredible stories. We have heard that the virus came from bats – that it might have been developed as a biological weapon – that is might have escaped a laboratory – and more. But now, when we know that it is just a normal mutation, that happens every year, it is clear that these wild stories fitted well to the unusual mortality rate of 3.4%, that needed an explanation. The explanation is that the WHO made it up. It is still unclear why. We know now for sure that there is not dangerous virus out there, killing us, COVID-19 is harmless. It is just the common cold.

What about all the hospitals filled with patients in ventilators, is this not proving, that we are under attack of a dangerous virus giving us lung-problems? No, it is not. Because the intensive units of the hospitals fills up with patients that should not be there; patients that has been send there because of new instructions for people with common cold and airway trouble. Normally these patients would just have stayed home in bed with their common cold, without any problems at all; now they are send with ambulance to intensive care. This is utterly unnecessary; it is political; what we see is created not by the virus, but by the politicians and the leaders of the health care sectors, following the WHOs irrational and dangerous instructions.

Hospital stories

The hospitals are filled with dying patients and dead bodies to such an extent that the bodies accumulates in the halls, because the dying old people are send to the hospitals.

What about the new and unexpected symptoms from COVID-19 many doctors are telling us about? We have discussed this earlier, and yes, there might be new symptoms, because we have a new, unusual situation people are reacting to. Human beings have a very strong physical reactions to mental beliefs; if you believe you have been infected with a deadly virus, you will experience this very different from a common cold, even with the same symptoms. Imagine you are travelling in Africa and the doctor tells you that you have attracted Ebola. That you are isolated, and people in space suits are looking after you. Scary, right? Now small symptoms become really unpleasant, because it is an indication of you death coming. The same with COVID-19. It scares people, and the experience changes into something very unpleasant. That is logic; it is not strange.

What about young people now also dying from COVID-19, All these stories have a very strong and convincing power. It happens that young people die. Because Corona viruses are so common such people are likely to test positive for Corona. This does not prove that they die BY Corona COVID-19! It is very difficult to establish a virus as the true cause of death; it takes a truly advances autopsy. We have no single story where medical experts have done such an analysis and concluded that this until this day healthy person was infected and died suddenly from Corona COVID-19! Nevertheless, this is how the media makes it look. Because this is the good story. Some young person with asthma or a young mentally ill patient on antipsychotic drugs dying is sad, but it is quite normal and not front-page stuff. You do not get all the information, you do not get the most likely explanation, for then there would be no story to begin with. That is how the media works. And this is why the media carry an enormous responsibility for the harm we have seen on people and society during the COVID-19 pandemic.

THINK BEFORE YOU BELIEVE

So now, when you meet the next story about "20 doctors in Uruguay dead by Corona" you will think twice before you buy into this story. You would like to know how they could be sure that it was Corona and not stress and exhaustion from working 100 hour in one go, or drugs that they abused (many doctors abuse opioids, central stimulants like amphetamine, and other drugs to make it through long shifts) that killed them. Alternatively, the ventilator they were put on because of the WHO instructions, or the antibiotic drugs they were given for the hospital infection they acquired. Now you want to know much more, before you accept the story as true.

If you fear for COVID-19 and see these stories in the media, you can buy into them and believe them; you can convince yourself that "Yes, there is really a dangerous new virus coming my way, Ill better take care not to attract it if I love my life".

The more you know, the more untrue the stories in the media look. Our three whistleblowers (see chapter 2) are all choked about the media and the stories they bring, and the naïve way people are receiving them and believing in them. If you know little, you are an easy target of manipulation. If you know a lot, you are naturally critical, because the story you hear needs to fit to all that you already know.

NEWS TRAVEL FAST

In these days of global media, stories travel fast all over the world. Good stories are picked up by all leading media, in all countries, like the stories about the Corona disaster in Italy, where so many people suddenly died. If people later hear that the average age of the Italian people reported to die from Corona is 81 years old, and that there is no more people dying this year than the two last years in Italy, people are getting confused: that cannot be true??? I heard they had a disaster where so many people died??? I even saw pictures of the overfilled morgues, and pictures of the military vehicles they used to help get rid of the bodies.

The same with the story of the catastrophe in New York, followed by brutal pictures of freezing trucks in the streets of New York filling up with the dead bodies. This is for many people a convincing prove that a new Corona virus with a crazy high mortality rate hitting New York. Except it is not.

Remember the story by Hans Christian Andersen (1805-1875) about one little feather becoming five hens:

> It's a dreadful story!" said a hen, and she said it in a part of town, too, where it had not taken place. "It's a dreadful story to happen in a henhouse. I'm afraid to sleep alone tonight; it's a good thing there are many of us on the perch!" And then she told a story that made the feathers of the other hens stand on end and the rooster's comb fall. It's quite true! …

What people fail to think of is how much of this is just normal fluctuation and situations created by the leader's bad decisions. Overfilled morgues in Italy happens every now and then because of the way the Italian health care system is made, where there is no overcapacity, so fluctuations in the number of dead, like under influenza pandemics, give this situations now and then. It is not so unusual; it is not for the first time in history this happens. But this is the idea you get from the news story. And why? Because that was how the story was angled.

In addition, if you suddenly move all the old people that normally are dying in the elderly homes to the hospitals, of course you then see an unusual accumulation of dead bodies in the hospitals and hospital morgues.

If you move patients to intensive care during a common cold where the oxygen tension is lower, these patients are almost sure to be put in a ventilator, so of course if you politically decide to do so, you will see much more people in ventilators. So now you have many more people in ventilators. Does it prove that we are under attack of an evil virus giving many more people serous lung problems? No, not at all. It proves that we have changed how the system works. That's all. But normal people do not think about, when the media reports the high number of people in respirators. They think: "Damn! I would not like to go there. I'll better be careful not to attract this nasty one! I'll better keep distance and stay at home."

If you take people who do not need a ventilator and give them a ventilator, you risk to harm them and this is what we see now – young people are ending up in ventilators they simply do not need, and getting infections, compression damage on their lung tissue etc. This is totally unnecessarily. It happens because of the instructions for treating COVID-

19, which happen to be a SARS virus, which means it attacks lung tissue, but this is not the same as it is dangerous! Most of thc 100 different viruses our immune system handles every year attacks the airways. If you know that, you will think very differently.

CONCLUSION

The conclusion is that the media have brought so many stories that have convinced people that we arc in the middle of a very dangerous viral pandemic; but the media have totally misinformed and mislead people. The media have explored the situation ruthlessly; they have had a feast, at the world's expense.

We have been working a lot with the media during the last three decades; for us it is not strange what is happening, it is just very sad. We understand how the media works, how the Corona virus works, and how people's minds works. It have been difficult to watch the theater of the world playing; we have been very sad to see the world being fooled. The WHO creates a story about the deadly Corona virus; a story that becomes self-confirming. This is also how our mind works: the moment we believe in a thing, this becomes confirmed in what we see. We are self-affirmative beings. We are interpreting our reality according to our beliefs.

Now that we know that the Corona COVID-19 virus is not dangerous at all, we have a big job to do explaining people how they were tricked to believe that the virus was dangerous. A big part of this is to teach people to be critical to the media, so they can be a little harder to manipulate next time the world goes totally crazy. We also need to teach people to be critical to authorities, because the authorities are not always serving our best interest. Sometimes other interests, like big money, comes into the play, which makes things skew and irrational. As we have seen in the COVID-19 pandemic in 2020.

Social media seriously harms your mental health.

REFERENCES

[1] Ventegodt S, Merrick J. A citizen's guide to survive Corona COVID-19 (SARS-CoV-2). Copenhagen: Quality-of-Life Research Center Press, 2020.

Chapter 4

WORLD HEALTH ORGANIZATION (WHO), HEALTH AND THE SWINE FLU

In the scientific community it is generally accepted that meta-analyses are more accurate than single studies and independent studies more trustworthy than industrial studies. It is therefore understandable that Cochrane reviews and similar meta-analyses based on rigid protocol and of independent origin, have the highest quality in medical research.

It is therefore unfortunate that Cochrane reviews seems systematically to conflict with the information and recommendations from the World Health Organization (WHO). A number of the drugs and vaccines recommended by WHO, especially the drugs used in psychiatry, are in Cochrane reviews found to be harmful and without significant clinical effect.

Since those recommendations are followed by many people, especially the doctors and leaders of the healthcare sectors in the 194 WHO-member states, it could indeed lead to patients getting the wrong medication. Many patients suffer severe adverse effects, because of taking drugs and vaccines recommended by the WHO, but not by the Cochrane researchers and other independent experts. When we say "many", the exact number is not known, but our estimate is 500 million patients worldwide, i.e., a large fraction of the patients in the developed world, and a substantial number in the third world.

To solve this serious public health problem it is recommended to revise the WHO-system, which in fact has been proven weak to the interests of the pharmaceutical industry. We therefore believe that the WHO's recommendations regarding medicine in its "list of essential medicines" and other drug directories are biased and not reliable as a source of information on medicine.

In this chapter we look into the 2009 Swine flu H1N1 scandal, where the close link between the WHO and the pharmaceutical industry was exposed. We hope that what we learned about the WHO in 2009 will be used when we make decisions in the crisis we have today.

INTRODUCTION

"So the potential significance of the call was clear to Fukuda: the start of a devastating pandemic, in which, according to WHO estimates, between 2.0 and 7.4 million could die -- assuming the pandemic was relatively mild. But if the new virus proved to be as aggressive as the one that triggered the Spanish Flu in 1918, the death toll could run to the tens of millions." Der Spiegel (1, 2)

April 29, 2009: The WHO raises its warning to phase 5, the last stage before a pandemic.

April 30, 2009: Egypt begins killing all domestic pigs in the country. French actress and animal rights activist Brigitte Bardot begs President Hosni Mubarak to stop the mass slaughter, but her appeals are unsuccessful.

May 4, 2009: In Mexico, football matches in the country's four highest-ranking leagues take place without spectators. The legislature in Germany 's western state of Saarland imposes a ban on kissing as a form of greeting. Der Spiegel (1, 2)

Oct. 9, 2009: Wolf-Dieter Ludwig, an oncologist and chairman of the Drug Commission of the German Medical Association, says: "The health authorities have fallen for a campaign by the pharmaceutical companies, which were plainly using a supposed threat to make money." Der Spiegel (1, 2)

The World Health Organization (WHO) is guiding the public health services of 194 member states and a number of other countries regarding their use of pharmacological drugs, vaccines and non-drug medicine (psychotherapy, physical therapy, alternative medicine (CAM). Ten years ago WHO changed its financial policy and allowed private money into its system, instead of only funding from the member states (3, 4). WHO has since been extremely successful in raising funds and is now receiving more than half of its yearly budget from private sources (3, 4). Bill Gates has for example given more than one billion dollars to the WHO (4). The new system of private funding of WHO has brought WHO much closer to the pharmaceutical industry.

This change in policy honoring rationality and science to serving the pharmaceutical industry and going for its money is what this chapter is about. We hope you are sitting down, because you might be up for a big surprise.

WHO director-general Margaret Chan from China (director 2006-2017) has been rated as the 30th most powerful woman in the world by Forbes Magazine (5) and this fact might give you an idea of the power we are talking about. More than half the population on planet Earth is more or less influenced by the advice and recommendations given by WHO. We estimate that 350 million patients – the sick population of the major cities of the wealthy member states - are receiving medical treatment with drugs partly or dominantly based on recommendations from the WHO.

DRUGS AND VACCINES

We believe that WHO is biased regarding pharmaceutical drugs. This is evident to us, when we compare the recommendations in the WHO's drug directories, i.e., "WHO's model list of essential medicines" (6) with the recommendations from independent researchers analyzing the positive and negative effects of drugs and vaccines, like for example Cochrane reviews.

Cochrane reviews are an acknowledged source of knowledge in medicine, because these meta-analyses come from the Cochrane organization's 3,000 independent physicians and researchers who in their unselfish service for humanity are documenting the effect of almost all the pharmaceutical drugs and vaccines and also of hundreds or more of different types of non-drug medicine, including a variety of alternative treatments (CAM) (7). The results from the Cochrane reviews, which most researchers regard as a much more reliable source of information on medicine than the data coming from the pharmaceutical industry itself, clash harshly with the recommendations of WHO in its drug directories. The Cochrane meta-analyses have systematically found less effect and more harm from the pharmaceutical drugs than the pharmaceutical industry does, when it documents its own products, also when the industry's own data is used (8).

Many drugs listed in the WHO drug directories, like "WHOs model list of essential medicines" (6), have no value as medicine according to Cochrane reviews, since the drugs are dangerous, often harmful, and without significant beneficial effects for the patient. You can even say that the lack of effect and the danger of the drugs are well documented!

An example of drugs harmful to patients include cytotoxic chemotherapy, which has a negative effect on the cancer patient quality of life and survival, as found by Ulrich Abel already in 1991 (9-11). Other examples are the lack of improvement of the mentally ill patients' mental state with anti-psychotic or anti-depressant drugs found in Cochrane reviews (12, 13), the documented lack of effect of the influenza vaccines (14) and of the anti-influenza medicines (15). These independent meta-analyses are of utmost importance and the results from such studies should be used in both the WHO's drug directories and the national drug directories, rather than the results and data from analyses coming directly from the pharmaceutical industry (8, 16).

Leaders of the Cochrane movement have openly criticized the pharmaceutical industry for buying and manipulating the researchers and cheating with the design and results of the randomized controlled trial (RCT)-test that documents the effects of their drugs (8). The former Danish director of the Nordic Cochrane Center openly addressed what he called "the criminal practices of the pharmaceutical industry" (8) and documented in his book the problem that "Big Pharma" already has taken patients lives and caused harm to patients from the use of poisonous, poorly documented and ineffective medicine (8).

The 2009 pandemic (Swine flu)

In 1988 Halfdan Mahler (1923-2016), Danish physician and WHO director general during 1973-1988 in the daily Danish newspaper Politiken warned the world against the power the pharmaceutical industry had over WHO: "the industry is taking over WHO", he said. But nobody believed him, because it was too difficult for the public to understand the complicated power games he talked about. Unfortunately he was right.

Recent scandals, like the Swine Flu scandal in 2009, has shown that WHO unfortunately has succumbed totally to the power of the pharmaceutical industry (1, 2, 17-59); we have also gained important insight in how the WHO-system works. Let us take a look at some of the facts that came to public knowledge during this scandal.

On June 11, 2009 the WHO declared that the world faced a horrible and deathly influenza pandemic (17, 19, 23, 27-29, 38, 41, 42, 58) with millions of people predicted to die in the worst disaster in modern time. All over the world more than two hundred countries prepared for the pandemic like the plaque or the Spanish Flu, which over the next few months could claim the lives of 40 million people or so - as it happened during the Spanish Flu in the cold and bitter years 1918-1919 following World War I. In June and July 2009 national borders were suddenly closed, thousands of public meeting places, like restaurants, cafes, and libraries in many countries were closed, and millions of travelers were stopped from entering a number of countries in Asia, if they had fewer or a common cold (27-29, 38, 41, 42, 58).

Many people travelling wasted hours on emergency health controls and physicians, hospitals and Ministries of Health panicked and started to send patients home from the hospitals. Many countries started to buy influenza vaccines or anti-influenza drugs and spend vast amounts of dollars (1, 2, 17-59). The pharmaceutical industry had good days indeed.

As the world reacted to the threat by continuing to buy incredible amounts of influenza vaccines and anti-influenza medicine a debate started in the scientific media, like the British Medical Journal (BMJ) (15-25) and slowly also in the public media worldwide (1, 2, 24-59). Suddenly WHO was accused of "crying wolf" (23) and supporting the pharmaceutical industry (1, 2, 14-25).

It turned out to be a false alarm and the Swine Flu epidemic in 2009 did not cause the many cases of deaths as first expected (12, 13, 15-25). Slowly it became known that the WHO actually knew this already BEFORE the director-general at the time Margeret Chan declared the pandemic. This can be seen by the fact that WHO changed the definition of a "pandemic" from meaning "millions of deaths" to mean a non-dangerous infection that spreads worldwide only one month before the WHO's declaration of the pandemic ((1, 2, 14-25, 28, 29).

PANIC AND A SCANDAL

In 2010 a number of representatives from governments all over the world as well as a number of international organizations, i.e., the Council of Europe agreed that WHO had caused an international panic and disaster by declaring the mildest flue ever, the A/H1N1 "Swine flu" influenza, to be a pandemic threatening mankind. The Council of Europe pointed in a dire report to the problem of WHO going private as the true cause of all the trouble (58). During 2010 the situation continued to develop and turned into a medical scandal of unknown proportions (1, 2, 17-59). Ineffective and dangerous medicines worth billions of dollars were sent for destruction. Close and secret links between the WHO and the pharmaceutical industry producing the vaccines was exposed. The Danish newspaper "Information" found that five researchers involving in advising WHO during the scandal had been paid around seven million Euro from the vaccine industry (38).

On top of that these vaccines and the anti-influenza medicine had already in Cochrane reviews been documented to be totally without value and burdening its users with a long list of adverse effects (1, 2, 14-25, 28, 29, 55).

Soon it was realized that thousands of patients suffered from a wide range of serious adverse effects: local inflammations, local or systemic muscle pain, vasculitis, neuritis (autoimmune nerve-inflammations), encephalitis, narcolepsy, and other chronic pains (19, 28, 29, 43-45, 49, 51, 58). The media then discovered that the adjuvants used in vaccines had many serious adverse effects that were mentioned to the citizens neither by the companies who sold the vaccines, nor by the governments buying and reselling the vaccines (1, 2, 17-59). It also turned out that the contracts the industry had made with the countries included a paragraph that the adverse effects were the buyer's full responsibility (1, 2, 17-25, 28-59).

In an interview the Polish health minister revealed everything about the horrible industrial contracts, where the pharmaceutical companies - helped by WHO - sold vaccines that were not even properly tested! The minister pointed to the fact that the test groups were extraordinary small – so small that the adverse effects of the vaccines could not even be evaluated (59). In spite of these horrible terms almost every country in Europe still signed the contracts, bought the drugs and vaccines in enormous quantities: two flu-shots per citizen (1, 2, 17-25, 28-59).

The media also brought WHO warning thoroughly and repeatedly and around July 2009 everybody knew about the coming catastrophe. One can easily understand the pressure on the many public health services and "better safe than sorry" seems to have been the mantra everywhere. To understand the kind of pressure and stress the states and the ministries of health were put under, you need to realize that not to buy the vaccines could easily, because of the close links between the industry and the press, mean the fall of a whole government.

This was what motivated the governments to sign sleeping contracts with the industry, and WHO played a vital role in this; sleeping means that the contract only become realized if WHO would declare a pandemic – which happened later. This way WHO pushed enormous quantities of vaccines and anti-influenza drugs to its 194 member states (1, 2, 17-59). How involved are WHO in the sales of pharmaceutical drugs in general? Well, for a start, WHO is negotiating the price of the medicine with the governments on behalf of the pharmaceutical companies (1, 2, 17-59). That was another thing that became publicly known during the scandal.

The scandal came with an after-match: During 2011, 2012, 1013 and 2014 many countries' patient-organizations have started court-cases against the governments, who had given them the ineffective and dangerous medicine (28, 29, 44, 51). It also became clear that it was the flu-vaccine-industry that had taken control over WHO and created a fake pandemic and the world wanted an answer to this question: Did WHO fail its responsibility as leader in international health in 2009 (1, 2, 14-23, 28, 29, 58)?

WHO agreed after a long period of total denial to make an investigation of itself; but after one year the internal WHO-rapport from the committee concluded that WHO had done nothing wrong at all. After the hearing of about 500 experts the WHO's investigation group concluded that WHO had done absolutely nothing wrong in 2009: "WHO performed well in many ways during the pandemic" (60).

Everybody who followed the development of the scandal and the exposure in the media - The Guardian, Der Spiegel, the BMJ and a number of other serious media - had to conclude that the biggest medical scandal ever was only possible, because something is wrong in the WHO-system (1, 2, 17-25, 28-59). It seems the history is repeating itself in 2019-2020 with the COVID-19 event.

FACTS ABOUT INFLUENZA

When the influenza comes it spreads all over via small drops with the virus in each, but out of all people infected only between 5-15% of the population develops the flu; 16% of these cases are influenza type A, B or C – and only 10% are of type A and B, which we can vaccinate against (14). This means that 1% of all gets the A or B influenza. If these people are vaccinated with the right type of flu, they can benefit from the vaccine. How many patients are helped of this 1% of the general population? Unfortunately only a small fraction, as the vaccine for influenza virus according to the big Cochrane meta-analysis is highly ineffective (14). So maybe one in a thousand can be helped to avoid a week in the bed, or get this year's flu shortened.

Unfortunately vaccinations are not free of adverse effects, as the adjuvant needed to provoke an immune response to a "dead" virion is provoking not only a response to the virus, but also to the body's own cells and molecules. Which gives a perfectly rational explanation for the many side effects we see from vaccination, both local and system, with local inflammation, local or systemic muscle pain, vasculitis, neuritis, encephalitis or narcolepsy as the severe adverse effects. The local adverse effects comes with every second vaccine or so, while the dire systemic effects are seen in one patient out of 1,000. If you vaccinate 1,000,000 people you will safe 1,000 from influenza, but you give 1,000 side effects, sometimes worse than the influenza itself. Such a negative balance between positive and negative effects will in a rational regime lead to the conclusion that the vaccine is not a rational medicine. It has no general use (14).

If the influenza is very mild – as the Swine flu A/H1N1 we had in the 2009 pandemic – there is no reason to fear it at all and even less reason to try to vaccine for it. Actually the pandemic H1A1 flu was the mildest flu we ever had – pandemic or epidemic. And it was even predictable from the statistics on the H1A1 flu that pandemics are getting milder and milder; all experts who were independent of the vaccine industry predicted that this pandemic would to be the mildest influenza pandemic ever (1, 2, 17-59).

So now compare this to the fact that WHO warned the world that many million people would die from it. Remember that WHO declared that we faced a deathly, horrible influenza pandemic, comparable to the Spanish flu in 1918-19, which killed about 40 million people. And consider the impact of this. In many countries the panic was total. In Egypt the government ordered all pigs slaughtered (56); in Mexico the government closed all restaurants and public places (56). In Asia the borders into China, Japan, Nepal and a number of other countries were closed for everybody with a fewer. A hundred million travelers had their travel prolonged with security checks for hours. Thousands of passengers with common colds were sent back home. In 2020 it became even worse with the COVID-19.

How was the vaccines sold?

The WHO declaration of pandemic in 2009 had an interesting consequence for a large number of pharmaceutical companies selling the vaccine and other types of flu medicine. The deeper the investigative journalist and people from independent organizations like the European Parliament investigated, the uglier the truth that was revealed. In the end an intimate cooperation between the pharmaceutical industry and WHO was exposed; a large number of people from the industry had been placed in secret advisory groups in WHO close to the Chinese director Margaret Chan (1, 2, 17, 18, 26-32, 34, 36, 38, 41, 43, 44, 54-56, 59). These people got in this way direct access to the control over the total WHO system.

So the world learned that the pharmaceutical industry was running WHO and it seems now in 2020 as the same is the case! Wow. So the industry itself declared the pandemic that forced all European countries and many more to buy enormous amount of ineffective and dangerous medicines (1, 2, 17-25, 28, 29, 31-59). But the scandal did not stop there. The contracts also contained paragraphs that transferred all responsibility for the adverse effects of the vaccine over to the governments of the countries (1, 2, 17-59). When the Council of Europe learned about this it caused extreme anger; WHO was subsequently criticized (60). In the end it turned out that the Cochrane experts and the Polish minister of health had been correct in their critique all along, when they said that the pharmaceutical industry and WHO together were selling vaccines and medicines that were not properly tested and dangerous (61-64).

In spite of an international scandal directly caused by WHO that made hundreds of countries pay billions of dollars and Euro from unnecessary vaccinations and medications, and in spite of thousands of victims for the serious adverse effects of these treatments, WHO concluded after the Swine flu scandal that all went well and happened according to the plans from 2005 (64) and that no errors had been made in the WHO system (65). We wonder what they will say in 2020?

CONCLUSION

With the Swine flu scandal the Genie came out and it was exposed that the pharmaceutical industry had gained control over the WHO system, leading to extreme bias towards the use of not only ineffective and unnecessary influenza vaccines and medicines, but also to the use of antipsychotics, antidepressant, antianxiety and other psychopharmaco-logical drugs, cytotoxic anti-cancer chemotherapy, and a number of other drugs, which according to independent meta-analyses and Cochrane reviews are found to be without significant beneficial effect – and often harmful.

In 2020 President Trump has also seen the light and stopped the annual 400 million dollars support of the WHO and we hope other countries will follow suit and instead strengthen national or regional collaborations.

We recommend a fundamental revision of the WHO-system that has proven itself weak to the interests of the pharmaceutical industry.

Acknowledgements

This chapter is an updated and changed version of an earlier paper with permission: Ventegodt S. Why the corruption of the World Health Organization (WHO) is the biggest threat to the world's public health of our time. J Integr Med Ther 2015;2(1):5.

References

[1] Bethge P, Elger K, Glüsing J, Grill M, Hachenbroch V, Puhl J, Von Rohr M, Traufetter G. Reconstruction of a mass hysteria: The Swine flu panic of 2009. Part 1. Der Spiegel 2010 Mar 12. URL: http://www.spiegel.de/international/world/reconstruction-of-a-mass-hysteria-the-swine-flu-panic-of-2009-a-682613.html.

[2] Bethge P, Elger K, Glüsing J, Grill M, Hachenbroch V, Puhl J, Von Rohr M, Traufetter G. Reconstruction of a Mass Hysteria: The Swine Flu Panic of 2009. Part 2. Der Spiegel 2010 Mar 12. URL: http://www.spiegel.de/international/world/reconstruction-of-a-mass-hysteria-the-swine-flu-panic-of-2009-a-682613-2.html.

[3] WHO's programbudget 2020-21. URL: https://apps.who.int/gb/ebwha/pdf_files/WHA72/A72_4-en.pdf.

[4] Voluntary contributors to the WHO. URL: https://www.who.int/about/finances-accountability/funding/voluntary-contributions/en/.

[5] Forbes. Margaret Chan. URL: http://www.forbes.com/profile/margaret-chan/.

[6] World Health Organization. List of recommended essential medicines. URL: http://www.who.int/medicines/publications/essentialmedicines/en/index.html.

[7] Committee on the Use of Complementary and Alternative Medicine by the American Public. Complementary and Alternative Medicine (CAM) in the United States. Washington, DC: National Academies Press, 2005.

[8] Gøtzsche P. Deadly medicines and organised crime: How Big Pharma has corrupted healthcare", New York: Radcliffe, 2013.

[9] Abel U. Chemotherapy of advanced epithelial cancer—a critical review. Biomed Pharmacother 1992;46:439-52.

[10] Abel U. [Chemotherapy of advanced epithelial cancer.] Stuttgart: Hippokrates Verlag, 1990. [German]

[11] Abel U. [Chemotherapie fortgesch-rittener Karzi-nome. Eine kritische Bestandsaufnahme.] Berlin: Hippokrates, 1995. [German]

[12] Adams CE, Awad G, Rathbone J, Thornley B. Chlorpromazine versus placebo for schizophrenia. Cochrane Database Syst Rev 2007;2:CD000284.

[13] Moncrieff J, Wessely S, Hardy R. Active placebos versus antidepressants for depression. Cochrane Database Syst Rev 2004;1:CD003012.

[14] Jefferson T, Di Pietrantonj C, Rivetti A, Bawazeer GA, Al-Ansary LA, Ferroni E. Vaccines for preventing influenza in healthy adults. Cochrane Database Syst Rev 2014;3:CD001269. doi: 10.1002/14651858.CD001269.pub5.

[15] Jefferson T, Jones MA, Doshi P, Del Mar CB, Hama R, Thompson MJ, et al. Neuraminidase inhibitors for preventing and treating influenza in healthy adults and children. Cochrane Database Syst Rev 2014;4:CD008965. doi: 10.1002/14651858. CD008965.pub4.

[16] Ventegodt S, Merrick J. A review of the Danish National Drug Directory: Who provides the data for the register? Int J Adolesc Med Health 2010;22(2):197-212

[17] Braillon A. The World Health Organization: No game of thrones. BMJ 2014 Jun 26. URL: http://www.bmj.com/content/348/bmj.g4265/rr/703675.

[18] Cohen D, Carter P. Conflicts of interest. WHO and the pandemic flu "conspiracies". BMJ 2010;340:c2912. doi: 10.1136/bmj.c2912.

[19] Cohen D, Carter P. WHO and the pandemic flu "conspiracies". BMJ 2009 Jun 4. URL: http://www.bmj.com/content/340/bmj.c2912.

[20] Doshi P, Jefferson T. WHO and pandemic flu. Another question for GSK. BMJ 2010;340:c3455. doi: 10.1136/bmj.c3455.

[21] JeffersonT, Doshi P. Multisystem failure: the story of anti-influenza drugs. BMJ 2014 April 10. URL: http://www.bmj.com/content/348/bmj.g2263.

[22] Jefferson T, Doshi P. WHO and pandemic flu. Time for change, WHO. BMJ 2010;;340:c3461.

[23] Law R. WHO and pandemic flu. There was also no new subtype. BMJ 2010;340:c3460. doi: 10.1136/bmj.c3460.

[24] Payne D. Tamiflu: The battle for secret drug data. BMJ 2012 Oct 29. URL: http://www.bmj.com/content/345/bmj.e7303.

[25] Watson R. WHO is accused of "crying wolf" over swine flu pandemic. BMJ 2010;340:c1904. doi: 10.1136/bmj.c1904.

[26] Zarocostas J. Swine flu pandemic review panel seeks access to confidential documents between WHO and drug companies. BMJ 2010;340:c2792. doi: 10.1136/bmj.c2792.

[27] Aagaard HL. [Vaccine... for og imod]. Berlinske Tidende 2009 Nov 10. URL: http://www.b.dk/danmark/vaccine...-imod. [Danish]

[28] ABC News. World Health Organization scientists linked to Swine flu vaccine makers. 2010 Jun 5. URL: http://abcnews.go.com/Health/SwineFlu/swine-flu-pandemic-world-health-organization-scientists-linked/story?id=10829940.

[29] BBC. Way opened for Pandemrix swine flu jab compensation. 2013 Sept 20. URL: http://www.bbc.com/news/health-24172715.

[30] Recearchgate. Biased experts, costly lies, and binary decisions. 2010 Jan. URL: http://www.researchgate.net/publication/46476997_Biased_experts_co.

[31] BBC. WHO swine flu experts 'linked' with drug companies. 2010 Jan. URL: http://www.bbc.com/news/10235558.
[32] Cohen D, Carter P. Key scientists advising the World Health Organization on planning for an influenza pandemic had done paid work for pharmaceutical firms that stood to gain from the guidance they were preparing. These conflicts of interest have never been publicly disclosed by WHO, and WHO has dismissed inquiries into its handling of the A/H1N1 pandemic as "conspiracy theories". BMJ 2010;340:c2912. URL: http://www.bmj.com/content/340/bmj.c2912.
[33] Editorial. The refusers. Australian journalist wins prestigious award for exposing flu vaccine scandal. 2011 Nov 28. URL: http://therefusers.com/refusers-newsroom/australian-journalist-wins-prestigious-award-for-exposing-flu-vaccine-scandal/.
[34] Edwards T. Big pharma probed for 'false' swine flu pandemic. The Week 2010 Jan 11. URL: http://www.theweek.co.uk/politics/17419/big-pharma-probed-%E2%80%98false%E2%80%99-swine-flu-pandemic.
[35] Ejbye AE, Korsgaard P. [Kun en ud af 100 har gavn af influenzavaccine]. Ekstra Bladet 2013 Dec 22. URL: http://ekstrabladet.dk/kup/sundhed/article4620514.ece. [Danish]
[36] Express. Swine flu scandal: Billions of pounds are wasted on vaccines. 2014 Nov 12. URL: http://www.express.co.uk/news/uk/156359/Swine-flu-scandal-Billions-
[37] Fletcher V. Swine flu scandal: Billions of pounds are wasted on vaccines. Express 2014 Oct 27. URL: http://www.express.co.uk/news/uk/156359/Swine-flu-scandal-Billions-of-pounds-are-wasted-on-vaccines.
[38] Galushko I. The reality behind the swine flu conspiracy. RT 2009 Dec 5. URL: http://rt.com/politics/reality-swine-flu-conspiracy/.
[39] Information. Can we trust WHO? [Tør vi stole på WHO?] 2009 Dec 12. URL: http://www.information.dk/218357. [Danish]
[40] Mercola J. Major victory with Swine flu scandal. Infowars 2009 Nov 19. URL: http://www.infowars.com/major-victory-with-swine-flu-scandal/.
[41] Neale T. World Health Organization scientists linked to Swine flu vaccine makers. ABC News 2010 Jun 5. URL: http://abcnews.go.com/Health/SwineFlu/swine-flu-pandemic-world-health-organization-scientists-linked/story?id=10829940.
[42] Petersen MH. Flu jabs linked to narcolepsia [Influenzavaccine koblet til narkolepsi.] MedWatch 2013 Jan 22. URL: http://medwatch.dk/Medicinal___Biotek/article5113322.ece. [Danish]
[43] Rappoport J. A new giant vaccine scandal exposes government lies and psyops. Jon Rappoport's Blog 2013 Jun 15. URL: https://jonrappoport.wordpress.com/2013/06/17/a-new-giant-vaccine-scandal-exposes-government-lies-and-psyops/.
[44] Editorial. Report condemns swine flu experts' ties to big pharma. The Guardian 2010 Jun 4. URL: http://www.theguardian.com/business/2010/jun/04/swine-flu-experts-big-pharmaceutical.

[45] Sample I. Swine flu vaccine can trigger narcolepsy, UK government concedes. The Guardian 2013 Sept 19. URL: http://www.theguardian.com/society/2013/sep/19/swine-flu-vaccine-narcolepsy-uk.

[46] Shanahan C. Law firm not expecting swine flu narcolepsy case in court before 2016. Irish Examiner 2014, Sept 15. URL: http://www.irishexaminer.com/ireland/law-firm-not-expecting-swine-flu-narcolepsy-case-in-court-before-2016-286331.html.

[47] Sørensen A. Vaccines has bad adverse effects. [Vaccine forbindes med alvorlige bivirkninger.] Berlinske Tidende 2009 Nov 14. URL: http://www.b.dk/danmark/vaccine-forbindes-med-alvorlige-bivirkninger. [Danish]

[48] Sørensen AB, Cuculiza M. Danish health authorities hides serious adverse effects. [Influenzavaccine: Sundhedsstyrelsen fortier alvorlige bivirkninger.] MX 2014 Oct, 20. URL: http://www.mx.dk/nyheder/danmark/story/22774533. [Danish]

[49] Sørensen AB, Cuculiza M. Flu jabs rarely protect you. [Influenza-vaccination beskytter dig sjældent. MX 2014 Oct 10. URL: http://www.mx.dk/nyheder/danmark/story/22497691. [Danish]

[50] Stein R. Reports accuse WHO of exaggerating H1N1 threat, possible ties to drug makers. Washington Post, 2010 June 4. URL: http://www.washingtonpost.com/wp-dyn/content/article/2010/06/04/AR2010060403034.html.

[51] Stenver D. Adverse effects of flu vaccines. [Bivirkninger ved influenzavaccination.] Sundhedsstyrelsen 2014 Oct 20. URL: http://sundhedsstyrelsen.dk/da/nyheder/2014/bivirkninger-ved-influenzavaccination. [Danish]

[52] Sundhedsstyrelsen. Influenza 2010 Nov 10. URL: https://sundhedsstyrelsen.dk/da/sundhed/smitsomme-sygdomme/influenza. [Danish]

[53] Tanjug RS. BELGRADE -- The Appellate Court has confirmed the Special Court's decision to declare itself incompetent to try suspects in the swine flue vaccines case. B92.net 2012 Jul 26. URL: http://www.b92.net/eng/news/crimes.php?yyyy=2012&mm=07&dd=2.

[54] Villesen K, Voller L. Secret commitee gives advices to WHO on Swine flu. [Hemmelig komité rådgiver WHO om svineinfluenza.] Information 2009 Dec 12. URL: http://www.information.dk/218354. [Danish]

[55] Voller L, Villesen K. WHO-advisers hides million-Euro contributions from the Pharmaceutical industry. [WHO-rådgiver skjuler millionbidrag fra medicinalindustrien]. Information 2009 Dec 11. URL: http://www.information.dk/218247. [Danish]

[56] Walsh F. WHO swine flu experts 'linked' with drug companies. BBC 2010 Jan 4. URL: http://www.bbc.com/news/10235558.

[57] Watson S. Baxter to develop swine flu vaccine despite bird flu scandal. Infowars 2009; Apr 27. URL: http://www.infowars.net/articles/april2009/270409Baxter.htm.

[58] Wikipedia. 2009 flu pandemic by country. URL: http://en.wikipedia.org/wiki/2009_flu_pandemic_by_country.

[59] William FE. Mega corruption at the WHO. Rense.com 2009 Sept 9. URL: http://rense.com/general88/megawho.htm.

[60] Council of Europe, Flynn P. The handling of the H1N1 pandemic: more transparency needed. 2010 Jun 4. URL: assembly.coe.int/Committee Docs/2010/ 20100604_H1N1pandemic_E.pdf.

[61] Youtube. Polish Health Ministry Mrs Ewa Kopacz gives speech in Polish Parliament. URL: https://www.youtube.com/watch?v=RhZesZe33cw.

[62] Gøtzsche PC. Psychiatry has gone astray. We would be much better off if we took away all psychotropic drugs from the market. The physicians are not able to handle them. [Psykiatri på afveje. Vi ville være langt bedre stillet, hvis alle psykofarmaka blev fjernet fra markedet. Lægerne er ikke i stand til at håndtere dem. Politiken 2014 Jan 6. [Danish]

[63] Interview with Epidemiologist Tom Jefferson: A whole industry is waiting for a pandemic. The world has been gripped with fears of swine flu in recent weeks. In an interview with SPIEGEL, epidemiologist Tom Jefferson speaks about dangerous fear-mongering, misguided, money-driven research and why we should all be washing our hands a lot more often. Der Spiegel 2009 Jul 21.

[64] World Health Organization. International health regulations. Geneva: WHO, 2005.

[65] World Health Organization. Report of the strengthening response to pandemics and other public-health emergencies. Report of the review committee on the functioning of the international health regulations (2005) and on pandemic influenza (h1n1) 2009. Geneva: WHO, 2012.

Chapter 5

DRUG AND TREATMENT GUIDANCE

The "WHO's model list of essential medicines" states on its first page: "The core list presents a list of minimum medicine needs for a basic health-care system, listing the most efficacious, safe and cost-effective medicines for priority conditions. Priority conditions are selected on the basis of current and estimated future public health relevance, and potential for safe and cost-effective treatment." We saw in 2009 that more than hundred nations bought for tens of billions of Euro and USDs of ineffective and harmful vaccines, because WHO gave totally wrong information about the Swine flu pandemic – first stating that the Swine flu which later became known as the mildest and least dangerous influenza ever – would kill millions of people - and then recommended its member states to buy a totally ineffective vaccines against the swine flu – making most countries buy two injections per every citizen of useless vaccines. Has this history and scandal repeated itself in the COVID-19 event of 2020?

INTRODUCTION

The World Health Organization (WHO) has for many years been a world leader in medicine and health and has guided its member states and a number of other countries in their choice of medicines, including drugs and vaccines. Most member states seem to follow the WHO's recommendation of medicine, i.e., as given in "WHO's model list of essential medicines"

(1). Therefore a great fraction of the world's physicians are following WHO's recommendations, and millions of patients are every years treated according to the recommendations summarized in WHO's drug directories.

Poverty sets a natural limit to the use of pharmaceutical drugs in many countries while non-drug medicine in general is available and according to recent Cochrane reviews and meta-analyses often effective (2). At the same time it is realized that all drugs has adverse effects consisting a potential threat to patients. In spite of this the use of pharmaceutical drugs is growing worldwide. We estimate that today about one billion patients are associated with doctors using pharmaceutical drugs. The treatment of these patients are directly influenced by the WHO's recommendation on pharmaceutical drugs.

Objective science

It is therefore of utmost importance that WHO's recommendations are based on the best and most objective science about the positive and negative effects of the available medicines, drugs as well as non-drug medicines. Recommendation of medicine must take into consideration all the different types of useful medicine there is for the different clinical conditions so that the physicians and the patients can chose the optimal treatment for the actual disease.

Sometimes there will only be one evidence-based treatment, like penicillin for syphilis or pelvic massage for female anorgasmia; but often the choice will often stand between different pharmaceutical drugs/ vaccines, and a number of evidence-based non-drug medicine/CAM treatments (2-8).

The "WHO's model list of essential medicines" (1) states on its first page: "The core list presents a list of minimum medicine needs for a basic health-care system, listing the most efficacious, safe and cost-effective medicines for priority conditions. Priority conditions are selected on the basis of current and estimated future public health relevance, and potential for safe and cost-effective treatment."

SHOULD WE BE ALARMED?

We have been alarmed to notice that the information on pharmaceutical drugs and vaccines in WHO's directory on essential medicines is in line with the pharmaceutical industry's own documentation of its products and often in conflict with data from independent research on drug efficacy and harm made by independent researchers in the Cochrane movement and meta-analyses of the positive and negative effects of the drugs from independent research projects (9-14).

This situation is highly problematic. First the WHO's constitution (15) makes it clear that WHO is obliged to deliver objective information to its member nation and the other nations following WHO's recommendation. As a consequence of this all new studies that contain new and relevant information about the relationship between benefit and harm of the drugs should be taken into consideration by the WHO and included in its recommendations.

When WHO's recommendations are not based on the appropriate valid science we are having the present horrible situation where a large number of the world's countries are buying ineffective and harmful medicine in the belief that it is good and efficient. We saw this in the large scale in 2009 where more than hundred nations bought for tens of billions of Euro and USDs of ineffective and harmful vaccines (16-26), because WHO gave totally wrong information about the Swine flu pandemic – first stating that the Swine flu which later became known as the mildest and least dangerous influenza ever – would kill millions of people - and then recommended its member states to buy a totally ineffective vaccines against the swine flu – making most countries buy two injections per every citizen of useless vaccines (16-26).

WHO IS IN BED WITH WHOM?

In this great scandal it was proven that the vaccine industry itself and people working for the industry and not independent researchers, i.e., the vaccine experts from the Cochrane collaboration had been advising WHO (16-26). WHO kept its close relations to the industry secret for the world which was harshly criticized by the European Council (27). The critique lead to the ridiculous situation that WHO made an investigation of itself and thereafter concluded that WHO had done nothing wrong: "WHO performed well in many ways during the pandemic…" and "The Committee found no evidence of malfeasance"(28 p. xvi).

Everybody who followed the revelation of the large scale scandal in the BMJ and other serious media - called the biggest medical scandal ever (16-26) – seems to agree that something is very wrong in the WHO-system when appraisal of WHO can be the only conclusion of WHOs own investigative rapport after causing that the whole world wasted billions of Euro and dollars on harmful and ineffective vaccines.

REFERENCES

[1] World Health Organization. URL: http://www.who.int/medicines/publications/essentialmedicines/en/index.html.

[2] Committee on the Use of Complementary and Alternative Medicine by the American Public. Complementary and Alternative Medicine (CAM) in the United States. Washington, DC: National Academies Press, 2005.

[3] Ventegodt S, Merrick J. Textbook on evidence-based holistic mind-body medicine: Basic philosophy and ethics of traditional Hippocratic medicine. New York: Nova Science, 2012.

[4] Ventegodt S, Merrick J. Textbook on evidence-based holistic mind-body medicine: Basic principles of healing in traditional Hippocratic medicine. New York: Nova Science, 2012.

[5] Ventegodt S, Merrick J. Textbook on evidence-based holistic mind-body medicine: Healing the mind in traditional Hippocratic medicine. New York: Nova Science, 2012.

[6] Ventegodt S, Merrick J. Textbook on evidence-based holistic mind-body medicine: Holistic practice of traditional Hippocratic medicine. New York: Nova Science, 2013.
[7] Ventegodt S, Merrick J. Textbook on evidence-based holistic mind-body medicine: Research, philosophy, economy and politics of traditional Hippocratic medicine. New York: Nova Science, 2013.
[8] Ventegodt S, Merrick J. Textbook on evidence-based holistic mind-body medicine: Sexology and traditional Hippocratic medicine. New York: Nova Science, 2013.
[9] Ventegodt S. Why the corruption of the World Health Organization (WHO) is the biggest threat to the world's public health of our time. J Integrative Med Ther 2015;2(1):5.
[10] Ventegodt S, Merrick J. The national laws on pharmaceutical drugs must be improved. Submitted to BMJ January, 2015.
[11] MB. Australian journalist wins prestigious award for exposing flu vaccine scandal. The Refusers 2011. URL: http://nhne-pulse.org/australian-journalist-wins-prestigious-award-for-exposing-flu-vaccine-scandal/.
[12] Franck L. Trust WHO. Oval Media Film 2018.
[13] A message from Oval Media, producers of trust WHO: TrustWHO filmmakers respond to Vimeo censorship, 2020 Apr 17. URL: https://www.youtube.com/watch?v=VjQGyqVN5RM.
[14] Gøtzsche P. Deadly medicines and organised crime: How Big Pharma has corrupted healthcare. New York: Radcliffe, 2013.
[15] World Health Organization. URL: pps.who.int/gb/bd/pdf/bd47/en/constitution-en.pdf.
[16] BBC. WHO swine flu experts 'linked' with drug companies. 2010 Jan 4. URL: http://www.bbc.com/news/10235558.
[17] Bethge P, Elger K, Glüsing J, Grill M, Hachenbroch V, Puhl J, Von Rohr M, Traufetter G. Reconstruction of a mass hysteria: The Swine flu panic of 2009. Part 1. Der Spiegel 2010 Mar 12. URL: http://www.spiegel.de/international/world/reconstruction-of-a-mass-hysteria-the-swine-flu-panic-of-2009-a-682613.html.
[18] Bethge P, Elger K, Glüsing J, Grill M, Hachenbroch V, Puhl J, Von Rohr M, Traufetter G. Reconstruction of a Mass Hysteria: The Swine Flu Panic of 2009. Part 2. Der Spiegel 2010 Mar 12. URL: http://www.spiegel.de/international/world/reconstruction-of-a-mass-hysteria-the-swine-flu-panic-of-2009-a-682613-2.html.
[19] The Guardian. Report condemns swine flu experts' ties to big pharma. 2010 Jun 4. URL: 2010. http://www.theguardian.com/business/2010/jun/04/swine-flu-experts-big-pharmaceutical.
[20] Cohen D, Carter P. Key scientists advising the World Health Organization on planning for an influenza pandemic had done paid work for pharmaceutical firms that stood to gain from the guidance they were preparing. These conflicts of interest have never been publicly disclosed by WHO, and WHO has dismissed inquiries into

its handling of the A/H1N1 pandemic as "conspiracy theories". BMJ 2010;340:c2912. URL: http://www.bmj.com/content/340/bmj.c2912.

[21] Jefferson T, Doshi P. WHO and pandemic flu. Time for change, WHO. BMJ 2010;340:c3461.

[22] Law R. WHO and pandemic flu. There was also no new subtype. BMJ 2010;340:c3460. doi: 10.1136/bmj.c3460.

[23] Doshi P, Jefferson T. WHO and pandemic flu. Another question for GSK. BMJ 2010;340:c3455. doi: 10.1136/bmj.c3455.

[24] Cohen D, Carter P. Conflicts of interest. WHO and the pandemic flu "conspiracies". BMJ. 2010;340:c2912. doi: 10.1136/bmj.c2912.

[25] Zarocostas J. Swine flu pandemic review panel seeks access to confidential documents between WHO and drug companies. BMJ 2010;340:c2792. doi: 10.1136/bmj.c2792.

[26] Watson R. WHO is accused of "crying wolf" over swine flu pandemic. BMJ 2010;340:c1904. doi: 10.1136/bmj.c1904.

[27] Council of Europe, Flynn P. The handling of the H1N1 pandemic: more transparency needed. 2010 Jun 4. URL: assembly.coe.int/Committee Docs/2010/20100604_H1N1pandemic_E.pdf.

[28] World Health Organization: Report of the strengthening response to pandemics and other public-health emergencies report of the review committee on the functioning of the international health regulations (2005) and on pandemic influenza (h1n1) 2009. Geneva: WHO, 2012.

Chapter 6

A REVIEW OF WORLD HEALTH ORGANIZATION'S RECOMMENDATIONS IN "WHO'S MODEL LIST OF ESSENTIAL MEDICINES": WHO PROVIDES THE DATA FOR THE DRUG REGISTER?

We have analyzed the WHO's drug directory (The WHO's model list of essential medicines) and found that it is based on the information from industrial drug trials instead of the more objective and reliable information on the drugs provided by meta-analyses made by researchers independent of the pharmaceutical industry, like the Cochrane collaboration. The consequence of this is a strong bias so a large fraction of the drugs are presented more beneficial and less harmful than they actually are. Whole classes of drugs that in independent meta-analyses have been found to be of little clinical value, or even harmful and of no value as medicine, are still listed in the WHO drug directories as beneficial drugs, including cytotoxic anti-cancer chemotherapy, the anti-depressive drugs, the anti-psychotic drugs, the influenza vaccines and the anti-influenza medicines. This means that WHO is misguiding its 194 member states leading to an estimated 500.000.000 patients being treated with pharmaceutical drugs which are often very harmful and often without any significant clinical benefit. To solve this serious problem, we have identified the core principles for rational listening of data regarding positive and negative effects of the pharmaceutical drugs. An outline of a standard list of positive and negative drug effects is suggested. Information on each drug should be provided with due regard to dose, indication of use, all clinically relevant outcomes, method of drug study used for documentation, including placebo type, and the quality of the study. We recommend the use of Number Needed to Treat (NNT) and Number Needed to Harm (NNH), Total Number Needed to Harm (NNH_{Total}), and Therapeutic Value ($TV= NNH_{Total}/NNT$). When more objective and reliable data exist, they should be preferred rather than more doubtful data from studies of lower quality. To make physicians and patients able to choose the optimal treatment WHO should also inform about evidence-based non-drug medicine.. We recommend a fundamental revision of the WHO-system that has proven itself weak to the interests of the pharmaceutical industry. We warn all governments, physicians and patients that the existing WHO drug directories are strongly biased and not reliable sources of information on drugs and vaccines.

INTRODUCTION

The World Health Organization (WHO) has for many years been a world leader in medicine and has guided its 194 member states and a number of other countries in their choice of medicines, including drugs and vaccines.

Most member states seem to follow the WHO's recommendation of medicine, i.e., as given in "WHO's model list of essential medicines" (1). Therefore, a great fraction of the world's physicians are following WHO, and millions of patients are every years treated according to the WHO recommendations summarized in the drug directories of WHO.

Poverty sets a limit to the use of pharmaceutical drugs in many countries while non-drug medicine is in general available and effective. In spite of this the use of pharmaceutical drugs is growing worldwide. We estimate that today the medical treatments of about one billion people – the people who live in the larger cities of the member states - are to some extend based on pharmaceutical drugs and influenced by the WHO's recommendation on pharmaceutical drugs.

It is therefore of utmost importance that WHO's recommendations are based on the best and most objective science about the positive and negative effects of the available medicine.

Any general recommendation of medicine must take into consideration all the different types of useful medicine there is so that the physicians and patients can chose the optimal treatment for the actual disease. The choice will often stand between different pharmaceutical drugs/vaccines, and a number of evidence-based non-drug medicine/CAM treatments (2-8).

The "WHO's model list of essential medicines" (1) states on its first page: "The core list presents a list of minimum medicine needs for a basic health-care system, listing the most efficacious, safe and cost-effective medicines for priority conditions. Priority conditions are selected on the basis of current and estimated future public health relevance, and potential for safe and cost-effective treatment."

We have been alarmed to notice that the information on pharmaceutical drugs and vaccines in the WHO's directory on essential medicines is in line with the pharmaceutical industry's own documentation of its products and often in conflict with data from independent research on drug efficacy and harm made by independent researchers in the Cochrane movement and meta-analyses of the positive and negative effects of the drugs from independent research projects.

This situation is highly problematic. First the WHO's constitution (9) makes it clear that the WHO is obliged to deliver objective information to its member nation and the other nations following the WHO's recommendation. As a consequence of this all new studies that contain new and relevant information about the relationship between benefit and harm of the drugs should be taken into consideration by the WHO and included in its recommendations.

When the WHO's recommendations are not based on the appropriate valid science we are having the present horrible situation where a large number of the world's countries are buying ineffective and harmful medicine in the belief that it is good and efficient. We saw this in the large scale in 2009 where more than hundred nations bought for tens of billions of EUROS and USDs of ineffective and harmful vaccines (10-21), because the WHO gave totally wrong information about the Swine flu pandemic – first stating that the Swine flu which later became known as the mildest and least dangerous influenza ever – would kill millions of people - and then recommended its member states to buy a totally ineffective vaccines against the swine flu – making most countries by two injections per every citizen of useless vaccines (10-21).

In this great scandal it was proven that the vaccine industry itself and people working for the industry and not independent researchers, i.e., the vaccine experts from the Cochrane organization had been advising the WHO (10-20). The WHO kept its close relations to the industry secret for the world which was harshly criticized by the European Council (19, 21).

The critique lead to the ridiculous situation that the WHO made an investigation of itself and thereafter concluded that the WHO had done nothing wrong: "WHO performed well in many ways during the pandemic" (12).

Everybody who followed the revelation of the large scale scandal in the BMJ and other serious media - called the biggest medical scandal ever (10-21) – seems to agree that something is very wrong in the WHO-system when appraisal of WHO can be the only conclusion of WHOs own investigative rapport.

Secondly, as there are often good evidence-based non-drug alternatives to treating with drugs, i.e., psychotherapy (23-25), physical therapy/bodywork/sexologic bodywork (26), and a variety of non-drug CAM methods (2-8), the physicians and patients must have objective and reliable information about the drugs as well as about the non-drug medicines, to be able to choose between a medical treatment with drugs and without drugs.

In many countries like the USA non-drug treatments are becoming increasingly popular (27), as the knowledge of the often quite serious adverse effects has increased and especially as the treatment with ineffective and harmful drugs has led to the accumulation of millions of chronic patients who has not been helped by drugs, and who therefore urgently need an alternative therapy (in Demark this is about 40% of the population (28)).

Without correct information from WHO and from the national health authorities that most often follows WHO's recommendations, the patients' and doctors' choice of medicine can never be rational.

We have, after the Swine flu scandal in 2009, become aware of weaknesses of the WHO system to resist the financial interests of the pharmaceutical companies (10-21). We have through this large-scale scandal come to understand how biases are introduced in the WHO-system and in the WHO's recommendations regarding pharmaceutical drugs as it is found in the WHO list of "essential medicines".

It is well known from the work of more than 3,000 researches in the Cochrane movement that a bias is always introduced when the pharmaceutical industry is documenting its own products; recently leaders of the Cochrane movement has accused the pharmaceutical industry of poisoning millions and killing hundreds of thousands of patients by selling poisonous and ineffective drugs which have not been properly tested (29). We know now after the Swine Flu scandal that this bias is a real threat to international health and health economy. The WHO and the national health organizations should be critical to the bias introduced by pharmaceutical industry but they are not.

This knowledge makes it extremely important that the member states immediately take action to make corrections in the WHO system to ensure that the correct data about medicine is delivered by WHO and the world's countries' health authorities; the serous misguidance of the world's millions of physicians and billions of patients which we have witnessed recently must be stopped.

The situation calls for immediate and strong action by WHO's member states who are the only entities empowered to change the state of affairs.

NATIONAL LAWS ON PHARMACEUTICAL DRUGS

In many countries in the developed world strict laws on the use of pharmaceutical drugs have been passed. In Denmark we have the Law on Pharmaceutical Drugs (30) that regulates the sale and marketing of drugs. The text begins with the purpose of the law: §1. The purpose of the law is to secure, that the citizens "1) have access to safe and effective pharmaceutical drugs of high quality", 2) has access to objective and adequate information about the pharmaceutical drugs and 3) is being protected from misleading commercials for pharmaceutical drugs and other illegal marketing of pharmaceutical drugs."

The law also informs when a drug cannot be on the market: §12. The Medicines Agency declines a marketing permit to a pharmaceutical drug, if: 1) the relationship between benefits and risks is un-favorable (Cmp. §2), 2) there is no therapeutic effect, or the therapeutic effect has not been sufficiently documented by the applicant for the permit, or 3) the medicine has not the specified qualitative or quantitative composition." §25 notify that the holder of a marketing permit must inform the Medicines Agency about any significant new information regarding the relation between benefits and risks of a drug.

EFFICACY AND HARM OF CLASSIC NON-DRUG MEDICINE

During the last three decades, sufficient research has been conducted to establish the number of patients needed to be treated for one to be cured (Number Needed to Treat, NNT) and the number of patients needed to be treated for one to be harmed (Number Needed to Harm, NNH) with non-drug holistic and complementary medicine (CAM) (2-8, 23-28).

The classic type of non-drug medicine, the holistic Hippocratic character medicine, was until recently in general use all over Europe and had been so for more than 2,000 years (31). In three reviews (32-34) we have estimated the general NNTs and NNHs for the most efficient non-drug medicine and found these numbers to be 2 and 64,000 respectively (NNT = 1-3 for the outcome "cured" and NNH = 64,000 for the only significant side effect found, which was brief reactive psychosis).

Research has during the last decades documented good clinical effect and safety of non-drug medical treatment for a long list of clinical conditions with NNTs about 2 and NNHs about 100.000 (see Table 1)(2-8). This means that most patients can be help without drugs and without side/adverse effects. WHOs recommendations to its member states do in no way reflect this fact.

NNT, NNH AND THERAPEUTIC VALUE

Since 1960, biomedical drugs have been developed for a long list of diseases and clinical conditions, of which many are out of clinical reach with non-drug medicine, like antibiotics for syphilis or meningitis. The general NNTs and NNHs of the pharmaceutical drugs has been established to be 20 and 3 respectively (NNT = 20 for the outcome "improved" (35), NNH = 3 for most common adverse effect.

Although most drugs have only one important effect, there are often several adverse effects, making the total likelihood to get one significant adverse reaction larger than the NNH for the most common adverse effect of the drug (NNT_{total} is often about 3 times the NNH of the most common adverse effect, or about $NNH_{total} = 1$, for the treatment of most serious physical and mental diseases). Recent reviews and Cochrane meta-analyses have documented a very problematic relationship between positive and negative effects for large groups of drugs, like the anti-depressants, the anti-psychotic drugs, anti-influenza drugs, and the influenza vaccines (27-34). We know from this that many drugs have problems in relation to the law as the drugs are not effective (only 5% of the patients are helped with most drugs (26)) and the benefits are often much smaller than the harm. Expressed in NNT and NNH, the therapeutic value NNT/NNH_{total} is less than one ($NNT/NNH_{total}<1$).

During the 1970s and 1980s, there was strong optimism about the pharmaceutical drugs, which in some European countries like Denmark has led to the nationalized medicine almost exclusively using pharmaceutical drugs; the use of which has been guided by national pharmaceutical drug directories. Unfortunately, biomedical drugs have failed to be curative for many diseases, and 40 years after the introduction of nationalized biomedicine in Denmark, almost every second Dane has a chronic disorder not cured by the drugs (18).

This situation has led to renewed interest for non-drug medicine all over the world. In Denmark we have seen an exponential development of the interest from about 10% of the population using complementary and alternative (CAM) and holistic medicine in 1990 to 20% using them in 2000 (35), with an estimated 40% of the population using it today. The chronic patients who are not helped much by pharmaceutical drugs go typically for classical non-drug medicine with a combination of talk and touch therapy.

CAM has been criticized for containing many rather inefficient methods like "flower medicine" (36) but many versions of the classical mind-body medicine has found to be evidence-based (2-8), and this method seems to be re-included in the curriculum of many American and European medical schools. A number of American universities are giving non-drug mind-body medicine an important place in the medical curriculum (37).

The WHO constitution, as well as national laws, insist that the public are informed well about medicine; this combined with the explosive growth in interest for non-drug treatments, makes it mandatory that the data on efficacy and harm from pharmaceutical medicine become known to the physicians, and the patients. WHO seems to focus mainly on drugs; this focus is itself a bias.

When it comes to drugs the WHO drug register is not helpful to people who wants the necessary data for evaluating the therapeutic value (expressed as NNT, NNH. NNH_{Total}, and TV) of a drug. These essential data are never given.

Today the WHOs list of Essential Medicines and most national drug directories are constructed in such a way that it is impossible to find the NNTs and NNHs for the drugs. Therefore nobody can see if a drug is only dangerous or of therapeutic value, and nobody can find out if a non-drug treatment is more efficient and safer than a drug-treatment – which will normally be the case. Remember here that non-drug medicine has no significant side effects (NNH=100.000 for most non-drug treatments), making it almost always the attractive choice for the informed patient.

Table 1. NNT-numbers for the best evidence-based non-drug treatments of physical, mental, existential and sexual health issues and working disability (mostly based on clinical studies using chronic patients as their own control (see 37-42 for reviews)

NON-DRUG MEDICINE for physical health	
Subjectively poor physical health	NNT=1-3
Coronary heart disease	NNT=1-2
Cancer (QOL, survival)	NNT=1-3, 2-7
Chronic pain	NNT=1-3
NON-DRUG MEDICINE for mental health	
Mental health problems in general	NNT=1-3
Schizophrenia	NNT=2-5
Major depression	NNT=1-3
Anorexia Nervosa	NNT=1-3
Anxiety	NNT=1-2
Social phobia	NNT=1-3
NON-DRUG MEDICINE for sexual dysfunctions	
Subjectively poor sexual functioning	NNT=1-2
Male erectile dysfunction	NNT=1-2
Female orgasmic dysfunction	NNT=1-2
Female lack of desire	NNT=1-3
Female dyspareunia	NNT=1-3
Vaginismus	NNT=1-3
Vulvodynia	NNT=1-2
Infertility (close ovarian tubes)	NNT=3
NON-DRUG MEDICINE for psychological and existential problems	
Subjectively poor quality of life	NNT=1-2
Low sense of coherence	NNT=1-3
Suicidal prevention (with decisions)	NNT=1
Low self-esteem	NNT=1-2
NON-DRUG MEDICINE for low working ability	
Subjectively poor working ability	NNT=2 (39)

The reason for WHO only promoting drugs is not clear, but it might be the same as the reason for promoting drugs which are not useful of medicine: A dominant influence from the pharmaceutical industry. It seems that WHO is not asking the NNT-numbers for the best evidence-based non-drug treatments of physical, mental, existential and sexual health issues and working disability (mostly based on clinical studies using chronic patients as their own control (37-42) pharmaceutical companies for the data on NNT and NNH, in spite of the knowledge of the importance of these numbers which is very strange. On the national level the national laws rarely force the pharmaceutical companies to inform the health authorities, doctors and patients about the NNT and NNH numbers. Neither WHO nor the National Medicines Agency seems to ask for the essential data on NNT, NNH, and NNH_{total} for the drugs.

The WHO member states must make it clear also to the director of WHO that the values of NNT and NNH are totally necessary for estimating the therapeutic value and usefulness of a drug. Without these numbers a rational choice of medicine can simply not be made.

The WHO member states MUST request the WHO to provide this essential information about the drugs to the public, and WHO must also be requested to document the value of the drugs on the WHO's list of "essential medicines" giving these numbers for each clinical condition.

One can argue that the fraction $TV=NNT/NNH_{total}$ is not a clear cut scientific expression of therapeutic value but this is far the best scientific expression of value we have today; and it is a fair measure. NNH_{total} and TV must be provided also.

The pharmaceutical industry had around 1950 many good measures for the positive effects which gave meaning to the RCTs (randomized clinical trials), including a number of very good, global measures (measuring the patients life all in all) of "quality of life" (like the happiness scale and the self-assessed quality-of-life scale still found in the QOL1 questionnaire (found in reference 38)) and of mental and physical health (outcomes like "self-rated health" and "the patient's experience to go from sick to cured") to less valuable indicators like "symptoms improved" and further down to the present day use of measures of "symptoms somewhat improved". This development has been motivated by an urge to improve the NNTs from around 100 for most drugs in 1950 to around 20 today (26). At the same time the measures for adverse effects have been made less and less sensitive, removing all global expressions of harm from the RCTs, making the NNHs larger. All this indicates that the fraction $TV=NNT/NNH_{total}$ is biased in favor of the pharmaceutical industry's products, but it is still the best measure we have - and when it comes down to it, the only scientific measure. But the global measures of quality of life and self-rated health are totally necessary in the evaluation of medical outcomes.

LISTING OF POSITIVE/NEGATIVE EFFECTS

A serious problem in providing accurate and reliable information about the effects of pharmaceutical drugs is the varying quality of the documentation of drug efficacy and harm. We therefore suggest a 10-step system for grading the evidence levels of the drug trials (see Table 2).

The documentation of the pharmaceutical companies themselves using the RCT procedure is known to be highly biased (39), which explains the significant difference between the documented efficacy of the drugs in industrial drug trials (RCTs) and in meta-analysis made by independent researchers at independent research institutions (40). This difference exists even when the same data is used.

The Cochrane meta-analyses finds systematically less effect and more harm from the pharmaceutical drugs than the pharmaceutical industry does, when it documents its own products, also when the industry's own data is used!

Well-known examples include the negative effects of chemotherapy on quality of life and survival found by Ulrich Abel (41-43), the lack of improvement of the mentally ill patients' mental state with anti-psychotic or anti-depressant drugs found in Cochrane reviews (44, 45), the lack of effect of the influenza vaccines (46), and of the anti-influenza medicines (47).

The indisputable higher qualities of independent meta-analysis make it of utmost importance that the results from such studies are used in both for WHO's and the national drug directories rather than the results and data from analyses coming directly from the pharmaceutical industries.

Table 2. Evidence Level 1-10 (quality) of drug trials. The reliability of the trial varies significantly with the level of analysis (RCT, review of RCTs, meta-analysis of RCTs, national study, cohort study) and the level of independency from the pharmaceutical industry. (1 is best and most reliable quality, 10 worst and least reliable)

1. Cohort studies of long term positive and negative effects of pharmaceutical drugs on the different categories of patients made by independent researchers at independent research centers.
2. Studies by independent researchers at independent research centers based on data from national studies using central registers made by independent researchers at independent research centers. If the health organizations of the state is influenced (i.e., infiltrated) by the pharmaceutical industry the data and the studies based on them will still be biased.
3. Meta-analyses of meta-analyses of RCTs made by independent researchers at independent research centers (studies including several meta-analysis). If the data comes from RCTs made by researchers related to the pharmaceutical industry, they are biased, and all analyses no matter how objective, will still be biased and not reliable.
4. Reviews of meta-analyses of RCTs made by independent researchers at independent research centers. If the data comes from RCTs made by researchers related to the pharmaceutical industry, they are biased, and all analyses no matter how objective, will still be biased and not reliable.
5. Meta-analyses made by independent researchers at independent research centers, i.e., the Cochrane reviews are as good as the data is. If the data comes from RCTs made by researchers related to the pharmaceutical industry, they are biased, and all analyses no matter how objective, will still be biased and not reliable. This is a problem for most Cochrane reviews.
6. Reviews of RCTs made by independent researchers at independent research centers, i.e., the Cochrane reviews are as good as the data is. If the data comes from RCTs made by researchers related to the pharmaceutical industry, they are biased.
7. Cohort studies of long term positive and negative effects of pharmaceutical drugs on the different categories of patients made by physicians, statisticians and other experts paid or in any other ways supported by the pharmaceutical industry are biased; they are made to serve the one who pays.
8. Data from central registers are good but studies made by physicians, statisticians and other experts paid or in any other ways supported by the pharmaceutical industry or made in institutions supported by or working together with the pharmaceutical industry are biased.
9. Meta-analysis of RCTs made by physicians, statisticians and other experts paid or in any other ways supported by the pharmaceutical industry are biased and not reliable.
10. RCTs are in general not reliable due to methodological problems; bias can too easily be introduced though the many phases of the procedure. RTCs sponsored by pharmaceutical companies are therefore always biased. RCTs made by organizations or national agencies which members are supported by or related to the pharmaceutical industry are biased. RCTs made by members of academic institutions who are supported by pharmaceutical companies are biased to some extent.

Another problem is that active pharmaceutical drugs often can be felt by the patient, breaking the blindness of the study and introducing a severe error due to the active placebo effect (48). It has been documented that the positive effects of the anti-depressive drugs found in drug trials with normal (passive) placebo disappeared when active placebo was used (45). If drug trials with active placebo exist, then the results from such trials must be reported instead of the results from drug trials using the incorrect placebo type.

There has been a strong tendency to not document the adverse effects of new drugs sufficiently, making the new drugs seem more efficient that the older drugs, with this tendency disappearing as times goes by and more and more adverse effects are registered, as we have seen with the anti-psychotic drugs (44). This is a severe problem as both physicians and patients are misled to believe that the new drugs are better, making these drugs used more often despite a far higher price and no true advantage. To avoid this problem it is important that global outcome measures of quality of life and self-assessed physical and mental health be included in all future drug trials; outcomes should be documented with global, validated, theory-based questionnaires (like QOL1 and QOL5 that has been developed for this purpose (38)). If a drug fails to improve global quality of life and either self-assessed physical or mental health, then that drug should not be approved because then the adverse effects are greater than the beneficial effects.

A problematic tendency is to report the positive and the negative outcomes differently. It has been shown that patients, physicians and politicians are less positive to treatments when they know the NNT numbers (49); therefore there has been a tendency to hide the NNT numbers and to replace them with horizontal risk measures, which gives the impression that the positive effect is for every patient, despite this obviously not being the case – only one patient in 20, 50 or 100 is helped by a normal pharmaceutical drug (35). At the same time, adverse effects are often reported with vertical risk measures like NNH, to give the impression that adverse effects are rare, in spite of the fact that in you count all adverse effects together (i.e., if you look at the NNH_{total}) every second patients or so is harmed with most pharmaceutical drugs.

The combination of horizontal effect measures for the positive effects with vertical effect measures for the negative makes the drugs look beneficial and harmless. This creates bias by itself. Not using the same measures for positive and negative effects makes it impossible to evaluate the relation between positive and negative effects, is a seriously violating of the intention of the Danish Law on pharmaceutical drugs, but this is nevertheless the normal practice even for the Danish national health authorities.

HOW TO REPORT EFFICACY AND HARM

Many problems follow from the inaccurate listing of positive and negative effects; a common problem is known as "dose-response-bias" where the dose of drug used for measuring the positive outcomes differs significantly from the dose of drugs used for measuring the negative outcomes (39). The only way to ensure that such a bias is not introduced is to place positive and negative effects in a list under the same dose.

Another problem is the confusion of outcomes, as when reduction of unwanted behavior (i.e., "hallucinatory behavior") is confused with improvement of mental health (the outcome "mental state"). Such confusions are common, making it necessary to strictly list all positive outcomes and the NNT for each.

If there is an industry-independent measure of NNT and NNH (Evidence level 1-3 in Table 1), these should replace the NNTs and NNHs provided by the pharmaceutical industry and its collaborators. If there are NNT-numbers and NNH-numbers from drug trials using active placebo, these should replace the NNTs and NNHs from studies using passive placebo. If there are several HHTs and NNHs from more than one study in the high evidence group level 1-3, then all these numbers should be provided; if there are several studies in the low evidence group 7-10, then all these should be provided but with a warning that they cannot be trusted.

In general, the patients and his/her physician should trust the higher NNT and the lower NNH as massive commercial interests induce bias in almost every single drug trial. The independent meta-analysis is still often based on the industrial RCTs, taking all the bias before statistical analysis with them into the meta-analysis. It is also important to be aware of the large, inherent problems of the RCT-test itself not to be over-optimistic of the treatment results from the pharmaceutical drugs (39). The RCT is so flawed amongst other reasons because it ignores the "active placebo effect", that its results are not scientifically valid (39).

It is of crucial importance that the drug directories follow the standard for medical science, with a complete and open reference system. As it is now, the references are not included in neither the WHO's nor the national drug directories. This is also the case in Denmark, where the references neither are in the most used register in book form "Medicine.dk" (50), nor in the electronic version on the homepage (51), nor on any side linked to the homepage, making it very difficult to realize what the source of the data really is; only by comparison of the actual data can you see that they are not from the independent meta-analysis, as they should be, but from other sources strongly biased in favor of the pharmaceutical drugs.

The WHO's drug directory of "Essential medicines" seems to be based only on industrial product resumes delivered by the pharmaceutical companies. We suspect that this result has been possibly due to the impact not only of the industry but also of a variety of international and EU-organizations which all to some extend also are influenced by the pharmaceutical industry.

The procedure WHO uses to determine which drugs should appear in its drug register is highly unclear, which is most regretful. It is also a mystery why WHO these days primarily recommends drugs and vaccines and not the many evidence-based non-drug treatments which often have much better benefit:harm ratios (TV-number).

Table 3. Structure of table for listing the positive and negative effects and therapeutic value of pharmaceutical drugs (revised version of Table 3 in (40))

Drug A, dose α				
A α 1. Indication: Disease D1				
		Short term	Medium term	Long term
Positive effects (Benefit)				
A α 1-B(1)				
Outcome 1:XXX.	NNT	X	X	X
Method:		a/b/c/d	a/b/c/d	a/b/c/d
Evidence level (1-10)	N	N	N	
	Reference	(1,2,3…)	(6,7,8…)	(12,13,14…)
A α 1-B(2)				
Outcome 2: XXX.	NNT	X	X	X
Method:		a/b/c/d	a/b/c/d	a/b/c/d
Evidence level (1-10)		N	N	N
	Reference	(21,22,23…)	(26,27,28…)	(32,33,34…)
ETC				
Negative effects (Harm)				
A α 1-H(1)				
Adverse effect 1: XXX.	NNH	X	X	X
Method:		a/b/c/d	a/b/c/d	a/b/c/d
Evidence level (1-10)		N	N	N
	Reference	(41,42,43)	(46,47,48)	(52,53,54)
A α 1-H(2)				
Adverse effect 2: XXX.	NNH	X	X	X
Method:		a/b/c/d	a/b/c/d	a/b/c/d
Evidence level (1-10)		N	N	N
	Reference	(61,62,63…)	(66,67,68…)	(72,73,74…)
A α 1-H(3)				
Adverse effect 3: XXX.	NNH	X	X	X
Method:		a/b/c/d	a/b/c/d	a/b/c/d
Evidence level (1-10)	N	N	N	
Reference		(81,82,83…)	(86,87,88…)	(92,93,94…)
A α 1-H (Death)				
Death	NNH	X	X	X
Method:		a/b/c/d	a/b/c/d	a/b/c/d
Evidence level (1-10)		N	N	N
	Reference	(121,122,123…)	(126,127,128…)	(132,133,134…)
A α 1-H (total)				
Total harm	NNH_{total}	X	X	X
Method:		a/b/c/d	a/b/c/d	a/b/c/d
Evidence level (1-10)		N	N	N
Reference		(221,222,223…)	(226,227,228…)	(232,233,234…)

Table 3. Structure of table for listing the positive and negative effects and therapeutic value of pharmaceutical drugs (Continued)

Therapeutic value (Benefit/Harm) Estimated therapeutic value for the treatment of disease 1 with drug A, dose α:				
	Therapeutic value **(NNT/NNH_{total})**	**Short term** **X**	**Medium term** **X**	**Long term** **X**
	A α 2. Indication: Disease D2			
		Short term	**Medium term**	**Long term**
	ETC			
	A α 3. Indication: Disease D3			
		Short term	**Medium term**	**Long term**
	ETC			
Drug A, dose β				
ETC				
Drug A, dose μ				
ETC				

Drug B, dose α				
ETC				

On the national level, only the pharmaceutical industry has the references to their own reports and evaluations of their own drugs; the Danish Medicine Agency refers people interested in the references back to the pharmaceutical companies (52), and this seems to be the situation in many countries, which is unacceptable.

Based on these considerations, we recommend that WHO's and the national pharmaceutical drug directories be made as follows. For each drug, the following data regarding the positive and negative effects must be listed. Table 3 gives an example of how such a table might be structured (from 40).

Positive effect(s)

- One table must be made for each specific treatment indication and for each recommended dose.

- For each dose, and each indication the table must include: The NNT for each outcome (i.e., "20% improvement", "50% improvement", "cured".
- For each NNT: information on the term used for the test: a) short term (0-6 month), b) intermediate (6-12 month) and c) long term treatment (12-60 month).
- For each NNT: information on the test method: a) RCT with active placebo, b) RCT with passive placebo, c) RCT with no treatment, d) Other test.
- For each specific treatment indication and for each recommended dose the improvement on global quality of life and self-rated mental and physical health must be listed.
- For each NNT the quality of the study (Evidence Level 1-10, in accordance with Table 2).
- Only clinically relevant outcomes should be listed. If a biomedical parameter or "diseases marker" is improved, and there is no data on the improvement on the patients' health, such data should not be listed in the national drug directory, as it is most likely that the patients are not benefiting from the intervention (78). As a 3%, 5%, or 10% improvement is clinically irrelevant to the patient who always wants to be cured, not slightly improved, such an outcome should not be included in the list of outcomes.
- Horizontal risk measures are normally used when the improvement has only this size and they therefore mislead patients and physicians to believe that a clinically insignificant effect like a 3% improvement has clinical significance and should therefore be avoided.
- If the information is not available, then information on the "missing info" must be found in the table.

Negative effects

- One table of adverse effects and events must be made for each specific treatment indication and for each recommended dose.
- For each specific treatment indication and for each recommended dose the negative impact on global quality of life and self-rated mental and physical health must be listed.
- For each dose, and each indication the table must include: The NNH for each adverse effect and adverse event (including suicide and sudden unexplained death), and the total likelihood for getting an adverse effect/event (NNH_{total}) (Table 3).
- For each NNH: information on the term used for the test: a) short term (0-6 month), b) intermediate (6-12 month) and c) long term treatment (12-60 month).
- For each NNH: information on the test method: a) RCT with active placebo, b) RCT with passive placebo, c) RCT with no treatment, d) Other test.
- If the information is not available, information on the "missing info" must be found in the table.

Therapeutic value

The therapeutic value is finally calculated as NNT/NNH_{total}.

DISCUSSION

We analyzed the WHO Drug Directory of "Essential medicine" (1) and found that it does not follow the above mentioned simple principles for listing positive and negative effects in drug directories. It simply recommends drugs totally without valid scientific documentation!

Whole classes of drugs that in independent meta-analyses have been found to be of little clinical value, or even directly harmful, are still listed in both the WHO and the national drug directories as beneficial drugs, i.e., anti-cancer chemotherapy, anti-depressive drugs, anti-psychotic drugs, vaccines and anti-influenza medicine (41-47).

We have found that several classes of drugs listed in the WHO-list of essential medicine including whole series of drugs should not be in that list; we estimate that at least half the listed drugs are presented as more efficient and less harmful than they are found to be in Cochrane meta-analyses and other more objective studies compared with the documentation provided by the pharmaceutical industry's own drug trials ("sponsored trials").

It seems that strong commercial and political interests have influenced how the drugs are presented both in WHO's and the national directories of the pharmaceutical drugs. It seems to be the standard procedure that the pharmaceutical industry provides the data which is then used by the WHO and the national authorities to make the drug directory that inform physicians and patients about the medicine.

Often the best quality of data from the meta-analyses made by independent researchers, which gives a much more nuanced picture of the effects than the often overwhelmingly positive results from the industrial drug trials, are totally ignored in the drug directories.

Taking the data directly from the pharmaceutical industry introduces a strong bias in favor of the drugs as we have seen above and lead to the marketing of drugs that are only poisonous and not beneficial, as we have seen grave examples of lately.

As a general rule, independent researchers, i.e., researchers from the Cochrane movement have noticed that the positive effects are smaller and the harmful effects more severe in the independent drug trials than in the documentation provided by the pharmaceutical industry and its collaborators.

In meta-analysis, the positive effects of many types of drugs, i.e., anti-cancer chemotherapy (41-43), anti-depressant (45), antipsychotic drugs (44), influenza vaccines (46) and anti-influenza medicines (47), have often been found to be almost non-existent, whereas the negative effects have been severe or even fatal.

Many drugs have been found to reduce the patients' health, quality of life and sexual performance, and to even shorten the patients' life in independent drug trials. We must always remember that pharmaceutical drugs are toxic drugs, that only should be used based on a scientifically well-documented positive effect. Careless use is always compromising the safety of the patient.

We have also found that different measures are used for positive and negative effects of the drugs, making it look like the drugs help every patient and only harm a few. This practice induces a strong bias in favor of the drugs and should be stopped immediately.

It is of the utmost importance that the most reliable and objective information it brought to the physicians and the patients, but we have noticed that this is not the case neither in the WHO system, nor in Denmark and many other countries following WHO.

It seems that the pharmaceutical industry has been able to influence the decision making process on product information and presentation of their data, to such an extent that the WHO directory of "Essential Medicine" and the national drug directories following the WHO's recommendations are not a reliable source of information on pharmaceutical drugs. We recommend that WHO's recommendations on drugs and vaccines are not to be followed until this problem has been solved.

To solve this problem, we suggest that the information on the positive and negative effects of the drugs listed in national drug directories in the future follow a rigid scheme. Only in this way can we avoid the introduction of bias in the drug directories, leading to the extremely problematic listing of harmful drugs as useful medicine, and the most problematic bias from the use of different measures for positive and negative effects, as mentioned above.

We estimate that about 25-50% of the drugs on the market today would be withdrawn (including almost all the psychopharmacological drugs) if high-quality studies were used instead of industrial studies. The drugs that should be removed from the market are the drugs that are only harmful to the patients and must be seen as a major health risk-factor on a national scale. Harmful drugs prescribed for diseases which can be treated more successfully with non-drug methods should not be on the market ether.

We estimate that 350.000.000 people or 5% of the total human population in the developed world are taking drugs that are only harmful and not beneficial, a large fraction of which will get more or less significant adverse effects and adverse events, some of which are likely to be fatal.

Many chronic patients, who are not helped much by drugs, are interested in a non-drug medical treatment, and the number of such patients has been constantly increasing the later decades as more and more patients have ended as chronic and "incurable" patients in countries who rely primarily on treatment with drugs; these patients need to know the NNTs and NNHs of all treatment alternatives to make a rational decision of which alternative treatment to choose.

Only the NNT and NNH numbers can give the patients comparable information about the different types of treatment. The horizontal measures for positive outcomes, which are the only measures provided today in the WHO and national drug directories, do not provide useful information for such a comparison and in general, horizontal measures stating that there is a small value for most patients from the treatment with a drug (small for all) is misleading.

The lack of clear information on the NNTs and NNHs of the drugs in the WHO and the national directories make the patients choices impossible; choices of crucial importance for their life quality and survival are left to guessing instead of being rational decisions based on facts, which is highly regrettable.

Many patients today are not getting the optimal treatment because of lack of information and especially wrong information given by the health authorities, and many patients are therefore misled to use drugs that in high-quality meta-analysis have been shown to only have harmful effects. This is a regular disaster for public health worldwide.

CONCLUSION

Today there are several sources of data on the efficacy and harm of the pharmaceutical drugs; some are provided by the pharmaceutical industry, often in studies of poor quality, whereas others are provided by independent researcher, often in high quality meta-analyses.

We have, in a number of concrete cases, found that data from the high-quality studies have not been used in the WHO's drug directory of "Essential medicine"; instead this list has been based directly on information provided by the pharmaceutical companies. As a result, the information on positive and negative effects (including NNTs and NNHs) are incorrect for large groups of pharmaceutical drugs in the WHO drug register. As many countries are following the WHO's recommendation, as we have seen it to be the case in our analysis of the national drug directory "Medicin.dk", we have an alarming situation where 194 WHO-member-states are passing wrong information on to millions of physicians therefore giving billions of patients a wrong and dangerous treatment.

While dangerous and ineffective drugs are praised as good and necessary medicine the important information on new life-saving treatment developed worldwide in the tradition of non-drug medicine methods for cancer and coronary heart diseases (53-55) with NNTs about 1 and NNHs about a million are not even mentioned by WHO to the member states.

The situation is highly alarming and must lead to immediate action against the WHO and all national health organizations following the WHO's recommendations.

We recommend that all present drug directories are considered seriously flawed and unreliable; only when sound principles for making the directories are taken into use can we rely on such a directory.

We have in this chapter suggested how a valid and useful drug directory can be created, based on the best and most objective medical science. It will only be valid as a guide in medicine if it is complemented by a similar list on all the evidence-based non-drug medical methods available.

REFERENCES

[1] World Health Organization. Essential medicines. URL: http://www.who.int/medicines/publications/essentialmedicines/en/index.html.

[2] Committee on the use of Complementary and Alternative Medicine by the American Public. Complementary and alternative medicine (CAM) in the United States. Washington, DC: National Academies Press, 2005.

[3] Ventegodt S, Merrick J. Textbook on evidence-based holistic mind-body medicine: Basic philosophy and ethics of traditional Hippocratic medicine. New York: Nova Science, 2012.

[4] Ventegodt S, Merrick J. Textbook on evidence-based holistic mind-body medicine: Basic principles of healing in traditional Hippocratic medicine. New York: Nova Science, 2012.

[5] Ventegodt S, Merrick J. Textbook on evidence-based holistic mind-body medicine: Healing the mind in traditional Hippocratic medicine. New York: Nova Science, 2012.

[6] Ventegodt S, Merrick J. Textbook on evidence-based holistic mind-body medicine: Holistic practice of traditional Hippocratic medicine. New York: Nova Science, 2013.

[7] Ventegodt S, Merrick J. Textbook on evidence-based holistic mind-body medicine: Research, philosophy, economy and politics of traditional Hippocratic medicine. New York: Nova Science, 2013.

[8] Ventegodt S, Merrick J. Textbook on evidence-based holistic mind-body medicine: Sexology and traditional Hippocratic medicine. New York: Nova Science, 2013.

[9] World Health Organization. Constitution. URL: pps.who.int/gb/bd/pdf/bd47/en/constitution-en.pdf.

[10] BBC. WHO swine flu experts 'linked' with drug companies. BBC 2010 Jan 4. URL: http://www.bbc.com/news/10235558

[11] The Guardian. Report condemns swine flu experts' ties to big pharma. Guardian 2010 Jun 4. URL: http://www.theguardian.com/business/2010/jun/04/swine-flu-experts-big-pharmaceutical.

[12] Cohen D, Carter P. Key scientists advising the World Health Organization on planning for an influenza pandemic had done paid work for pharmaceutical firms that stood to gain from the guidance they were preparing. These conflicts of interest have never been publicly disclosed by WHO, and WHO has dismissed inquiries into its handling of the A/H1N1 pandemic as "conspiracy theories". BMJ 2010;340:c2912. URL: http://www.bmj.com/content/340/bmj.c2912.

[13] Jefferson T, Doshi P. WHO and pandemic flu. Time for change, WHO. BMJ 2010 Jun 29;340:c3461.

[14] Law R. WHO and pandemic flu. There was also no new subtype. BMJ 2010;340:c3460. doi: 10.1136/bmj.c3460.

[15] Doshi P, Jefferson T. WHO and pandemic flu. Another question for GSK. BMJ 2010;340:c3455. doi: 10.1136/bmj.c3455.

[16] Cohen D, Carter P. Conflicts of interest. WHO and the pandemic flu "conspiracies". BMJ 2010;340:c2912. doi: 10.1136/bmj.c2912.

[17] Zarocostas J. Swine flu pandemic review panel seeks access to confidential documents between WHO and drug companies. BMJ 2010;340:c2792. doi: 10.1136/bmj.c2792.

[18] Watson R. WHO is accused of "crying wolf" over swine flu pandemic. BMJ 2010;340:c1904. doi: 10.1136/bmj.c1904.

[19] Council of Europe and Flynn P. The handling of the H1N1 pandemic: more transparency needed. Council of Europe 2010 Jun 4. URL: assembly.coe.int/ CommitteeDocs/2010/20100604_H1N1pandemic_E.pdf

[20] World Health Organization: Report of the strengthening response to pandemics and other public-health emergencies report of the review committee on the functioning of the international health regulations (2005) and on pandemic influenza (h1n1) 2009. Geneva: WHO, 2012.

[21] Leichsenring F, Rabung S, Leibing E. The efficacy of short-term psychodynamic psychotherapy in specific psychiatric disorders: a meta-analysis. Arch Gen Psychiatry 2004;61(12):1208-16.

[22] Leichsenring F. Are psychodynamic and psychoanalytic therapies effective? A review of empirical data. Int J Psychoanal 2005;86(Pt 3):841-68.

[23] Leichsenring F, Leibing E. Psychodynamic psychotherapy: a systematic review of techniques, indications and empirical evidence. Psychol Psychother 2007;80(Pt 2):217-28.

[24] Bø K, Berghmans B, Mørkved S, Van Kampen, M. Evidence-based physical physical therapy for the pelvic floor. Bridging science and clinical practice. New York: Elsevier Butterworth Heinemann, 2007.

[25] Chopra D, Ornish D, Roy R, Weil A. Alternative' Medicine Is Mainstream. The evidence is mounting that diet and lifestyle are the best cures for our worst afflictions. Wall Street Journal. Jan 9 2019

[26] Kjøller M, Juel K, Kamper-Jørgensen F. [Folkesundhedsrapporten Danmark 2007]. Copenhagen: Statens Inst Folkesundhed, 2007. [Danish] [Public Health Report Denmark]

[27] Gøtzsche P. Deadly medicines and organised crime: How Big Pharma has corrupted healthcare", New York: Radcliffe, 2013.

[28] Lov om lægemidler med noter og stikordsregister, 2. Udg. Lov nr. 1180 af 12. December 2005, som ændret ved lov nr. 538 af 8. Juni 2006 og lov nr 1557 af 20 december 2006 samt ændring ved lov nr 534 af 17. Juni 2008. Copenhagen:, Danish Medicine Agency, 2010. [Act on Medicines with Notes and Index, 2nd Ed. Act No. 1180 of December 12, 2005, as amended by Act No. 538 of June 8, 2006 and Act No. 1557 of December 20, 2006, and Amendment by Act No. 534 of June 17, 2008]

[29] Jones WHS. Hippocrates, Vol. I–IV. London: William Heinemann, 1923-1931.

[30] Ventegodt S, Andersen NJ, Kandel I, Merrick J. Effect, side effects and adverse events of non-pharmaceutical medicine. A review. Int J Disabil Hum Dev 2009;8(3):227-35.

[31] Ventegodt S, Omar HA, Merrick J. Quality of life as medicine: Inter-ventions that induce salutogenesis. A review of the literature. Soc Indicat Res 2011;100(3):415-33..

[32] Ventegodt S, Andersen NJ, Kandel I, Merrick J. Effect, side effects and adverse events of non-pharmaceutical medicine. A review. Int J Disabil Hum Dev 2009;8(3):227-35.

[33] Smith R. The drugs don't work. BMJ 2003;327:0-h.

[34] Susan M. Review shows no evidence that individualised herbal treatments are effective. BMJ 2007;335:743.

[35] Wetzel MS, Eisenberg DM, Kaptchuk TJ. Courses involving complementary and alternative medicine at US medical schools. JAMA 1998;280(9):784-7.

[36] Lindholt, JS, Ventegodt S, Henneberg EW. Development and validation of QoL5 for clinical databases. A short, global and generic questionnaire based on an integrated theory of the quality of life. Eur J Surgery 2002;168(2):107-13.

[37] Ventegodt S, Andersen NJ, Brom B, Merrick J, Greydanus DE: Evidence-based medicine: Four fundamental problems with the randomised clinical trial (RCT) used to document chemical medicine. Int J Adolesc Med Health 2009;21(4):485-96.

[38] Ventegodt S, Merrick J. A review of the Danish National Drug Directory: Who provides the data for the register? Int J Adolesc Med Health 2010;22(2):197-212

[39] Abel U. Chemotherapy of advanced epithelial cancer—a critical review. Biomed Pharmacother 1992;46:439-52.

[40] Abel U. [Chemotherapy of advanced epithelial cancer.] Stuttgart: Hippokrates Verlag, 1990. [German]

[41] Abel U. [Chemotherapie fortgesch-rittener Karzi-nome. Eine kritische Bestandsaufnahme.] Berlin: Hippo-krates, 1995. [German]

[42] Adams CE, Awad G, Rathbone J, Thornley B. Chlorpromazine versus placebo for schizophrenia. Cochrane Database Syst Rev 2007;2:CD000284.

[43] Moncrieff J, Wessely S, Hardy R. Active placebos versus antidepressants for depression. Cochrane Database Syst Rev 2004;1:CD003012.

[44] Jefferson T, Di Pietrantonj C, Rivetti A, Bawazeer GA, Al-Ansary LA, Ferroni E. Vaccines for preventing influenza in healthy adults. Cochrane Database Syst Rev 2014;3:CD001269. doi: 10.1002/14651858.CD001269.pub5.

[45] Jefferson T, Jones MA, Doshi P, Del Mar CB, Hama R, Thompson MJ, et al. Neuraminidase inhibitors for preventing and treating influenza in healthy adults and children. Cochrane Database Syst Rev. 2014;4:CD008965. doi: 10.1002/14651858. CD008965.pub4.

[46] Boutron I, Estellat C, Guittet L, Dechartres A, Sackett DL, Hróbjartsson A, Ravaud P. Methods of blinding in reports of randomized controlled trials assessing pharmacologic treatments: A systematic review. PLoS Med 2006;3(10):e425.

[47] Christensen PM, Kristiansen IS. Number-Needed-to-Treat (NNT): Needs treatment with care. Basic Clin Pharmacolol Toxicol. 2006;99(1):12-6.

[48] Pedersen C, Bjerrum L, Dalhoff KP, Friis H, Hendel J. Medicin.dk 2010. København: Informatum, 2010. [Danish]

[49] Medicine Denmark. URL: www.medicine.dk.

[50] Personal communication. Regulatory coordinator Rikke Bradstrup Haladyn, Danish Medicine Agency, 2009 Dec 14.

[51] Ornish D, Brown SE, Scherwitz LW, Billings JH, Armstrong WT, et al. Can lifestyle changes reverse coronary heart disease? The lifestyle heart trial. Lancet 1990;336(8708):129-33.

[52] Ornish D, Scherwitz LW, Billings JH, Brown SE, Gould KL, et al. Intensive lifestyle changes for reversal of coronary heart disease. JAMA1998;280(23),2001-7.

[53] Spiegel D, Bloom JR, Kraemer HC, Gottheil E. Effect of psychosocial treatment on survival of patients with metastatic breast cancer. Lancet 1989;2(8668):888-91.

SECTION TWO:
PSYCHO-IMMUNOLOGY AND SUSTAINABILITY IN MEDICINE

Chapter 7

The Psychosomatic Work of Dean Ornish: The Power of Mind in Disease

Dean Ornish at the Preventive Medicine Research Institute in Sausalito, California, United States has created an intensive holistic treatment for coronary heart patients and cancer patients with improved diet (low fat, whole foods, plant-based), exercise, stress management, and psychological, emotional, and social support, which has proven to be safe and efficient. We analyze in this chapter the rationale behind his cure in relation to contemporary holistic medical theory. In spite of a complex treatment program, the principles seem to be simple and in accordance with holistic medical theories, stressing the healing power of self-confidence, self-exploration and self-insight, leading to a life with more focus on love, sex, intimacy, friendship and social closeness.

Introduction

If you want to understand the power of the human psyche in disease you might like to study the research of Dean Ornish in clinical holistic medicine (1). Ornish has focused on heart disorders and cancer – first he conducted "The Lifestyle Heart Trial" and subsequently the "Prostate

Cancer Trial". In the "Heart Trial", Ornish documented that the most efficient and lasting way to cure a patient with a heart disorder was by lifestyle intervention (2-4). He would intervene, not only on the physical level, but also on the emotional, mental and spiritual levels, with love and spirituality as the most important components (5). The tradition of holistic medicine goes all the way back to the Hippocratic physicians (6); Dean Ornish seems to work in this tradition. In the same way as the traditional holistic doctors, Ornish believes that love and sexuality are major healing powers: "I happen to think that healing energy and erotic energy is just two different forms of the same thing" (1).

Dean Michael Ornish, MD (born 16 July 1953), is the president and founder of the not-for-profit Preventive Medicine Research Institute in Sausalito, California, United States, as well as a clinical professor of medicine at the University of California, San Francisco. Eighty percent of patients are clinically cured and pain-free after one month (NNT = 1). When patients understand the association between lifestyle and health and change the way they think, feel and live, they heal. Ornish has shown us that it really is that simple, and also applies when it comes to the most severe physical diseases, such as coronary vessel stenosis in the heart and prostate cancer. It normally takes heart patients less than a month to re-open an almost closed coronary artery (2-4), which is very quick. How efficient is his medicine then? Well, according to published statistics, about 80% of his heart patients are cured by the intervention, both in the short-term (1-3 months) and in the long-term (three years) (1, 4). Looking at his prostate cancer patients, we find the same pattern (1, 7).

Therefore, if you accept the publications of his holistic healings of extremely ill patients in the Lancet, JAMA and other highly esteemed journals, there can be no doubt: Ornish and his team have found the key to fast and efficient healing. According to most of the published statistics, 80% of patients are clinically cured and pain free in one to three month after the initiation of treatment (4), which is a truly miraculous medicine.

The Number Needed to Treat (NNT) in his clinical trials is one, both in his heart disease trial and his cancer trial – this is truly remarkable. His holistic medicine is actually so good that most people do not believe in his results. Acknowledgment by Medicare shows that they do believe in Dean Ornish. Medicare has acknowledged his method, which means that US citizens can be cured by holistic medicine paid by the government.

In the academic world, a complementary and alternative medicine (CAM) revolution is happening. Numerous hospitals have launched CAM programs. George Washington University in Washington, DC, has a CAM clinic, and the University of California Los Angeles (UCLA) has had a CAM clinic for a decade. The integrative hospital programs at Columbia-New York Presbyterian utilize mind-body medicine. Memorial Sloan-Kettering Cancer Center in New York has developed an integrative medicine center. Other academic medical centers that offer integrative clinics include the University of Arizona, Dartmouth, Duke, Harvard, the University of Maryland, the University of Minnesota, Stanford and Tufts (8). Interestingly, what drives this development seems to be money (8). One angioplasty costs $31,000 and one bypass surgery $46,000 – and these procedures will often have to be repeated – while a life-saving, one-off holistic medicine intervention at Dean Ornish's clinic costs only $7,000. In Europe, the cost of a chronic patient being treated repeatedly is often hundreds of thousand Euros.

Would we not like to get cured for 5,000 Euros in Europe? Of course, we would. But we are, in general, not informed about this possibility; huge national savings and not appreciation of the magical results for the patients, seems to be what has made Dean Ornish become acknowledged and highly respected in the US. Has Dean Ornish's holistic medicine significant side effects? We all know that surgery has side effects, such as wound infections and sudden deaths from reactions to anesthetics. In general, we know that drugs always have some adverse effects. It is, therefore, also remarkable that holistic mind- body-medicine the way it is practiced by Dean Ornish – at least according to all the research Ornish has published in the field – has no known significant side effects.

Psychosomatic (holistic) medicine is not really Ornish's invention: it has been used for two millennia (6). It was actually the great medicine every physician in Europe used before the industrial age; holistic medicine is known to have no side effects. The Hippocratic doctors found this very important: "First do no harm".

Ornish has declared himself a "non-drug, non-surgery doctor". We would describe him as a "quality of life doctor", as he heals his patients through making them happy. More accurately, he helps them to improve their own happiness as holistic medicine is about self-awareness, self-knowledge and self-insight.

Among doctors and experts in Europe, few seem to be aware of what Dean Ornish has accomplished. Most national health authorities in European countries seem to know little about the great benefits and safety of holistic medicine documented by Dean Ornish. Ornish has showed us that this medicine, the classical medicine of Europe, is not obsolete, is not old fashioned and tired. It is powerful, highly efficient, and totally safe for patients. It is the kind of medicine we need today and in the future.

Ornish says that what truly heals is trust in each other, closeness, intimacy, love and a healthy sexuality. Notice that the political actions that are taking as a response to the WHO-Corona-scare campaign is exactly going against these social needs, making it more difficult for the world's population the be happy and healthy.

A SCIENTIFIC EXPLANATION

Statistically, one of two living in the developed world will die from a cardiovascular disease. Most "heart conditions" are due to a constriction in the coronary arteries from atherosclerosis. Keeping heart and blood vessels healthy are therefore very important to our life expectancy and well-being. Within the last three decades, holistic medicine has achieved a break-through in the understanding and treatment of heart conditions and their psychosomatic treatment. With this new angle on body and soul, it is possible to make even very advanced, life-threatening heart disease disappear, when the patients work on themselves. Many scientific measurements have shown that the constricted coronary arteries are able to physically open up again. The pioneer within this field and a great source of inspiration is Dean Ornish.

Ornish et al. already in 1983 (9) published a study to evaluate the short term effects of intervention (stress management training and dietary changes) in patients with ischemic heart disease (IHD), who received the intervention and 23 controls. After 24 days the experimental group had a 44% mean increase in duration of exercise, a 55% mean increase in total work performed, a 20.5% mean decrease in plasma cholesterol and a 91.0% mean reduction in angina episodes. It was a break-through for holistic medicine in 1990, when Ornish et al. (2) demonstrated that patients through change of beliefs, behavior and experience can make their constricted coronary arteries expand again.

This was a one- year follow-up study of 28 patients (with 20 controls), who changed their life, relations, and lifestyle radically. They began to work with their emotions and sexuality, they started to eat low fat, vegetarian diet; they stopped smoking and drinking, and they worked in a purposeful manner to let rid of stress through stress management training (mindfulness meditation) and moderate exercise.

Artery lesions analyzed by quantitative coronary angiography showed regression in stenosis diameter and overall 82% of the experimental group had an average change towards regression, even in severe coronary atherosclerosis after one year without use of lipid reducing drugs.

Ornish's key tools are love, intimacy and a new more positive life philosophy. The treatment regime affects many aspects of life. As far as we can see, the regime is designed to give the patient a feeling of being more whole, close, happy and healthy. It addresses the patient's perceptions and consciousness. To us, this points to the real cause of cardiovascular disease – and of most other disorders and ailments – our self-created, non-optimal perception of ourselves, our lives and our bodies. In chapter 10 we will talk about the traditional Hippocratic psychosomatic medicine, which also is holistic, meaning that it addresses all aspects of life.

In 1998 these pilot studies were further expanded with 194 in the experimental and 139 in the control group (3, 9). It was found that the experimental group (with the training and changes listed above) was able to avoid revascularization for at least three years by making comprehensive lifestyle changes at substantial low cost without increase in cardiac morbidity or mortality. At this five year follow-up (4) 48 patients with moderate to severe coronary disease were randomized to an intensive lifestyle change group or to the usual care group and 35 completed the five-year follow-up quantitative coronary angiography at two tertiary care university medical centers. More regression of coronary atherosclerosis occurred after five years than after one year in the experimental group, while the control group showed coronary atherosclerosis progression and more than twice as many cardiac events.

The study in 2003 with 440 patients (10) (mean age 58 years, 21% women) with coronary artery disease at baseline and at three and twelve month follow-up showed significant improvements due to the intervention program for both genders and in both the medical and psychosocial sphere. The improvement in women was similar to than in the men, which is important because women in general have higher morbidity and mortality after a heart attack, angioplasty or bypass surgery.

Atherosclerosis

Atherosclerosis is not a phenomenon that can be understood in a purely mechanical manner the way we understand lime scale in a coffee maker (11-13). Blood vessels are damaged, because the cells do not work the way they should, but "scamp" and build delicate and sickly vessels. According to holistic medicine the cells are scamping, because their work is disrupted.

The single most important, disrupting or interrupting factor seems to be our repressed feelings acting as informational "blockages". They are identifiable in the patient's body as, i.e., muscle tensions and tender "trigger points", sites in the body that become especially tender, when we restrain our feelings. These trigger points are also popular "points of attack" in the treatment for the holistic body therapist by acupressure or other techniques.

Our favorite approach is direct interaction with the patient's consciousness, where gestalts are identified and integrated. Thc classical cure is a combination of talk therapy, bodywork to make feelings and emotions appear in consciousness, combined with emotional, relational, and physical exercises. We believe body therapy like acupressure and massage are needed less, when the patient is cooperative and willing to work emotionally with himself.

Conversation is the most effective tool therapeutic we know. The grand tradition of holistic medicine works by helping the patient to come present in their bodies, feel his difficult feelings, "blockages" and old life pain sitting in his body as memory.

Then the patient is helped to understand the association between body and soul in order to formulate difficult feelings. Finally, the patient will acknowledge his inappropriate conclusions and decisions in life, which have given the problems in the body up to the present.

As soon as we acknowledge the irrationality of the perceptions and viewpoints we harvest through life's events, we can let go of them and change our perspective to a happy and trusting philosophy of life, where we openly and honestly feel life as it is, and accept it as a joy and a gift.

Patients with a heart condition need a program focusing on improving the quality of life with a combination of life philosophical tuition, training and supervision. Dean Ornish use the expression "opening the heart" – physically, emotionally and spiritually and the clever backbone of his course of treatment (and one that we used in our research clinic in Copenhagen) is an individual program that combines holistic medical treatment with a personal development program for the patient to carry out on his or her own. The patient, who has experienced heart problems before is offered "secondary prevention" in the form of a personal development program that should counteract any future heart conditions.

Discussion

Ornish and his team have shown that when patients with heart conditions caused by severe atherosclerosis change their mind and their lives and start to reflect, feel, meditate, and relate, the constricted blood vessels can expand again. In the controls, the blood vessels continued to constrict and soon these patients will need bypass surgery to graft new vessels in their hearts.

Often the vessels opened in surgery will also narrow and block in time. A new lifestyle seems to be the only lasting solution to this problem.

So far the most troubling problem seemed to be that the success of Ornish and team to induce these healings have not been repeated by other medical teams. It is well known that the charisma of a therapist can be so enormous that this therapist can make almost all cures work, even when treating the patient with poisonous drugs like arsenic, which was often used as medicine only a century ago. Dean Ornish is known to be a man of such charisma and maybe it is him more that his treatments that actually cure the patients.

In order to test this it was urgently needed that multi-center studies be made using Ornish program for "opening the hearth", which in fact has been done with the study in 2003. This study examined both medical and psychosocial aspects of 440 patients (with mean age 58 years and 21% women) with coronary artery disease at baseline and a three and 12 month follow-up. All were part of a multi-center Lifestyle Demonstration Project, where the participants improved diet (low fat, whole foods, plant-based), exercised, learned stress management, and received social support. Partners were also asked to participate in order to maximize the effect on the family unit, and increase the focus on sexuality as a factor in healing.

Both genders had significant improvements in their diet, exercise and stress management practices. These improvements were maintained over 12 month course of the study. Both women and men also showed significant medical (e.g., plasma lipids, blood pressure, body weight, exercise capacity) and psychosocial (e.g., quality of life) improvements.

This multi-center study showed that a multi-component lifestyle change program can be successfully implemented and repeated at various sites.

It seems that the results of the clinical work of Dean Ornish as a whole on patients with coronary heart disease is fairly well explained by contemporary holistic medical theory (13-24). When a person heals emotionally and these emotions are connected to blockages in the heart region of the body, all tissues might be affected in this region and the coronary vessels being the weakest link is breaking down first. When the person integrate the feelings giving informational disturbance to the tissues the tissues will heal, and thus the coronary vessels can open again as the cells aging receive correct information on structure and functioning from the information system of the body (25, 26).

ACKNOWLEDGEMENTS

This chapter is based on: Ventegodt S, Merrick J. A citizen's guide to survive Corona COVID-19 (SARS-CoV-2). Copenhagen: Quality-of-Life Research Center Press, 2020.

REFERENCES

[1] Ornish D. TED speaker. URL: https://www.ted.com/speakers/dr_dean_ornish.

[2] Ornish D, Brown SE, Scherwitz LW, Billings JH, Armstrong WT, et al. Can lifestyle changes reverse coronary heart disease? The Lifestyle Heart Trial. Lancet 1990;336:129-33.

[3] Ornish D, Scherwitz LW, Billings JH, Brown SE, Gould KL, et al. Intensive lifestyle changes for reversal of coronary heart disease. JAMA 1998;280:2001- 7.

[4] Ornish D. Avoiding revascularization with lifestyle changes: the multicenter lifestyle demonstration project. Am J Cardiol 1998;82(10B):72T-6.

[5] Ornish D. Love and survival. The scientific basis for the healing power of intimacy. New York: Harper Collins, 1999.

[6] Jones WH. Hippocrates. Vol I-IV. London: William Heinemann, 1923-31.

[7] Frattaroli J, Weidner G, Dnistrian AM, Kemp C, Daubenmier JJ, Marlin RO, et al. Clinical events in prostate cancer lifestyle trial: results from two years of follow-up. Urology 2008;72(6):1319-23.

[8] Faass N. Integrating complementary medicine into health systems. Gaithersburg, MD: Aspen, 2001.

[9] Ornish D, Scherwitz LW, Doody RS, Kesten D, McLanahan SM, Brown SE, et al. Effects of stress management training and dietary changes in treating ischemic heart disease. JAMA 1983;249(1), 54-59.

[10] Koertge J, Weidner G, Elliott-Eller M, Scherwitz L, Merritt-Worden TA, Marlin R, et al. Improvement in medical risk factors and quality of life in women and men with coronary artery disease in the Multicenter Lifestyle Demonstration Project. Am J Cardiol 2003;91(11):1316-22.

[11] Pischke CR, Weidner G, Elliott-Eller M, Ornish D. Lifestyle changes and clinical profile in coronary heart disease patients with an ejection fraction of <or=40% or >40% in the Multicenter Lifestyle Demonstration Project. Eur J Heart Fail 2007;9(9):928-34.

[12] Ornish, D. Dr. Dean Ornish's program for reversing heart disease. New York: Ballantine Books, 1990.

[13] Antonovsk, A. Health, stress and coping: New perspectives on mental and physical well-being. San Francisco, CA: Jossey-Bass,1979.

[14] Antonovsky, A. Unraveling the mystery of health. San Francisco, CA: Jossey-Bass, 1987.

[15] Antonovsky A, Sagy S. The development of sense of coherence and its impact on responses to stress situations. J Soc Psychol 1986;126:213-25.

[16] Antonovsky A. The structure and properties of the sense of coherence scale. Soc Sci Med 1993;36(6):725-33.

[17] Maslow, A. Toward a psychology of being. Princeston, NJ: Van Nostrand, 1962.

[18] Frankl, V Man´s search for meaning. New York: Simon Schuster, 1997.

[19] Ventegodt S, Andersen NJ, Merrick J. Editorial: Five theories of human existence. ScientificWorldJournal.2003;3:1272-6.

[20] Ventegodt S. The life mission theory: A theory for a consciousness-based medicine. Int J Adolesc Med Health 2003;15(1):89-91.

[21] Ventegodt S, Merrick J, Andersen NJ. QOL philosophy III: Towards a new biology. ScientificWorldJournal 2003;3:1186-98.

[22] Ventegodt S, Andersen NJ, Merrick J. Holistic medicine III: The holistic process theory of healing. ScientificWorldJournal 2003;3:1138-46.

[23] Ventegodt S, Andersen NJ, Merrick J. Holistic medicine IV: The principles of the holistic process of healing in a group setting. ScientificWorldJournal 2003; 3:1294-1301.

[24] Ventegodt S, Merrick, J., Andersen NJ. Quality of life theory I. The IQOL theory: An integrative theory of the global quality of life concept. ScientificWorldJournal 2003;3:1030-40.

[25] Freeman AM, Morris PB, Barnard N, Esselstyn CB, Ros E, Agatston A, et al. Trending cardiovascular nutrition controversies. J Am Coll Cardiol 2017;69(9):1172-87. doi: 10.1016/j.jacc.2016.10.086.

[26] Freeman AM, Morris PB, Aspry K, Gordon NF, Barnard ND, Esselstyn CB, et al. A clinician's guide for trending cardiovascular nutrition controversies: Part II. J Am Coll Cardiol 2018;72(5):553-68.

Chapter 8

BRAIN AND CONSCIOUSNESS

The most complicated structure of the known universe is the human brain. We can give up on understanding it, or we can try. A theory of the human brain does not last long, for they are often not very good and new theories follows and take over the attention. We can do two things here, we can give up, or we can take the fight for understanding. If you are not up for big mind-struggles this day, you might like to skip over chapter 8 and 9, which is about a theory of the immune system, not much more digestible than the theory in this chapter on the brain. If you take the challenge and try to read it, do not despair. It might be that our ideas are not that good, so if something seems wrong; it is likely to be wrong. Just forgive us, and jump to next chapter.

In this chapter 7, we look at the brain's structure and function from a philosophical perspective. Although the brain at micro-level, with its trillions of ultra-thin nerve fibers, is one of the most complicated structures in the known universe, you can still grasp its composition if you go up to the level of the cell. How this structure functions is not quite clear. You can understand its function at fiber level, because it is fairly simple, and you can understand it at cell level, but it is already vague.

Roughly speaking, you can envision a single nerve cell as a tiny, independent computer whose behavior is dependent on continuous calculations of all input. At organ level, the function can be understood as an extremely complex pattern machine. Finally, the brain's function can be understood at the cognitive level as what provides consciousness through its ability to keep order in our complicated reality.

The superior function of the brain is to connect the real us, our higher self, to the surrounding world. The brain has been developed so that it can create all possible complex patterns. The connectivity seems to imply that the patterns of the human brain are 1000-dimensional. It is our vision that these complicated patterns arise from basic patterns in the quantum matter of which everything is created.

In our opinion, our consciousness' special utilization of a patterned aspect of nature is what lies behind inscrutable statements like "Man is created in God's image". We suggest that these patterns in matter are the basic, creative force that influences all living organisms. Unfortunately, science has only just begun to understand these patterns. The Bible's description of the origin of man is two people eating from the Tree of Knowledge and as punishment they are expelled from the Garden of Eden.

What does that mean? It means that, as conscious creatures, we no longer were an unproblematic, harmonious part of the world around us. The great question is why this consciousness about the world, provided by the brain, is not a gift that makes life better instead of getting us expelled from the Garden of Eden. We think that our real problem is the fact that we are still not in control of our consciousness. Instead of it serving us, we have become its slaves.

If we come to understand brain and consciousness in order to solve this basic problem of our existence, we shall again be able to become a coherent part of the world, both as individuals and as a species. We share the vision that such an understanding of the problems of consciousness will make medical science holistic and will bring quality of life, health, and the ability to function to its patients.

INTRODUCTION

The problem addressed in this paper is one of the most complex in biology and medicine and one that has been the subject for intense scientific exploration during the last several decades with many amazing new discoveries. There is a literature so vast that it can hardly be studied in detail by any researcher, and nobody seems to be able to read all the articles published in fine journals like Behavioral and Brain Sciences. A number of nice introductions, like Kandel and Schwartz' great book "Principles of neural science" (1), have been published during this period covering a number of aspects from philosophical to anatomical and physiological (1-13). So what can we contribute to this huge body of knowledge on the brain and consciousness?

Let us start with the very simple consideration that science is an interpretation of reality. When we describe the brain, we must make some initial choices about how to conceive mind, consciousness, understanding, and the project of science itself. So in this chapter, we step back to look at the fundamentals. What do we know, from a philosophical and abstract perspective? What are the axioms we choose to believe in, so we can get on with the scientific exploration? In our opinion, this process of stepping back and looking at the greater picture is much too seldom done in our science, where we are so busy producing scientific papers full of models, theories, and data from measurements. It is so important in medical scientific research and of value to our patients that we know direction, reason, and the problems connected to consciousness, that we find it valuable to stop and think, abstractly and vaguely, about the connection between consciousness and brain (14). We hope that the reader shares this opinion.

DEVELOPMENT

About 10,000 years ago something very strange happened here on Earth. Some rather primitive ape-men developed the ability to describe the world in a very detailed way using an abstract language. They developed mental consciousness. According to archaeological discoveries, the leap to modern man has been under way for about 100,000 years, starting with the mastery of fire and the use of very primitive tools. But not until a common description of the world appeared was it possible to work out social rules in tribal communities, develop a number of specialized techniques, and develop the very complicated townships, which appeared for the first time around then.

How may we understand the evolution of humankind and the emergence of consciousness? A good place to start is the study of the human brain, which is quite unique. How was the brain developed and what were the forces that spurred this development? It is our personal vision that complicated basic patterns in the quantum matter (8, 15), of which everything is created, has served as a template, because the brain has been developed so that it can create all possible complex patterns, as we shall see. In our opinion, our special utilization of a patterned aspect of nature (16, 17) is what lies behind inscrutable statements like "Man is created in God's image". As we see it, these patterns in matter are the basic, creative force that influences living organisms. Unfortunately, science has only just begun to understand these patterns (18-20).

We shall look at the brain's structure and function. Although the brain at micro-level, with its trillions of ultra-thin nerve fibers, is one of the most complicated structures in the known universe, you can still grasp its composition if you go up to the level of the cell (21-25). How this structure functions is not quite clear. You can understand its function at fiber level, because it is fairly simple (1) and you can understand it at cell level, but it is already vague (26-30). Roughly speaking, you can envision a single nerve cell as a tiny, independent computer whose behavior is dependent on continuous calculations of all input. At organ level, the function can be understood as an extremely complex pattern machine. Finally, the brain's function can be understood at the cognitive level as what provides consciousness through its ability to keep order in our complicated reality (7, 31-34). The superior function of the brain is to connect us to the surrounding world, at least for the brains of a size we can manage to study (35). Apparently, the brain systematizes all our experiences and verbal inputs into that map of reality. This map is not just a static depiction; it contains time so that our plans and strategies for realizing our innermost dreams are also part of this map (14).

The Bible's description of the origin of man is two people eating from the tree of knowledge and as punishment they are expelled from the Garden of Eden. What does that mean? It means that, as conscious creatures, we no longer were an unproblematic, harmonious part of the world around us. We were no longer as one with the animals and plants of the Garden of Eden. The great question is why this consciousness about the world provided by the brain is not a gift that makes life better instead of getting us expelled from Eden (36-38). We think that our real problem is the fact that we are still not in control of our consciousness (39). Instead of it serving us, we have become its slaves. If we solve this basic problem of our existence (40), we shall again be able to become a coherent part of the world, both as individuals (41, 42) and as a species.

THE BRAIN IS A PUZZLE

The brain is one of science's greatest puzzles. We have only just begun to understand how the brain is able to interpret data from the eyes and the ears, how the motor patterns that coordinate the body's scores of muscles are arranged during walking, how we can recognize a particular face among billions, and speak ten different languages with thousands and thousands of words, as some people are able (1). And we have not even begun to understand what it means to understand. How is man able to design things like the theory of relativity, quantum mechanics, and mathematics?

Today there are many models that are vaguely starting to explain some of the things that take place in the brain's layer of nerve cells, e.g., "neural networks", and promising models of the creation of very complex patterns from the repetition of simple processes (19). But really, it is not very impressive when you think of the creativity and efficiency of our brains. Without insight into matter itself and biology, we shall never be able to understand the basic principles behind the brain and consciousness. Let us introduce the problem of the brain with a couple of examples of the mysterious connection between brain and consciousness. It once happened that a university student with practically no brain was used in a brain-scan test (43). When he was still a fetus, the main part of the cerebral substance had been replaced by water. Usually, this condition — hydrochephalus, with water in the head — leads to severe mental disability, but this person managed to reach university level without obvious mental deficiencies. His brain consisted of an edge of tissue only millimeters or a few centimeters thick, lining the cranium. The traditional explanation claims that normally we only use 10% of the brain and therefore the student possessed exactly the amount that was needed. But if we observe the functions of a normal brain, we will see that every brain cell is working more or less constantly. If we could manage with 10%, we probably would not have developed our large brain. And still, there is something wrong, because apparently there are some who can manage with such a small brain.

An experiment with cats showed similar results (43). During a test, a researcher surgically removed most of a cat's brain apart from the areas that covered vital reflexes. He had the cat walk around on the tables during a large conference with neurologists and people in brain research and challenged the assembly to correctly diagnose the cat. Nobody was able to guess that the cat had no brain, because it behaved almost normally. It comes as something of a surprise that our knowledge of life is born by life itself, but if we remember everything that Hydra was able to do without a brain, it does not appear so shocking after all (4). This is just meant as a warning against too quick and simple conclusions.

THE STRUCTURE OF THE BRAIN

In our attempts to understand the brain and consciousness, let us enter the brain and see what takes place in there, starting with the brain structure. Our main interest is the cerebrum cortex, which was especially developed in our transition from ape to man. The human brain consists of a bisected cerebrum weighing approximately one kilogram and situated inside the head. The cerebral cortex consists of about 25,000,000,000 brain cells that constantly receive messages from thousands of the other cells, and they in turn communicate with thousands of other cells in an extremely complicated and ramified pattern. There is an incredible proliferation of cerebral connections within the brain. Neural connections run from numerous cells to the other half of the brain or to distant parts within their own hemisphere. Therefore, it hardly seems likely that the brain is functionally bisected into two essentially different halves, which is the opinion of several neuropsychologists. Despite the anatomical bisection, it is actually a closely knit whole with only minor areas possessing well-defined and isolated functions. All these brain cells are interconnected through an almost incredible mass of neural fibers, nearly 1,000,000 km, which would circumvent the Earth 25 times. The brain can contain all these impulses because they are only one thousandth of a millimeter thick.

PHYSIOLOGY OF THE BRAIN

Neural impulses run from one nerve cell to another. Apart from a few details, the opinion today is that we fully understand the distribution of the neural signal from one nerve cell to the next. The next level of understanding is the cell. The cell deals with incoming signals by adding them up one by one (the actual summary function is dependent on the individual cell and can be very complicated). Thus the cell can be seen as a computer that calculates the input received and forwards new signals when the result is correct. There is little doubt that the cell has such a summary function, but we are convinced that this function is continuously modified by the biological system through biological information. At levels above the cell level, it becomes almost impossible to follow what happens in the brain, because the brain produces functional patterns of nearly infinite complexity, which are also modeled by input from life's information in a way that is not understood at all (44). The effect, however, is that information is transferred from the depth of the organism to the brain and this is a decisive input to our dreams and intuitive awareness of the world. We imagine that brain patterns can be directly regulated by the organism's information system, as in dreaming. This is parallel to the way the self-organization of the cell's molecules is governed by the cell's biological information system (38). Much research has been carried out in the individual subareas of the cerebrum cortex, especially the optical cortex, which is the area that interprets vision. The hope is to pick up how the brain is able to see and thus to produce artificial, electronic eyes for use in military surveillance, for example. Science has advanced somewhat towards analyzing how optical impressions are gradually led to higher and higher of complexity. Unfortunately, scientists lose the threads just where it starts to get interesting, when the optical impressions received from the retina are about to make sense (1). A large number of areas with fixed functions are known, but most of the cerebrum cortex is integrative, that is, occupied with interpreting information received by the brain. The frontal lobe deals with the highest integrative levels, the top of the pyramid of consciousness, and keeps track of space, time, and abstract ideas (1).

IS THE BRAIN A COMPUTER?

At some time in the future, a very fast computer (perhaps 1,000 times faster than the ones we know today) may be able to copy the ability of the human brain to organize the world. But the experience of meaning and consciousness only come from life itself. Therefore, a computer can never become conscious or understanding in an intelligent way the way a human being is. Many scientists and other people try to reduce the brain and consciousness to something inorganic. Especially among physicists, the so-called "neural network" is a hot research subject. However, these fairly simple physical models only bear passing resemblance to the human brain. The dynamic we know as "thought" is not analogous to the lifeless physical models that are on the market today, however sophisticated they may be.

In his book "The user illusion " (45), the author Tor Nørretranders has described the brain as a complicated calculator that more or less creates consciousness as a by-product of the process that reduces the complex to the simple (seemingly a misinterpretation of the Libet's famous experiments) (46). In our opinion this is a materialistic reduction of all those fantastic things that take place in the human brain. Such a description disregards the fact that the brain is a living organ in a living organism, and it does not do justice to consciousness at all. We hold the view that the foundation of consciousness and awareness stems from life itself, from the communication between all the cells of the organism, and not just from the brain. Therefore, the brain does not actually create consciousness; it just provides it with the particular quality or mental order we call reason.

The brain bridges the gap between the depth of life and the world around us; nerve cells communicate with each other and the other cells in the body in two ways. First, like any other cell, through an exchange of biological information of an unknown nature (14, 37) which, at conception, provides the brain with its shape and structure (5). Second, through chemical and electrical communication where electrical neural impulses can be transported along neural fibers and jump from cell to cell via chemical synapses. Hormone-like substances secreted by the brain itself that are called neuropeptides also chemically influence nerve cells. In order to understand the function of the brain, both forms of communication — the one that disseminates biological information and the one that communicates chemical-electrical signals — are needed. This is because the brain bridges the gap between life inside the organism and the outside world (14). The first form of communication, which may be called the basic biological communication that makes the brain an integrated organ in the organism, creates the bridge towards the inside. The bridge towards the outside, to the outside world, is built with the help of the other form of communication, the electrical and chemical, that is well suited for sensing via the sensory organs.

One might say that the brain receives the signals about our inner dreams and wishes (the biological potentials) through the former kind of communication, while the information about the outside world is received through the latter. The brain's real business appears to be the production of electrical patterns that are so like the biological patterns (whose nature today is unknown but probably not electrical, more like quantum mechanical) that the description of reality can bridge the gap between the inside and the outside. In this way, meaning is created of all the input we receive from the outside through our sensory organs, a meaning, which, popularly speaking, occurs when sense perceptions from the outside agree with the organism's inner biological order.

What the brain is doing is organizing reality. It handles all sense perceptions and impressions that over time pass our way and reorganizes these sense perceptions into plans and strategies for the future in accordance with our inner dreams and wishes.

Reason and Intuition

The result of the brain's activity is the order of reason. The whole world has been neatly arranged and described to the smallest detail in time and space. Still, this order is somehow artificial, a reduction of an infinitely complicated reality into something that is easy for us to comprehend and relate to. As organisms we are able directly to experience reality — in principle. We use our wholeness instead of our brain and senses. Such a direct experience ought to provide us with a much more dynamic and correct picture of reality. However, the picture is so chaotic and disorderly that it does not make much sense to our reason, which is practically drowning in the flood of information.

It is this direct access to reality that we usually call intuition, a sure knowledge situated at a level that is lower than that of the model of the world, which is created by language and reason. We possess two sources of knowledge. One is through the senses, where the impressions become a certain, well-organized picture of reality with the help of the brain's organizing process. All the things that we learn can be stored in a neat and well-organized way in this picture, which produces our map of reality. Usually, we call this organizing faculty reason. Our other source of knowledge is intuition. Here awareness takes hold of the reality of life, both on the inside and outside, in a more direct but far less organized way. In this way, intuition is directly connected to the information system living matter uses. Through this information system, our intuition can draw upon all the information contained in the recipe for a human being, as well as all the knowledge life acquires through its intense dialog with other living beings at all the levels that make up the world. People can function at his optimum only when both intuition and reason are cultivated and in balance, that is, when reason gives intuition ample space and when intuition does not cover subjects that are better handled by reason.

AWARENESS

The nature of human awareness is mysterious. Let us distinguish between consciousness and awareness. To us, consciousness is a cultivated form of awareness. Consciousness is connected to the brain in the shape of reason, while awareness is connected to life itself. The awareness of the individual cells coalesces and makes up the raw material for the organism's overall awareness.

There are people who can relate how they witnessed operations performed on them although they were fully anesthetized. What makes it difficult to disregard such stories is the fact that what the patients purported to have experienced, while their brain was fully anesthetized, such as dialogs and other events, actually did take place. Something or other in their being was aware, even though the brain was anesthetized. Apparently in these cases man is aware without being conscious and without the senses being active. We may think of awareness as a faculty that can grab hold of multitudinous things. When the cells' united awareness gets hold of the brain, it lets us experience the outside world through our senses and through the organized interpretation we call our map of reality, that is, our reason's consciousness of the world. This is different from the direct, spontaneous, and unreflective experience of the world that the brain receives when awareness grabs hold of reality directly and without consulting the brain and the senses. Awareness is the ability produced by being fully and completely present in your life.

DREAMS

When we sleep, half the time is spent dreaming. Actually, we also sometimes dream when we are awake, but daydreams, imaginings, and other creative thought processes are of a more fragile quality, because our brain is already using most of its energy on maintaining the awareness of the world that is descriptive of the ordinary waking state.

But at night, when our senses are disconnected from the world, the brain is set free and is able to carry out the creative process we call dreaming. Probably this process is not qualitatively different from daydreaming or having visions about the good life, but night dreams are still of a different nature than daydreams. In our dreams we get much closer to our body, our life, and our organism. When we are disconnected from the outside world, we become temporarily free and are able to shape our pictures in the brain according to our profound desires and potentials. The dreaming state can be registered with electrodes attached to the brain. We see that the brain works in different, characteristic rhythms (high-frequency alpha and beta waves and low-frequency delta and theta waves).

During the night we have periods with very active dreams (with extremely high-frequency brain waves) and periods without dreams (with extremely low-frequency brain waves). We think that what happens here is that awareness swings from being mostly in the brain to being mostly in the body when you go from dreaming to not dreaming. An interpretation of this can be that the natural course of sleep is about fusing brain and body and brings the map in harmony with the inner life just like the daily, outer activity is about bringing the map in harmony with the outside world. In this way, we try every night to heal ourselves and create the sound bridge between the depth of life and the outside world (14).

Dreams in the Freudian and Jungian tradition (47) are understood to be about our conflicts and existential problems. A lively debate occurs inside us when what we have learned about the world is inconsistent with life itself. Subconsciously we try to become whole, healthy, happy, and well-balanced people. Therefore, dreams hold an enormous potential for healing and curing. When we dream and really relax it seems that all parts of our organism are tied together a little better, as if disorders and breaches in our existence are healed. It is important to notice that this conception of dreams as a bridge to our soul or genuine self (higher self, wholeness) is not shared with all researchers in the cognitive traditions.

THE WORLD IS MODELED ON THE PATTERNS OF THE BRAIN

To understand what happens in the brain, it should also be mentioned that a quarter of the energy of the human organism is spent on keeping the brain going 24 hours a day. Nerve tissue has a formidably high metabolism. Every nerve cell is constantly sending signals to others, the brain as whole never rests. Now, what is the brain doing with all these nerve fibers and all that energy? Apparently it produces very advanced patterns that are the templates we use for shaping our whole description of the world. To get an idea of just how complicated these patterns are, you can think of the patterns in water, where impulses are only moved from one molecule to the next in two or three dimensions. The surface of water, with its two dimensions, produces rings and the like. With three dimensions, you can see various types of whirls and spindrifts. The ramifications in the brain make the brain's patterns 1,000-dimensional. The patterns are further complicated by the fact that each area of the brain (each nerve cell) communicates not only with its neighbor, but also with distant areas all over the brain that again react back to the first place via a number of intermediate steps. However, it does not become really complex until the brain starts working and keeps feeding every nerve cell with its own and other brain cells' output. Such iterative processes where the same simple process is repeated time and again in almost the same way have led to the most complex patterns (just think of the many levels of spirals and patterns of the Mandelbrot fractal, or whirls in the water or clouds in the sky) (18, 19). So what happens when the processes in question are patterns in the brain's incredibly complicated network?

Then it no longer seems strange that our brain can model and create all the various shapes, phenomena, processes, and basic qualities of the outside world that we use for constructing our interpretation of reality. However, it is still shocking that our head is able to contain such an incredibly extensive and dynamic model of the whole world. One of the real mysteries is memory — that all these impressions, experiences, and phenomena can be stored in the brain and recalled in an orderly way almost immediately. On the other hand, perhaps it is no stranger than the recipe for the human being that is stored in the biological material. The principle of storage is probably exactly the same. Life's ability to handle information is almost unfathomable.

THE BRAIN CREATES ORDER

The brain organizes reality for the person and it creates order from a chaotic reality. The brain can organize every received element of reality into groups of elements that have common properties. In this way all the elements of reality are organized hierarchically, so that elements combine at still higher levels to finally produce our abstract concepts of the world. You could say that reality is arranged into a "pyramid of consciousness" with everything concrete forming the broad foundation and the few, extensive concepts at the top of the pyramid.

Everything we know is organized according to properties. Some examples are kitchen utensils, others vehicles. The kitchen utensils can be subdivided into pots and pans, while the means of transportation can be subdivided into cars, bicycles, etc. In the same way all the processes that exist in reality are categorized as being creative, destructive, for maintenance, or for transformation. All phenomena can be grouped according to certain specific qualities like shape and color, or according to abstract qualities such as value, meaning, structure, etc. The whole of reality is organized into main areas through concepts such as "matter" (the physical, chemical, or inorganic, dead), "life" (the organic), "consciousness" (the psychological, ethical, philosophical, and religious), and "society" (economy, law, and politics) as well as a number of other concepts.

This order is the leading principle in what we call reason, but the actual structure behind this order, the system in which reason acts, is still not understood, neither philosophically nor scientifically. This profusion of concrete phenomena and processes that characterize our world is gathered into an ordered description of the world through abstract concepts and principles. When you add it all up, it becomes the map of reality. This map is constructed through an ingenious combination of the brain's ability to create order in the world with the help of self-organizing patterns and life's ability to add meaning to such patterns.

Conclusion

Thus our mind contains a description of the world that is very complicated and that is made up of endless numbers of these extremely complicated patterns that are added together in order to produce faces, flowers, and trees and even products such as metal surfaces. Everything that we have experienced in life, all the pencils we have used and the glasses of water we have lifted, has been boiled down into a very complicated and dynamic description of the reality contained in our brains. We just have to see the reflection of the sun in a glass to acknowledge that we are facing a water tumbler. How can this be? It is because we have seen so many glasses that now we master visual perception almost completely. What makes our description of the world really effective is that we are able to sprinkle our personal history, all our previous experiences and interpretations, over every new environment or locality that we enter.

Thus every sensation is tinged with those like it that we have seen before, and almost any scene immediately becomes a whole and meaningful picture with people, furniture, trees, or whatever. This is very practical and you do not really need to spend much energy on what you are actually seeing, because you are able get a sense of it very well purely by reflex. You only need a few sensory clues and everything you have learned and experienced about the world becomes present again. Now we are able to understand what is the evolutionary purpose of the brain: To create order out of the chaos of reality.

With a sound model of the world, we become incredibly efficient at perceiving, ordering, and acting in the world. Thus, through this ability man has become the master of matter and has been able to invent zippers and space shuttles. The problem is that, concurrent with mastering matter, we have lost our grip of our soul (48-51). We have lost our way in the mental maps of the world (44, 52). If we come to understand brain and consciousness and solve this basic problem of our existence, we shall again be able to become a coherent part of the world, both as individuals and as a species. We share the vision that such an understanding of the problems of consciousness will make medical science holistic and will bring quality of life, health, and the ability to function to its patients.

ACKNOWLEDGEMENTS

This chapter is an updated and revised version of an earlier paper with permission: Ventegodt S, Anderson NJ, Merrick J. Quality of life philosophy IV. The brain and consciousness. ScientificWorldJournal 2003;3:1199-209.

REFERENCES

[1] Kandel ER, Schwartz JH. Principles of neural science. New York: Elsevier, 1985.
[2] Williams PL, Warwick R. Grays anatomy, 36th ed. Edinburgh: Churchill Livingstone, 1980.
[3] Barr ML, Kiernen JA. The human nervous system. An anatomical viewpoint. Philadelphia, PA: Harper Row, 1983.
[4] Alberts B, Bray D, Lewis J, Raff M, Roberts K, Watson JD. Molecular biology of the cell, 3rd ed. New York: Garland, 1994.
[5] Sadler TW. Langman's medical embryology. Baltimore, MD: Williams Wilkins, 1985.
[6] Luria AR. Functional organization of the brain. Sci Am 1970;222(3):66–72.
[7] Marr D. A theory for cerebral neocortex, Proc Royal Soc London 1970;176: 161–234.
[8] Schrødinger E. What is Life? The physical aspect of the living cell. Cambridge: Cambridge University Press, 1944.
[9] Rumelhart DE, McClelland JL. Parallel distributed processing: Explorations in the microstructure of cognition. Cambridge, MA: MIT Press, 1975.
[10] Prigogine I, Stengers I. Order out of chaos: Man's new dialogue with nature. New York: Bantam Books, 1984.
[11] Popper KR, Eccles JC. The self and its brain. Berlin: Springer, 1977.
[12] Purves D, Lichtman JW. Principles of neural development. Sunderland, MA: Sinauer, 1985.
[13] Edelman GM. The mindful brain. Cambridge, MA: MIT Press, 1978.
[14] Ventegodt S. Quality of life: Seizing the meaning of life and becoming well again. Copenhagen: Forskningcentrets Forlag, 1995. [Danish]
[15] Symonds N. What is life? Schrødingers influence on biology. Quart Rev Biol 1986;61(2):221–6.
[16] Meinhardt H. Models of biological pattern formation. London: Academic Press, 1982.
[17] Jensen RV. Classical chaos. Am Sci 1987;75:168–81.
[18] Mandelbrot BB. Fractal geometry of nature. San Francisco, CA: WH Freeman, 1982.
[19] Wolfram S. A new kind of science., Champaign, IL: Wolfram Media, 2002.
[20] Peitgen HO, Richter PH. The beauty of fractals. Berlin: Springer, Berlin, 1986.

[21] Szentagothai J. The "module concept" in cerebral cortex architecture. Brain Res 1975;95(2–3):475–96.

[22] Szentagothai J. The neuron network of the cerebral cortex: A functional interpretation. Proc Royal Soc London Ser B Biol Sci 1978;201(1144):219–48.

[23] Szentagothai J. The modular architectonic principle of neural centers. Rev Physiol Biochem Pharmacol 1983;98:11–61.

[24] Szentagothai J. Specificity versus (quasi-) randomness in cortical connectivity. In: Brazier MAB, Petche H, eds. Architectonics of the cerebral cortex. New York: Raven Press, 1978:77–97.

[25] Szentagothai J. Too much and too soon. A lifetime of inquiry into the functional organization of the nervous system. Acta Biol 1982;33(2–3):107–26.

[26] Babloyantz A. Self-organization phenomena resulting from cell-cell-contact. J Theor Bio 1977;68:551–61.

[27] Babloyantz A, Kaczmarek LK. Self-organization in biological systems with multiple cellular contact. Bull Math Biol 1979;41:193–201.

[28] Kohonen T. Self-organization and associative memory. Berlin: Springe, Berlin, 1984.

[29] Rumelhart DE, Geoffrey EH, Williams RJ. Parallel distributed processing: Explorations in the microstructure of cognition. Cambridge, MA: MIT Press, 1986.

[30] Jones WP, Hoskins J. Back-propagation. A generalized delta learning rule. Byte Mag 1987;Oct:155–62.

[31] Mountcastle VB. An organizing principle for cerebral function: The unit module and the distributed system. In: Edelman GM, ed. The mindful brain. Cambridge MA: MIT Press, 1978:17–49.

[32] Rockel AJ, Hions RW, Powell TPS. The basic uniformity in the structure of the neocortex. Brain 1980;103:221–4.

[33] Edelman GM. Cell adhesion molecules in the regulation of animal form and tissue pattern. Ann Rev Cell Biol 1986;2:81–116.

[34] Marr D. A theory of cerebellar cortex. J Physiol London 1969;202(2):437–70.

[35] Strausfeld NJ. Altas of an insect brain. Berlin: Springer, 1976.

[36] Ventegodt S, Andersen NJ, Merrick J. Quality of life philosophy I. Quality of life, happiness, and meaning in life. ScientificWorldJournal 2003;3:1164-75.

[37] Ventegodt S, Andersen NJ, Kromann M, Merrick J. Quality of life philosophy II. What is a human being? ScientificWorldJournal 2003;3:1176-85.

[38] Ventegodt S, Andersen NJ, Merrick J. Quality of life philosophy III. Towards a new biology: understanding the biological connection between quality of life, disease, and healing. ScientificWorldJournal 2002;3:1186-98.

[39] Ventegodt S. The life mission theory. A theory for a consciousness based medicine. Int J Adolesc Med.Health 2003;15:89–91.

[40] Ventegodt S, Andersen NJ, Merrick J. Holistic medicine III. The holistic process theory ofhealing. ScientificWorldJournal 2003;3:1138-46.

[41] Ventegodt S, Merrick J, Andersen NJ. Quality of life as medicine. A pilot study of patients with chronic illness and pain. ScientificWorldJournal 2003;3: 520–32.

[42] Ventegodt S, Merrick J, Andersen NJ. Quality of life as medicine II. A pilot study of a five day "quality of life and health" cure for patients with alcoholism. ScientificWorldJournal 2003;3:842–52.

[43] Hultborn H, University of Copenhagen. Personal communication.

[44] Ventegodt S, Merrick J, Andersen NJ. Quality of life theory II. Quality of life as the realization of life potential: a biological theory of human being. Scientific WorldJournal 2003;3:1041–9.

[45] Nørretranders T. The user illusion. New York: Viking Press, 1998.

[46] Ventegodt S. The philosophy of life that heals. Copenhagen: Forskningscentrets Forlag, 1999. [Danish]

[47] Jung CG. Man and his symbols. New York. Anchor Press, 1964.

[48] Antonovsky A. Unravelling the mystery of health. How people manage stress and stay well. San Francisco, CA: Jossey-Bass, 1987.

[49] Maslow A. Toward a psychology of being. Princeton, NJ: Van Nostrand, 1962.

[50] Frankl V. Man's search for meaning. New York: Pocket Books, 1985.

[51] Ventegodt S, Merrick J, Andersen NJ. Quality of life theory I. The IQOL theory: an integrative theory of the global quality of life concept. ScientificWorldJournal 2003;3:1030-40.

[52] Ventegodt S, Merrick J, Andersen NJ. Quality of life theory III. Maslow revisited. ScientificWorldJournal 2003;3:1199–209.

Chapter 9

OUR IMMUNE SYSTEM

Can we trust our immune system? Can it take care of us? Can it protect us against all the different viruses, bacteria and parasites we encounter through life? The whole Corona hype has been turning around one postulate: that our natural immunity is not strong enough to protect us against the new Corona COVID-19 virus. People who know little about immunology can be very scared when they hear that a new virus is attacking them. People who know about the amazing work of our immune system are much less scared; if you know that our immune system without any problems take care of about 100 new mutations of viruses every year, most of the time without you even noticing, you are not scared of a new mutation. Why would you be? There is nothing but new mutations coming all the time. The body wins over them almost every single time without us even noticing it. People who never heard about Corona viruses before can also be scared of that – a new virus, called Corona! Again, if you know that 15% of all the viruses attacking us are Corona viruses, you just relax: It is the common cold. It is not dangerous. It was not dangerous last year, the year before, or the year before that. So why would it be dangerous this year, or the next? The immune system is the most important defense against dangerous attacks from the outside world and a strong immune response is necessary for a human to stay healthy. In this chapter, the immunological self-nonself recognition is discussed from the view of the holistic paradigm. The biological immunological self-nonself discrimination is discussed in context to the mental, conscious self-nonself discrimination and the possible informational connections between these two levels are discussed. Immunological self-nonself discrimination and the relation to non-genetic somatic diseases, like infectious diseases, are discussed. We hypothesize that these diseases could be a consequence of incorrectly adjusted immunological self-nonself discrimination due to unsolved social, psychological, emotional, sexual and/or existential problems. To say it simple: If you have problems on the level of conscious, this disturbs the body so you can become sick. If you are having a symptomatic disease when you meet a Corona virus, it might be because you suffer from fear, worries, stress or maybe emotional problems.

INTRODUCTION

A key problem in immuno-regulation today is the self-nonself discrimination, characterized by the ability of the organism to react toward the nonself-antigens and to avoid to react against self-antigens. By the 1970s it had become increasingly clear, that the immune-regulation was taking place at a systemic level. At that time, however, there was no general conceptual handling of biological systems at a systemic level. The existing cybernetic analyses were summarized as a network of interactions. A number of network theories appeared to describe biological systems, e.g., network theories of gene expression in eukaryotes (1), for the function of the cerebellum (2), and later also for the function of the cerebrum (3, 4).

However, the Danish immunologist Niels Kaj Jerne (1911-1994) (5) developed an immunological network model trying to explain the capability of a body to discriminate between organismic self and nonself through its immune system (5). We have discussed Jerne's immunological network model in Ventegodt et al. (6) and came to the conclusion that Jerne's network was not able to explain the crucial immunological self-nonself discrimination essential for a body to stay fit and survive, and for people with non-genetic, somatic diseases, to be able to overcome their illnesses and stay fit.

In this chapter we give our explanation of how the immune system can be able to discriminate between self and nonself in the human body. We discuss the immunological self-nonself discrimination in the view of the holistic paradigm (7-13). Because of the very complicated mechanism behind the immunological self-nonself discrimination, there have been some attempts to explain this mechanism. But no model proposed in the past has been sufficient enough to be able to explain such mechanisms in a satisfactory way. On the other hand, we think the holistic paradigm is able to give scientists a tool to explain the immunological self-nonself discrimination in a more satisfactory way then the past models, because it predicts an interaction between the psychical level (through the consciousness and the intent), and the immunological-systemic level.

In this chapter we will discuss the immunological self-nonself discrimination and its interaction with the mental self-nonself discrimination that follows the holistic paradigm as a consequence of the interaction between the intent and the systemic fractal levels of a human body, and thereby, which are under tight control from the super orbital of the individual human being (8). Morphogenetic analyses show that biological system function like sensitive control systems, which naturally have the ability to evaluate the placement of the cells and correct this, if it is wrong. This ability of biological systems is the foundation of the self-nonself discrimination.

Psycho-neuro-immunology is a rather new discipline. It aims to expounding the control of the psyche through the immune system and brain. Self-nonself discrimination is a crucial point of this control. Besides the morphological self-nonself discrimination, this new science deals with immunological-systemic self-nonself discrimination and mental self-nonself discrimination. The psychoneuroimmunologists believe the immune defense of the body can be conditioned in a pavlovian way, because the mental self-nonself discrimination is able to influence the immunological-systemic self-nonself discrimination. These two kinds of self-nonself discrimination are only seen as the specific expressions of the self-nonself discrimination of the organism pertaining to the brain and the immune system respectively, explaining the close affinity between these two different ways of discrimination.

The immunological-systemic self-nonself discrimination is governed by the biological information carried by the quantum field of the organism (the "super orbital"). The super orbital is united by all quantum chemical energies of a body and following the holistic paradigm it is the source of the consciousness and thereby of the intention (8). The super orbital follows the holistic paradigm governing everything in a biological body that demands an energetic source, including all biochemical and biophysical functions (8). Following the holistic paradigm this means that the immunological-systemic self-nonself discrimination is tuned by the super orbital/read consciousness (8). The intention that is sourced from the super orbital interacts with the energies of positional information of the fractal levels that exists in a human body (8). These fractal levels (7) represent the different levels of the building plane of the body as, e.g., the cells, the organs (build by the cells), the tissues (gathered by the organs) and the complete organic body (gathered by the tissues). The immunological-systemic self-nonself discrimination is directed through the interaction between the intention and the systemic fractal levels (meaning all the fractal levels represented in the body).

The consciousness that sources the intention is also the source of the mind and the psyche. The psyche is representing the mental self-nonself discrimination. Because of the psychological relation between the consciousness, the intension, the mind and the psyche, and thereby the clear connection between the intension and the positional information of the systemic fractal levels of the human body, there is also a connection between the mental self-nonself discrimination and the immunological-systemic self-nonself discrimination that interacts in a united co-operation to fine tune the body to be fit and capable of survival.

Following the holistic paradigm the interaction between the physical body and the consciousness is very tightly coupled. This gives the individual human being the possibility through his consciousness and his intention (9), to govern the positional information (10, 11) of the systemic fractal levels (7) in a way so that he is able to control the coordination between the mental self-nonself discrimination and the immunological-systemic self-nonself discrimination.

This means that these two kinds of self-nonself discrimination perform a very close interaction between these two different ways of the human body and mind to discriminate between itself and the outside world. How effective this discrimination is depends on the interaction between the intention and the systemic fractal levels (8). This interaction makes the holistic paradigm very powerful, because it makes it possible for the individual human being to adjust his immune system after his immediate psychological state. Following the holistic paradigm this means that the interaction between the intention and the positional information of the systemic fractal levels also are directly dependent of the individual human being's immediate psychically state. Thereby, the human self-nonself discrimination becomes an important part of the united system that controls the most important mechanisms leading to fitness and survival, namely human self-nonself discrimination and adult human metamorphosis (12, 13), but the self-nonself discrimination can also lead to decay, self-destruction and dead, because a sick mind can direct a human being's immune system to attack his own body.

Therefore, it is of an immensely importance for a human being to be able to fine tune his immunological self-nonself discrimination to be as optimal as possible, because only in this way he will be able to maintain the appropriate fitness necessary for survival, the main function of the evolution (12). Without the capability of being able to fine tune the immunological self-nonself discrimination the human being would probably never have been created.

We think this is the case, because by this capability the immunological-systemic self-nonself discrimination, in a way, side by side with the naturally selection proposed by Charles Darwin (14) and the "metamorphous top down" evolution described by Hermansen et al. (12) is responsible for the evolutionary mechanisms that leads towards fitness and survival and probably towards further evolutionary development of the human being (12). By this, the immunological-systemic self-nonself discrimination becomes a key function of human fitness and survival, but also a key function of the evolution.

The “metamorphous top down” evolution, as mentioned in Hermansen et al. (12), is coupled to adult human metamorphosis (12, 13), because the last one is a reminiscent of the first (12). Following the holistic paradigm, this means that the interaction between the immunological-systemic self-nonself discrimination and the adult human metamorphosis, in the human body, both have the mission of getting the individual human being capable of staying fit for fight and capable of survival, and to cooperate to insure the farther evolution of the human being.

Table 1. Development of immunological ideas according to Jerne (5)

Aims	Periods	Pioneers /Types of theory	Notions
Application	1870-1890	Pasteur Metchnikoff	Immunization Phagocytosis
Description	1890-1910	Bering Ehrlich	Antibodies Cell receptors
	1910-1930	Bordet Landsteiner	Specificity Haptens
Mechanisms	1930-1950	Sub-cellular	Antibody synthesis Antigen template
	1950-1970	Cellular	Selection Clones
System analysis	1970-1990	Multi-cellular	Network Cooperation and suppression

Immunology has been a scientific discipline for about 120 years. According to Niels Jerne it has been developed through a number of phases, each based on specific ideas (see Table 1). It is a plausible hypothesis that choices of self-nonself discrimination throughout life are the cause of such diseases. If this is the case the elucidation of the mechanisms will provide both a therapy and a generally preventive medicine for these diseases. Of cause it is not yet possible to understand the fundamental mechanisms behind immunological self-nonself discrimination. However, following the holistic paradigm it is given that the intention has an essential influence on the immunological self-nonself discrimination, and thereby that the consciousness is deeply involved in the human health. A bad intention will lead to malfunction of the body's building plane and structures (8) and give the immune response, and capability to distinguish between self and nonself, bad conditions for optimal activity, while a good intention will involve a fit and sound body capable of survival. In such a body the conditions for the immunological self-nonself discrimination are optimal and capable of helping the body to stay fit. Such a body involves a kind of positive feedback mechanism, where a more fit body makes the conditions for the self-nonself better. This makes an even fitter body etc. On the other hand a bad intention involves a kind of negative feedback. Such persons that involve a negative feedback are very vulnerable to attack from bacteria, vira and other parasites, and thereby the non-genetic, somatic diseases often confront them. However, by the help of a therapist such persons can reverse a negative feedback to a positive feedback and by this activate the adult human metamorphosis (12, 13) and strengthen the immunological self-nonself discrimination leading to fitness and survival.

Table 2. Results of imbalance in the self-nonself discrimination

Origin of stimulus	Too low a discrimination	Too high a discrimination
Outer stimulus	Infection	Hyperreactivity
Inner stimulus	Neoplasm	Autoimmunity

Such mechanisms are much more complicated than this. For instance, for humans in a negative feed-back cycle the etiology of the non-genetic, non-traumatic somatic diseases probably can be explained by too weak or too strong a self-nonself discrimination (see Table 2) and why the choices of the self-nonself discrimination could be the cause of somatic diseases. If this is the case, it will provide both a therapy and a generally preventive medicine against such diseases. Therefore it is most important to focus the future research on such problems and realize that a better understanding of the self-nonself discrimination could be the key to a better health (15-17).

Discussion

In our quest for a new understanding of the mysterious connection between life, matter and consciousness (6-13, 15-17), we have now turned our interest towards the immune system. The structure held responsible for the structure and quality of human immune response is called the "immune system", but the problem is that it might not be a separate organ in the same way as the kidney or brain, but a much more integrated cell population completely depending on the state and informational conditions of the local tissue.

Our motivation for the exploration of the immune system is our finding that quality of life, health and ability primarily is determined by our consciousness (18). This discovery has lead us to the interesting possibility that guided shifts in the state of consciousness and the development of self-insight with a more positive, responsible and constructive philosophy of life can be used to strengtehn the human immune response and help cure patients, i.e., by reducing the number of recidivant infections.

We have made a series of papers setting the strategy for alleviating healing many different physical, mental, existential, and sexual diseases and health problems (19-59). We also know that the discriminative ability of the immuse system is closely connected to the patient recovering his experience of "sense of coherence" (SOC) (60-66). SOC is actually the experience that one conscious being is connected to the whole universe though our physical and mental existence (67); to bring the patient back to be an integrated part of the world seems to be the fundamental idea of all medicine, the tratition going all the way back to Hippocrates and his students (67).

CONCLUSION

The self-nonself discrimination is characterized by the ability of the organism to react toward the nonself-antigens and to avoid to react against self-antigens.

When 80% of the passengers on a Diamond Princess (see chapter 2) did not test positive for COVID-19 when tested for antibodies in their blood, it was most likely not because they did not get exposed to the virus, but because their immune system was so good that the non-specific immune system that only uses the self-nonself discrimination took care of the virus. Therefore antibodies were not needed at all.

This is so amazing when you think about it. Because this is what happens to almost all of the 100 viruses that attacks a healthy person every year. And the organism still learn and remember the virus, and in this way build its immunity to similar virus when they come in the future.

No model proposed in the past has been able to explain the mechanisms behind the self-nonself discrimination satisfactory; but we think the holistic paradigm is able to give an appropriate explanation of the immunological self-nonself discrimination because it predicts an interaction between the psychical level and the cellular.

Following the holistic paradigm, the "informational field" or "quantum super orbital" where consciousness resides, is governing everything in a biological body that demands an informational source. This means that the immunological-systemic self-nonself discrimination is tuned by the consciousness (sourced by the field or "super orbital").

The immunological-systemic self-nonself discrimination is directed through the interaction between the intention and the systemic fractal levels, and the intention is sourced from the consciousness (read super orbital). Also a connection between the psychological self-nonself discrimination and the immunological-systemic self-nonself discrimination exists, that interacts in a united co-operation to fine tune the body to be fit and capable of survival. All this activity is governed from the super orbital of the human wholeness. Following the holistic paradigm the interaction between the intention and the positional information of the systemic fractal levels are directly dependent on the individual human being's immediate psychically state. Thereby, the human self-nonself discrimination becomes an important part of the united system that controls the most important mechanisms leading to fitness and survival, namely human self-nonself discrimination.

It is of an immensely importance for a human being to be able to fine tune his immunological self-nonself discrimination to be as optimal as possible, because only in this way he will be able to maintain the appropriate fitness necessary for survival, the main function of the evolution.

The immunological-systemic self-nonself discrimination becomes a key function of human fitness and survival, but also a key function of the evolution. Therefore, the interaction between the immunological-systemic self-nonself discrimination and the adult human metamorphosis, in the human body, both have the mission of getting the individual human being capable of staying fit for fight and capable of survival, and to cooperate to insure the farther evolution of the human being.

At last, following the holistic paradigm it is a plausible hypothesis that choices of self-nonself discrimination throughout life are the cause of non-genetic, somatic diseases. If this is the case the elucidation of the mechanisms will provide both a therapy and a generally preventive medicine for such diseases.

REFERENCES

[1] Davidson EH, Britten RJ. Regulation of gene expression: possible role of repetitive sequences. Science 1979;204(4397):1052-9.

[2] Marr D. A theory of cerebellar cortex. J Physiol 1969;202(2):437-70.

[3] Ballard R. General practice management of stabilised schizophrenics. Aust Fam Physician 1986;15(12):1616-21.

[4] Jones WP, Hoskins JC. Back propagation: A generalized delta learning rule. ByteMagazine 1987:155-62.

[5] Jerne NK. Towards a network theory of the immune system. Ann Immunol (Inst. Pasteur) 1974;125C:373–89.

[6] Ventegodt S, Hermansen TD, Rald E, Nielsen ML, Clausen B, Merrick J. Human development XVII: Jerne's anti-idiotypic network theory cannot explain self-nonself discrimination. J Altern Med Res 2009;1(4):439-44.

[7] Ventegodt S, Hermansen TD, Flensborg-Madsen T, Rald E, Nielsen ML, Merrick J. Human development VII: A spiral fractal model of fine structure of physical energy could explain central aspects of biological information, biological organisation, and biological creativity. ScientificWorldJournal 2006;6:1434-40.

[8] Hermansen TD, Ventegodt S, Flensborg-Madsen T, Nielsen ML, Merrick J. Human development VIII: A theory of "deep" quantum chemistry and cell consciousness. Quantum chemistry controls genes and biochemistry to give cells and higher organisms consciousness and complex behavior. ScientificWorldJournal 2006;6:1441-53.

[9] Ventegodt S, Andersen NJ, Merrick J. Quality of life philosophy V. Seizing the meaning of life and becoming well again. ScientificWorldJournal 2003;3:1210-29.

[10] Ventegodt S, Hermansen TD, Flensborg-Madsen T, Nielsen ML, Merrick J. Human development IV: The living cell has information-directed self-organisation – and consciousness. Scientific WorldJournal 2006;6:1132-8.

[11] Ventegodt S, Hermansen TD, Flensborg-Madsen T, Nielsen ML, Merrick J. Human development VI: Supra-cellular morphogenesis - the origin of biological and cellular order. ScientificWorldJournal 2006;6:1424-33.

[12] Hermansen TD, Ventegodt S, Merrick J. Human development X: Explanation of the macro-evolution: top down evolution materialises consciousness. The origin of metamorphosis. ScientificWorldJournal 2006;6:1656-66.

[13] Ventegodt S, Hermansen TD, Kandel I, Merrick J. Human development XX: A theory for accelerated, spontaneous existential healing (salutogenesis): Human adult metamorphosis. J Altern Med Res 2009;1(4):465-74.

[14] Darwin C. The origin of species. New York: Gramercy, 1995.

[15] Hermansen TD, Ventegodt S, Rald E, Clausen B, Nielsen ML, Merrick J. Human development I: 20 fundamental problems of biology, medicine and neuro-psychology related to biological information. ScientificWorldJournal 2006;6:747-59.

[16] Ventegodt S, Hermansen TD, Nielsen ML, Clausen B, Merrick J. Human development II: We need an integrated theory for matter, life and consciousness to understand life and healing. ScientificWorldJournal 2006;6:760-6.

[17] Ventegodt S, Hermansen TD, Rald E, Flensborg-Madsen T, Nielsen ML, Clausen B, Merrick J. Human development III: Bridging brain-mind and body-mind. Introduction to "deep" (fractal, poly-ray) cosmology. ScientificWorldJournal 2006;6:767-76.

[18] Ventegodt S, Flensborg-Madsen T, Andersen NJ, Nielsen M, Mohammed M, Merrick J. Global quality of Human development XVIII 451life (QOL), health and ability are primarily determined by our consciousness. Research findings from Denmark 1991-2004. Soc Indicat Res 2005;71:87-122.

[19] Ventegodt S, Merrick J. Clinical holistic medicine: Applied consciousness-based medicine. ScientificWorldJournal 2004;4:96-9.

[20] Ventegodt S, Morad M, Merrick J. Clinical holistic medicine: Classic art of healing or the therapeutic touch. ScientificWorldJournal 2004;4:134-47.

[21] Ventegodt S, Morad M, Merrick J. Clinical holistic medicine: The "new medicine", the multi-paradigmatic physician and the medical record. ScientificWorldJournal 2004;4:273-85.

[22] Ventegodt S, Morad M, Merrick J. Clinical holistic medicine: Holistic pelvic examination and holistic treatment of infertility. ScientificWorldJournal 2004;4:148-58.

[23] Ventegodt S, Morad M, Hyam E, Merrick J. Clinical holistic medicine: Use and limitations of the biomedical paradigm ScientificWorldJournal 2004;4:295-306.

[24] Ventegodt S, Morad M, Kandel I, Merrick J. Clinical holistic medicine: Social problems disguised as illness. ScientificWorldJournal 2004;4:286-94.

[25] Ventegodt S, Morad M, Andersen NJ, Merrick J. Clinical holistic medicine Tools for a medical science based on consciousness. ScientificWorldJournal 2004;4:347-61.

[26] Ventegodt S, Morad M, Merrick J. Clinical holistic medicine: Prevention through healthy lifestyle and quality of life. Oral Health Prev Dent 2004;1:239-45.

[27] Ventegodt S, Morad M, Hyam E, Merrick J. Clinical holistic medicine: When biomedicine is inadequate. ScientificWorldJournal 2004;4:333-46.

[28] Ventegodt S, Morad M, Merrick J. Clinical holistic medicine: Holistic treatment of children. ScientificWorldJournal 2004;4:581-8.

[29] Ventegodt S, Morad M, Merrick J. Clinical holistic medicine: Problems in sex and living together. ScientificWorldJournal 2004;4:562-70.

[30] Ventegodt S, Morad M, Hyam E, Merrick J. Clinical holistic medicine: Holistic sexology and treatment of vulvodynia through existential therapy and acceptance through touch. ScientificWorldJournal 2004;4:571-80.

[31] Ventegodt S, Flensborg-Madsen T, Andersen NJ, Morad M, Merrick J. Clinical holistic medicine: A pilot on HIV and quality of life and a suggested treatment of HIV and AIDS. ScientificWorldJournal 2004;4:264-72.

[32] Ventegodt S, Morad M, Merrick J. Clinical holistic medicine: Induction of spontaneous remission of cancer by recovery of the human character and the purpose of life (the Life Mission). ScientificWorldJournal 2004;4:362-77.

[33] Ventegodt S, Morad M, Kandel I, Merrick J. Clinical holistic medicine: Treatment of physical health problems without a known cause, exemplified by hypertension and tinnitus. ScientificWorldJournal 2004;4:716-24.

[34] Ventegodt S, Morad M, Merrick J. Clinical holistic medicine: Developing from asthma, allergy and eczema. ScientificWorldJournal 2004;4:936-42.

[35] Ventegodt S, Morad M, Press J, Merrick J, Shek DTL Clinical holistic medicine: Holistic adolescent medicine. ScientificWorld Journal 2004;4:551-61.

[36] Ventegodt S, Solheim E, Saunte ME, Morad M, Kandel I, Merrick J. Clinical holistic medicine: Metastatic cancer. ScientificWorldJournal 2004;4:913-35.

[37] Ventegodt S, Morad M, Kandel I, Merrick J. Clinical holistic medicine: a psychological theory of dependency to improve quality of life. ScientificWorldJournal 2004;4:638-48.

[38] Ventegodt S, Merrick J. Clinical holistic medicine: Chronic infections and autoimmune diseases. ScientificWorldJournal 2005;5:155-64.

[39] Ventegodt S, Kandel I, Neikrug S, Merrick J. Clinical holistic medicine: Holistic treatment of rape and incest traumas. ScientificWorldJournal 2005;5:288-97.

[40] Ventegodt S, Merrick J. Clinical holistic medicine: Chronic pain in the locomotor system. ScientificWorldJournal 2005;5:165-72.

[41] Ventegodt S, Merrick J. Clinical holistic medicine: Chronic pain in internal organs. ScientificWorldJournal 2005;5:205-10.

[42] Ventegodt S, Kandel I, Neikrug S, Merrick J. Clinical holistic medicine: The existential crisis – life crisis, stress and burnout. ScientificWorldJournal 2005;5:300-12.

[43] Ventegodt S, Gringols G, Merrick J. Clinical holistic medicine: Holistic rehabilitation. ScientificWorldJournal 2005;5:280-7.

[44] Ventegodt S, Andersen NJ, Neikrug S, Kandel I, Merrick J. Clinical holistic medicine: Mental disorders in a holistic perspective. ScientificWorldJournal 2005;5:313-23.

[45] Ventegodt S, Andersen NJ, Neikrug S, Kandel I, Merrick J. Clinical holistic medicine: Holistic treatment of mental disorders. ScientificWorldJournal 2005;5:427-45.

[46] Ventegodt S, Merrick J. Clinical holistic medicine: The patient with multiple diseases. ScientificWorldJournal 2005;5:324-39.

[47] Ventegodt S, Clausen B, Nielsen ML, Merrick J. Clinical holistic medicine: Advanced tools for holistic medicine. ScientificWorldJournal 2006;6:2048-65.

[48] Ventegodt S, Clausen B, Merrick J. Clinical holistic medicine: The case story of Anna: I. Long term effect of child sexual abuse and incest with a treatment approach. ScientificWorldJournal 2006;6:1965-76.

[49] Ventegodt S, Clausen B, Merrick J. Clinical holistic medicine: the case story of Anna. II. Patient diary as a tool in treatment. ScientificWorldJournal 2006;6:2006-34.

[50] Ventegodt S, Clausen B, Merrick J. Clinical holistic medicine: The case story of Anna. III. Rehabilitation of philosophy of life during holistic existential therapy for childhood sexual abuse. ScientificWorldJournal 2006;6:2080-91.

[51] Ventegodt S, Merrick J. Suicide from a holistic point of view. Scientific WorldJournal 2005;5:759-66.

[52] Ventegodt S, Clausen B, Omar HA, Merrick J. Clinical holistic medicine: Holistic sexology and acupressure through the vagina (Hippocratic pelvic massage). ScientificWorldJournal 2006;6:2066-79.

[53] Ventegodt S, Clausen B, Merrick J. Clinical holistic medicine: Pilot study on the effect of vaginal acupressure (Hippocratic pelvic massage). ScientificWorldJournal 2006;6:2066-79.

[54] Ventegodt S, Thegler S, Andreasen T, Struve F, Enevoldsen L, et al. Clinical holistic medicine: Psychodynamic short-time therapy complemented with bodywork. A clinical follow-up study of 109 patients. ScientificWorldJournal 2006;6:2220-38.

[55] Ventegodt S, Thegler S, Andreasen T, Struve F, Enevoldsen L, et al. Clinical holistic medicine (mindful, short-term psychodynamic psychotherapy complemented with bodywork) in the treatment of experienced impaired sexual functioning. ScientificWorldJournal 2007;7:324-9.

[56] Ventegodt S, Thegler S, Andreasen T, Struve F, Enevoldsen L, et al. Clinical holistic medicine (mindful, short-term psychodynamic psychotherapy complemented with bodywork) improves quality of life, health, and ability by induction of Antonovsky-salutogenesis. ScientificWorldJournal 2007;7:317-23.

[57] Ventegodt S, Thegler S, Andreasen T, Struve F, Enevoldsen L, et al. Clinical holistic medicine (mindful, short-term psychodynamic psychotherapy complemented with bodywork) in the treatment of experienced physical illness and chronic pain. ScientificWorldJournal 2007;7:310-6.

[58] Ventegodt S, Thegler S, Andreasen T, Struve F, Enevoldsen L, et al. Clinical holistic medicine (mindful, short-term psychodynamic psychotherapy complemented with bodywork) in the treatment of experienced mental illness. ScientificWorldJournal 2007;7:306-9.

[59] Ventegodt S, Thegler S, Andreasen T, Struve F, Enevoldsen L, et al. Self-reported low self-esteem. Intervention and follow-up in a clinical setting. Scientific WorldJournal 2007;7:299-305.

[60] Flensborg-Madsen T, Ventegodt S, Merrick J. Sense of coherence and physical health. A Review of previous findings. ScientificWorldJournal 2005;5:665-73.

[61] Flensborg-Madsen T, Ventegodt S, Merrick J. Why is Antonovsky's sense of coherence not correlated to physical health? Analysing Antonovsky's 29-item sense of coherence scale (SOCS). ScientificWorldJournal 2005;5:767-76.

[62] Flensborg-Madsen T, Ventegodt S, Merrick J. Sense of coherence and health. The construction of an amendment to Antonovsky's sense of coherence scale (SOC II ScientificWorldJournal 2006;6:2133-9.

[63] Flensborg-Madsen T, Ventegodt S, Merrick J. Sense of coherence and physical health. A cross-sectional study using a new SOC scale (SOC II). Scientific WorldJournal 2006;6:2200-11.

[64] Flensborg-Madsen T, Ventegodt S, Merrick J. Sense of coherence and physical health. Testing Antonovsky's theory. ScientificWorldJournal 2006;6:2212-9.

[65] Flensborg-Madsen T, Ventegodt S, Merrick J. Sense of coherence and health. The emotional sense of coherence (SOC-E) was found to be the best-known predictor of physical health. ScientificWorldJournal 2006;6:2147-57.

[66] Ventegodt S, Flensborg-Madsen T, Andersen NJ, Merrick J. Life mission theory VII: Theory of existential (Antonovsky) coherence: a theory of quality of life, health and ability for use in holistic medicine. ScientificWorldJournal 2005;5:377-89.

[67] Jones WHS. Hippocrates. Vol. I–IV. London: William Heinemann, 1923-31.

Chapter 10

PRACTICAL PSYCHO-IMMUNOLOGY

The classical or traditional doctor has for more than two thousand years worked to support the individuals in finding, growing and developing good health. You can say that in the end of the day, it is all about getting rid of negative beliefs we have accumulated since early childhood. Interestingly all pre-modern cultures have rituals, ceremonies and spiritual leaders to help their people live in truth, happiness, and good health. Modern doctors trained in chemistry smile at the traditional healers and their old ways. The practical side of psycho-immunology is working, is working well, and has been working for at least the last 2,400 years. If we go to the medical papyri, it seems that the famous Egyptian medicine was a psychosomatic medicine working the same way. One can only speculate if the classical Greek medicine was originally inherited from the Egyptians.

INTRODUCTION

The theories presented in chapter 8 and 9 might be good, or they might be bad. They might be meaningful and helpful to some people in search of a deeper understanding of biology; and they might look like pure nonsense to other people. We include them to inspire you to think deeper about the mysteries of the body, and its organs, and especially about the brain and the immune system and the mystical connection between these two organs.

Theories about brain function and immunological function will always follow the language of its time, and therefore they are ever changing. When new concepts are introduced in one science, like mathematics (the fractals), physics (the fields), chemistry (protein-super-orbitals) or biology (biological information systems), they are right away taken into the existing theories of the brain and the immune system, where we still need good explanations and thus, the theories are evolved, upgraded, modernized, and hopefully improved. Every 10 years the theories come in a new version, in a new dress of concepts and ideas. Because of their ever-changing nature, these theories are not so much worth. They are funny, but they are not true.

STABLE THEORIES

Is there something more stable, more permanent, and more useful than theories then, we can rely on, and use as guidance, when we need it? Yes there is. For thousands of years there have been a medical practice, where simple and effective principles have guided the doctor in his treatment of patients.

The classical psycho-somatic holistic medicine, often called the Hippocratic medicine after the doctor that first described it scenically (Hippocrates from Cos 460-370 BCE) (1), tells us how to find balance, strengthen our physical and mental health, prevent health problems, and fight diseases like infections when they happen. You can call it practical psycho-immunology if you want.

It is a wonderful, simple method, which focuses on getting rid of emotional disturbances and false beliefs. The perfect healthy human being is empty of thoughts, present, happy, and one with reality, one with what is.

Love and sexuality is the most important if you want to stay healthy; you need to understand yourself well enough to perform well in both these aspects. You need to find your strength and talents, and you need to speak truth and follow your words with your actions.

These simple advises – be happy, live close to people, enjoy your work, your partner and your family and don't worry – seems to be the core of the practical side of psycho-immunology and psychosomatics.

THE CLASSIC PHYSICIAN

The classical doctor has for more than two thousand years worked to support the individuals in finding, growing and developing these things. In the end of the day, it is all about getting rid of negative beliefs we have accumulated since early childhood.

Interestingly all pre-modern cultures have rituals, ceremonies and spiritual leaders to help their people live in truth, happiness, and good health. Modern doctors trained in chemistry smile at the traditional healers and their old ways. But as we shall see in the next chapter, there is not so much to smile of. The practical side of psycho-immunology is working, is working well, and has been working for at least the last 2,400 years. If we go to the medical papyri, it seems that the famous Egyptian medicine was a psychosomatic medicine working the same way. One can only speculate if the classical Greek medicine was originally inherited from the Egyptians (2, 3).

> "The physician must be able to tell the antecedents, know the present, and foretell the future — must mediate these things, and have two special objects in view with regard to disease, namely, to do good or to do no harm." Hippocrates (460-370 BCE)

ACKNOWLEDGEMENTS

This chapter is based on: Ventegodt S, Merrick J. A citizen's guide to survive Corona COVID-19 (SARS-CoV-2). Copenhagen: Quality-of-Life Research Center Press, 2020.

REFERENCES

[1] Jones WHS. Hippocrates. Vol. I–IV. London: William Heinemann, 1923-1931.

[2] Ventegodt S. Comparison of the medical principles of the ancient Egyptian and the ancient Greek medicine based on the medical Papyri and Corpus Hippocraticum. J Altern Med Res 2020;12(2):in press.

[3] Ventegodt S The traditional Hippocratic holistic mind-body medicine: The Hippocratic Oath and its sacred promise of professional closeness. J Altern Med Res 2020;12(2):in press.

Chapter 11

THE TRADITIONAL HIPPOCRATIC HOLISTIC MIND-BODY MEDICINE

In this chapter, we review the Corpus Hippocraticum and argue that the traditional European mind-body medicine, which was used all over Europe during the last 2,400 years, was already well developed at the time of Hippocrates. Most likely, it had its roots in the ancient Egyptian medicine, as this medicine shared many similarities. Hippocrates has been called "the father of medicine" due to the production of about 70 scientific books on medicine he and his students wrote about 400 BCE, but Hippocrates inherited his hospital from his father who had inherited it from his father. At Hippocrates' time, there were about 100 holistic hospitals in the civilized European world, indicating that the medicine was old and well developed already then. Hippocrates stated in the Corpus Hippocraticum that his medicine is very effective and very safe, as it can help most patients back to health successfully, independently of the physical or mental illness that brings them to his clinic. He is also helping his patients with chronic pains, sexual problems, infertility and many other clinical conditions. During the past 30 years, a great number of scientific studies in mind-body medicine all over the world have documented the safety and effectivity of the traditional mind-body medicine for the serious diseases like coronary artery stenosis, cancer, depression and the major psychoses. Finally, the traditional medicine is a human-to-human medicine, which is cheap and sustainable and helps raising consciousness of our true values, while pharmaceutical medicine brings a major burden to the global ecosystem that cannot continue, if we want humankind to survive in the future.

"If you are not your own doctor, you are a fool." Hippocrates 460-370 BC (1)

INTRODUCTION

2,400 years ago a medical student had to swear a holy oath to begin his studies. We still today know the exact wording of this oath:

> I swear by Apollo Physician, by Asclepius, by Hygieia, by Panacea, and by all the gods and goddesses, making them my witnesses, that I will carry out, according to my ability and judgment, this oath and this indenture.
>
> To hold my teacher in this art equal to my own parents; to make him partner in my livelihood; when he is in need of money to share mine with him; to consider his family as my own brothers, and to teach them this art, if they want to learn it, without fee or indenture; to impart precept, oral instruction, and all other instruction to my own sons, the sons of my teacher, and to indentured pupils who have taken the physician's oath, but to nobody else.
>
> I will use treatment to help the sick according to my ability and judgment, but never with a view to injury and wrong-doing. Neither will I administer a poison to anybody when asked to do so, nor will I suggest such a course. Similarly I will not give to a woman a pessary to cause abortion. But I will keep pure and holy both my life and my art. I will not use the knife, not even, verily, on sufferers from stone, but I will give place to such as are craftsmen therein.
>
> Into whatsoever houses I enter, I will enter to help the sick, and I will abstain from all intentional wrong-doing and harm, especially from abusing the bodies of man or woman, bond or free. And whatsoever I shall see or hear in the course of my profession, as well as outside my profession in my intercourse with men, if it be what should not be published abroad, I will never divulge, holding such things to be holy secrets.

> Now if I carry out this oath, and break it not, may I gain for ever reputation among all men for my life and for my art; but if I break it and forswear myself, may the opposite befall me (1)

Today every medical student in the western world is asked to take the "Hippocratic oath"; but if you study the many modern versions of the oath you will find that the oath the modern student swear has almost nothing to do with the original Hippocratic Oath.

In this chapter, we will show you the tragic state of todays alienated medicine, and explain you why the traditional Hippocratic medicine worked and healed the patients, while our modern pharmaceutical medicine does very little for the patients. The tragedy lies in the fact that we have lost the healing doctor. We have lost the closeness in medicine which made it possible for the doctor to help.

We have lost our medical roots. We have completely forgotten what traditional European medicine (2-12) is all about. That is a shame, because we have a matchless medicine that takes care of the whole human being and can help us with all human problems - whether it be about the body, mind, spirit, emotions, relationships, sex or working life (2-26). At the same time it is safe (19-24) and sustainable (25-27). The classic medicine is a gift to humanity; is has made the doctor a timeless icon. We cannot afford to lose it.

The traditional holistic medicine is several thousand years old. 2,400 years ago, all medical students at Hippocrates holistic hospital swore a sacred oath, promising closeness with their teacher, each other and their patients:

> To hold my teacher in this art equal to my own parents; to make him partner in my livelihood; when he is in need of money to share mine with him; to consider his family as my own brothers, and to teach them this art, if they want to learn it, without fee or indenture (1)

HUMAN TO HUMAN MEDICINE

When you think about it, it is quite a huge promise that the medical students had to give their teacher. The students became part of the teacher's family through the oath; as all the physician's students swore this oath they all became brothers and sisters. It simply cannot get any closer.

Today we talk about "professional distance" in medicine, without realizing that this is a new thing that came into medicine in the twentieth century together with the use of the chemical drugs as medicine - a medical practice that of course does not need human proximity.

However, the whole foundation of the traditional European medicine is human closeness, because only in close proximity can we be there for each other, understand each other, and help each other. Understanding of your patient as a human being was seen as crucial: "It is far more important to know what person the disease has than what disease the person has" (1).

Traditional medicine is a human-to-human medicine. In other words, traditional medicine is about love: "Where there is love for medicine, there is love for man," Hippocrates said (1). As you know, love brings an experience of closeness, togetherness and unity between people. Love is therefore the complete opposite of distance.

Because the doctor comes so close to the patient, the doctor's oath also promised not to abuse this closeness: "Into whatsoever houses I enter, I will enter to help the sick, and I will abstain from all intentional wrong-doing and harm, especially from abusing the bodies of man or woman, bond or free." (1)

It is important to understand that adhering to the sexual boundaries does not contradict physical or emotional closeness, as many people today believe. The holistic doctor can be very close and intimate with the patient, e.g., the traditional practice of massaging the patients' entire body including the genitals (16) and still respect and keep the sexual boundary. It is precisely this balance between intimacy and sexuality that is the central theme of Hippocrates' medical oath, and this is a central part of the medical arts that the student of holistic medicine must be trained for a substantial time to learn: "The life so short, the craft so long to learn." (1)

HIPPOCRATES MEDICINE

Hippocrates' medicine had a general rule for all treatment, known as: "First, do no harm". In order to avoid harm to the patient, the future physician promised at the time of Hippocrates, as part of the doctor's oath, that he would never use chemical drugs and that he would also refrain from practicing surgery:

> Neither will I administer a poison to anybody when asked to do so, nor will I suggest such a course… But I will keep pure and holy both my life and my art. I will not use the knife… (1)

Both chemical substances (called "poisons" in the oath) - to which the Greeks had access at the time by virtue of plant extracts and minerals extracted - and surgery were banned in Hippocratic medicine. The Greeks knew that the drugs were toxic and that surgery was often harmful. Therefore, these things were too harmful to be usable by a doctor. Again and again you can read Hippocrates' caution against the dangerous in poor medical practice:

> "When it comes to illness, a habit does one of two things: help, or at least do no harm!" (1) and now and then this is said even stronger: "Whenever a doctor cannot do good, he must be kept from doing harm" (1).

There are only two basic tools allowed in Hippocrates' holistic human-to-human medicine: talk therapy and therapeutic touch. Many passages from the about 70 books that came from Hippocrates medical school called "Corpus Hippocraticum" (1) described these two techniques, i.e.:

"Anyone wishing to study medicine must master the art of massage" (1)

"The way to health is to have an aromatic bath and a scented massage every day (1)

Divine is the task to relieve pain" (1).

"It has often appeared, while I have been soothing my patients, as if there was a singular property in my hands to pull and draw away from the affected parts aches and diverse impurities, by laying my hand upon the place, and extending my fingers toward it" (1)

About the art of conversation, Hippocrates said, "The chief virtue that language can have is clearness" (1). The pervasive theme of Corpus Hippocraticum is that the doctor practices a love-medicine, with the doctor himself being the medicine. Throughout the text of the Corpus, Hippocrates speaks that being a good doctor is indistinguishable from being a good person. Famous quotes on this states that there is no art of medicine, there is no art of living, there is only the Art: "Where there is love for medicine, there is love for man" (1). "Cure sometimes, treat often, comfort always" (1) and "Some patients, though conscious that their condition is perilous, recover their health simply through their contentment with the goodness of the physician" (1).

The Greek doctors had a clear understanding of the role of the physician as a human being, which, by virtue of the close contact between the doctor and the patient, can help activate the patient's inner self-healing powers:

"The doctor is treating, but nature is healing" (1)

"The natural healing force within each of us is the greatest force in getting well" (1)

"Natural forces within us are the true healers of disease" (1)

Because the self-healing powers are understood and well known by the holistic physician, he can also prevent illness. Hippocrates said: "The function of protecting and developing health must rank even above that of restoring it when it is impaired." (1), and "The greatest medicine of all is teaching people how not to need it" (1).

Illness is seen as something understandable, a natural consequence of a wrong and unbalanced way of life:

> "Illnesses do not come upon us out of the blue. They are developed from small daily sins against Nature. When enough sins have accumulated, illnesses will suddenly appear" (1)
>
> "If anyone wants good health, one must first ask if he is willing to let go of what is the cause of his illness. Only then is it possible to help him" (1)
>
> "Before you heal someone, ask him if he's willing to give up the things that make him sick" (1)
>
> "If someone wishes for good health, one must first ask oneself if he is ready to do away with the reasons for his illness. Only then is it possible to help him" (1)

THE MESSAGE

Hippocrates also has a strong message to his patient: "If you are not your own doctor you are a fool" (1). If you get sick you must fight with his doctor: "The art has three factors, the disease, the patient, the physician. The physician is the servant of the art. The patient must cooperate with the physician in combatting the disease." (1). Only when the patient learns from the disease can the treatment work: "A wise man should consider that health is the greatest of human blessings, and learn how by his own thought to derive benefit from his illnesses" (1).

How good was Hippocrates medicine in 400 BCE? Try to see what Hippocrates said in response to this question:

> "Medicine in its present state is, it seems to me, by now completely discovered, insofar as it teaches in each instance the particular details and the correct measures. For anyone who has an understanding of medicine in this way depends very little upon good luck, but is able to do good with or without luck. For the whole of medicine has been established, and the excellent principles discovered in it clearly have very little need of good luck" (1).

A modern human being will smile at Hippocrates' perfect confidence in the medical arts in 400 BCE, but that smile may stiffen when you understand what medical science Hippocrates was actually sitting with.

Hippocrates from the island of Kos in Greece was the most famous medical school of his time. Hippocrates is a historical person and Plato called him "the mighty Hippocrates". Hippocrates has been called "the father of medical science", and the 70 books in the Corpus that he and his students wrote became dogma in medical science. Corpus Hippocraticum stood as the highest medical authority right up to the time chemistry took over around 1950. It was 2,350 years anyway.

Hippocrates was called the medicine father, but Hippocrates did not invent the traditional European holistic mind-body medicine. The teaching hospital in Kos was inherited from his father, who in turn had inherited it from his father. The ruins of the hospital can still be seen in Kos, and the foundation shows a 10,000 m^2 large and impressive building. The hospital had a large spa area, a temple, and numerous treatment rooms as well as living rooms for the hospital's patients, doctors and medical students.

THE OLD MEDICINE

Holistic medicine was already old in the time of Hippocrates; the historical sources showed that at that time there were about 100 holistic hospitals in the civilized world, which at that time in Europe were around the Mediterranean area (28). The roots of medicine are unknown, but judging from its spread, it is probably at least 2,000 years older than Hippocrates.

My guess is that it goes back to ancient Persia and before that to ancient Egypt, which according to the sources also had a well-developed, psychosocial, spiritual medicine not very different from the Hippocratic medicine (29). A major difference seems though to be the use of pharmaceutical drugs recommended in the original papyri, which are not found useful by the Greek doctors in the Hippocratic tradition (1, 29).

Does it make any sense that Hippocrates wrote that the doctors of his time knew all the important diseases and had good cures for them all? We know that Hippocrates knowledge of anatomy and physiology was modest; chemistry was not well developed and biology had not yet been established as a science. So how could medical art be developed enough to help all patients?

TESTING HIPPOCRATES' MEDICINE

For the past 30 years, we have been scientifically testing Hippocrates psychosocial medicine at a number of centers all over the world, and the conclusion may surprise. The holistic, psycho-social mind-body medicine has been found highly effective in most physical diseases (15, 19-26), including cardiovascular diseases and cancer, as, i.e., the American doctor Dean Ornish has shown (30-33). Existential conversational therapy focusing on emotion and sexuality can cure virtually all mental disorders, as German Falk Leischenring's many meta-analyses have documented (34-38). The combination of conversation therapy and body therapy showed healing rates typically of over 80% (NNT = 1 – compare that to pharmaceutical drugs with NNTs often around 20! (39)) and typical treatment times of 6-12 month (2-26, 30-38). Hippocratic medicine seems to work amazingly well, and it has been doing so ever since Hippocrates, and probably millennia before him.

Hippocrates was spiritual. The basis for all the work of helping people lies in a special human view, namely the idea that we all basically derive from the same consciousness, and therefore basically are the same. Hippocrates put it this way:

> "The soul is the same in all living creatures, although the body of each is different" (1) and he also said: "There is one common flow, one common breathing, all things are in sympathy "(1).

About the love between man and woman, Hippocrates said:

> "Male and female have the power to fuse into one solid, both because both are nourished in both and also because soul is the same thing in all living creatures, although the body of each is different" (1).

For Hippocrates, being present and knowing nature and the great common consciousness and living in accordance with what this understanding entails the same as being a holy man. Only by being devoted to the divine in one self can one truly understand medicine and the inner reality of man:

> "Holy things are only revealed to holy people" (1).

SPIRITUALITY

The spiritual element is very strong in Hippocratic medicine. The study of medicine commits the student to a pure and spiritual life; as the Hippocratic Oath says:

> "I will keep both my life and my [medical] art sacred" (1).

Hippocrates' books return again and again to the importance for the future doctor of proximity with both nature and man, and oneness with the great spirit:

> "First of all a natural talent is required; for when nature opposes, everything else is in vain; but when nature leads the way to what is most excellent, instruction in the art takes place" (1).

> "The things that are sacred must only be shared with pure and holy persons; sharing them with ordinary people is not legal until these have been inaugurated in the mysteries of science" (1).

Plato wrote that "...according to the Aeskiepiad Hippocrates, it is impossible to understand the body without understanding the whole". Hippocrates was not only a doctor, he was an asclepiad, which can best be translated by "priest-doctor". The Greek priest of the time was quite far from the ecclesiastical. There was no single God in ancient Greece, but a number of Gods, each of whom stood for principles in the universe and human nature, which one must understand and respect, to live the good, happy and healthy life.

In spite of all spirituality, or perhaps precisely because of it, Hippocrates saw himself as a scientist and spoke harshly against superstition and ignorance:

> "Science is the father of knowledge, but opinion breeds ignorance" (1) he said and he rejected the direct influence of the gods on the human:" Prayers, amulets, and sacred songs work only through the patient's faith" (1).

He was mad at the doctors of his own time that refused to respect and follow tradition:

> "Foolish the doctor who despises the knowledge acquired by the ancients" (1)
>
> "Physicians are many in title but very few in reality." (1).

Hippocrates was a strong supporter of observation, which is the foundation of science:

> "We must turn to nature itself, to the observations of the body in health and in disease to learn the truth" (1).

It was precisely this clear attitude that made Hippocrates a scientist.

It is not only the body, but also the patient's mind that must be observed. Because Hippocrates placed the ultimate responsibility for the major physical and mental illnesses on the patient's own mind:

> "All the most acute, violent and deadly diseases, and those that are most difficult to understand for the inexperienced, are due to the mind" (1)
>
> "Men ought to know that from the mind and from the mind only arise our pleasures, joys, laughter, and jests as well as our sorrows, pains, griefs and tears. ... It is the same thing that makes us mad…" (1)

> "And men ought to know that from nothing else but thence [from the mind] come joys, delights, laughter and sports, and sorrows, griefs, despondency, and lamentations. And by this, in an especial manner, we acquire wisdom and knowledge, and see and hear, and know what are foul and what are fair, what are bad and what are good, what are sweet, and what unsavory... And by the same organ we become mad and delirious, and fears and terrors assail us... All these things we endure from the mind, when it is not healthy... In these ways I am of the opinion that the mind exercises the greatest power in the man. This is the interpreter to us of those things which emanate from the air, when it happens to be in a sound state" (1)

It seems, therefore, that Hippocrates believed that precisely because the good doctor is a loving and deeply spiritual man who has completely surrendered to a life in harmony with the forces of nature, he is able to objectively observe his fellow man. It is apparently paradoxical that it requires deep spirituality to observe objectively. But looking deeper into it, I think it makes a lot of sense: Only from a deep and tranquil place within ourselves can we be a neutral witness to the body, mind and flow of life of which we are all a part. This is a philosophical position that I share with Hippocrates.

Allow me to end this paper on the Hippocratic medicine with a few gold-nuggets from the Corpus, pointing to the importance of healthy living, using similarity in healing, creating a new cure for every new patient, and sometimes stepping back and letting nature take its course:

> To do nothing is sometimes a good remedy (1)

A wise man ought to realize that health is his most valuable possession (1)

> Walking is man's best medicine (1)

Opposites are cures for opposites (1) – This refers to the famous *principle of similarity* often quoted in Latin as "similia similibus curentur" which translates to "the same cures the same".

> For extreme illnesses extreme treatments are most fitting (1)

CONCLUSION

The art of medicine had an outstanding status even amongst the earliest of human civilizations and many of the Egyptian papyri was dedicated to medicine describing bodywork and massage and even the complicated spiritual anatomy of the system of circulation of sexual energy, so much used in the Hippocratic medicine.

Many modern people believe that our natural science has brought development and effectivity to medicine, but in this article, we notice that 400 BCE the doctor Hippocrates and his students found medicine to be highly effective and most diseases and clinical conditions treatable and even curable.

If we look at the statistics for modern pharmaceutical treatment, with NNT numbers from 5-100 (39) this is definitely not the case; and if we look at the number of diseases or the fraction of patients modern medicine can cure, we need to admit that our modern pharmaceutical medicine has only little to offer patients today. If we look at the side effects of drugs, experts in evaluation of treatment effect have recently concluded that our medicine most likely does more harm than good (40, 41).

During the last three decades, a number of studies have proven the old psychosomatic medicine highly effective against most of the problems seen in the medical clinic. There is no reason to believe that these methods were less effective at Hippocrates time; and as the spiritual medicine of Egypt was based on similar principles as the Hippocratic medicine, we have reason to believe that the high standing of the ancient Egyptian doctors was due to highly effective cures given by the ancient Egyptians priest healers.

In conclusion, the traditional, holistic, mind-body medicine seems to have triumphed through seven millennia; the sad state of modern medicine where human help has been substituted with chemical interventions must be seen as a symptom of the materialistic worldview and the market mechanisms values (power and money) are dominating today's world.

But the world is changing, and there is a growing understanding of the destructive consequences of our materialistic culture and its habits of trying to solve things without engaging feeling and consciousness. Our global ecosystem is breaking down, and there is no place in the future for an unsustainable pharmaceutical industry with a turnover of 1,7 trillion dollars a year (with a 4-doubling every 10 years (42)) that leads to massive pollution of both the human inner and outer environment – including all living organisms on the planet (25-27).

Let us stand together to save the world. Let us change our ways, also in medicine, and go back to what was safe, effective and sustainable. We need the holistic mind-body medicine more than ever. Luckily, it is not lost, just a bit forgotten. Let us raise consciousness and follow life; let us wake up and serve the ocean of life we came from, so we can be forgiven by the Universe for our collective crimes against nature and be allowed another millennium as human species.

REFERENCES

[1] Jones WHS. Hippocrates. Vol. I–IV. London: William Heinemann, 1923-1931.

[2] Ventegodt S, Merrick J. Principles of holistic psychiatry. A textbook on evidence-based holistic medicine for mental disorders. New York: Nova Science, 2011.

[3] Ventegodt S, Merrick J. Sexology from a holistic point of view. A textbook of classic and modern sexology. New York: Nova Science, 2011.

[4] Ventegodt S, Merrick J. Textbook on evidence-based holistic mind-body medicine: Basic philosophy and ethics of traditional Hippocratic medicine. New York: Nova Science, 2012.

[5] Ventegodt S, Merrick J. Textbook on evidence-based holistic mind-body medicine: Basic principles of healing in traditional Hippocratic medicine. New York: Nova Science, 2012.

[6] Ventegodt S, Merrick J. Textbook on evidence-based holistic mind-body medicine: Healing the mind in traditional Hippocratic medicine. New York: Nova Science, 2012.

[7] Ventegodt S, Merrick J. Textbook on evidence-based holistic mind-body medicine: Holistic practice of traditional Hippocratic medicine. New York: Nova Science, 2013.

[8] Ventegodt S, Merrick J. Textbook on evidence-based holistic mind-body medicine: Research, philosophy, economy and politics of traditional Hippocratic medicine. New York: Nova Science, 2013.

[9] Ventegodt S, Merrick J. Textbook on evidence-based holistic mind-body medicine: Sexology and traditional Hippocratic medicine. New York: Nova Science, 2013.

[10] Ventegodt S, Kandel I, Merrick J. Principles of holistic medicine. Philosophy behind quality of life. Victoria, BC: Trafford, 2005.

[11] Ventegodt S, Kandel I, Merrick J. Principles of holistic medicine. Quality of life and health. New York: Hippocrates Sci Publ, 2005.

[12] Ventegodt S, Kandel I, Merrick J. Principles of holistic medicine. Global quality of life. Theory, research and methodology. New York: Hippocrates Sci Publ, 2005.

[13] Ventegodt S, Thegler S, Andreasen T, Struve F, Enevoldsen L, Bassaine L, et al. Clinical holistic medicine: Psychodynamic short-time therapy complemented with bodywork. A clinical follow-up study of 109 patients. TSW Holistic Health Medicine 2006;1:256-7.

[14] Ventegodt S, Thegler S, Andreasen T, Struve F, Enevoldsen L, Bassaine L, et al. Clinical holistic medicine (mindful, short-term psychodynamic psychotherapy complemented with bodywork) in the treatment of experienced impaired sexual functioning. ScientificWorldJournal 2007;7:324-9.

[15] Ventegodt S, Thegler S, Andreasen T, Struve F, Enevoldsen L, Bassaine L, et al. Clinical holistic medicine (mindful, short-term psychodynamic psychotherapy

complemented with bodywork) in the treatment of experienced physical illness and chronic pain. ScientificWorldJournal 2007;7:310-6.

[16] Ventegodt S, Thegler S, Andreasen T, Struve F, Enevoldsen L, Bassaine L, et al. Clinical holistic medicine (mindful, short-term psychodynamic psychotherapy complemented with bodywork) in the treatment of experienced mental illness. ScientificWorldJournal 2007;7:306-9.

[17] Ventegodt S, Thegler S, Andreasen T, Struve F, Enevoldsen L, Bassaine L, et al.. Self-reported low self-esteem. Intervention and follow-up in a clinical setting. ScientificWorldJournal 2007;7: 299-305.

[18] Ventegodt S, Clausen B, Merrick J. Clinical holistic medicine: Pilot study on the effect of vaginal acupressure (Hippocratic pelvic massage). TSW Holistic Health Medicine 2006;1:136-52.

[19] Allmer C, Ventegodt S, Kandel I, Merrick J. Positive effects, side effects, and adverse events of clinical holistic medicine. A review of Gerda Boyesen's nonpharmaceutical mind-body medicine (biodynamic body-psychotherapy) at two centers in the United Kingdom and Germany. Int J Adolesc Med Health 2009;21(3):281-97.

[20] Ventegodt S, Andersen NJ, Kandel I, Merrick J. Comparative analysis of cost-effectiveness of non-drug medicine (nonpharmaceutical holistic, complementary and alternative medicine/CAM) and biomedicine (pharmaceutical drugs) for all clinical conditions. Int J Disabil Hum Dev 2009;8(3):243-58.

[21] Ventegodt S, Andersen NJ, Kandel I, Merrick J. Effect, side effects and adverse events of non-pharmaceutical medicine. A review. Int J Disabil Hum Dev 2009;8(3):227-35.

[22] Ventegodt S, Andersen NJ, Merrick J, Greydanus DE. Effectiveness of traditional pharmaceutical biomedicine versus complementary and alternative medicine in a physician's general practice. J Altern Med Res 2010;2(2):179-86.

[23] Ventegodt S, Merrick J. A review of side effects and adverse events of non-drug medicine (nonpharmaceutical complementary and alternative medicine): Psychotherapy, mind-body medicine and clinical holistic medicine. J Complement Integr Med 2009;6(1):1-29. doi:10.2202/1553-3840.1156.

[24] Ventegodt S, Merrick J. Meta-analysis of positive effects, side effects and adverse events of holistic mind-body medicine (clinical holistic medicine): experience from Denmark, Sweden, United Kingdom and Germany. Int J Adolesc Med Health 2009;21(4):441-56.

[25] Ventegodt S. Comparative analysis of the world's ten major medical systems based on data from evidence-based medicine (preferably metaanalyses): Which types of medicine are effective for a majority of clinical conditions, safe, affordable, and sustainable? J Altern Med Res 2019;11(2):in print.

[26] Ventegodt S. A comparative analysis of the environmental consequences of the world's different types of medicine: Consciousness-based holistic medicine versus pharmaceutical medicine. J Altern Med Res 2019;11(1):67-78.

[27] Ventegodt S. Is there a university brave enough to host the "First International Conference on Sustainable Medicine"? J Altern Med Res 2019;11(1):3-5.

[28] Ventegodt S, Merrick J. Reflections from a study tour to Hippocrates' Asklepieion on the island of Kos. J Altern Med Res 2012; 4(2):221-3.

[29] Allen JP. The art of medicine in Ancient Egypt. New York: Metropolitan Museum Art, 2005.

[30] Ornish D. Avoiding revascularization with lifestyle changes: The Multicenter Lifestyle Demonstration Project. Am J Cardiol 1998;82(10B):72T-6.

[31] Ornish D, Brown SE, Scherwitz LW, Billings JH, Armstrong WT, Ports TA, et al. Can lifestyle changes reverse coronary heart disease? Lancet 1990;336(8708):129–33.

[32] Ornish D. Love and survival. The scientific basis for the healing power of intimacy. New York: Harper Collins, 1999.

[33] Frattaroli J, Weidner G, Dnistrian AM, Kemp C, Daubenmier JJ, Marlin RO, et al. Clinical events in prostate cancer lifestyle trial: Results from two years of follow-up. Urology 2008;72(6):1319-23.

[34] Leichsenring F, Leibing E. Psychodynamic psychotherapy: a systematic review of techniques, indications and empirical evidence. Psychol Psychother 2007;80(Pt 2):217-28.

[35] Leichsenring F, Rabung S, Leibing E. The efficacy of short-term psychodynamic psychotherapy in specific psychiatric disorders: a meta-analysis. Arch Gen Psychiatry 2004;61(12):1208-16.

[36] Leichsenring F, Rabung S, Leibing E. The efficacy of short-term psychodynamic psychotherapy in specific psychiatric disorders: a meta-analysis. Arch Gen Psychiatry 2004;61(12):1208–16.

[37] Leichsenring F, Rabung S. Effectiveness of long-term psychodynamic psychotherapy: A meta-analysis. JAMA 2008;300(13):1551-65.

[38] Leichsenring F. Are psychodynamic and psychoanalytic therapies effective?: A review of empirical data. Int J Psychoanal 2005;86(Pt 3):841-68.

[39] Smith R. The drugs don't work. BMJ 2003;327(7428):0-h.

[40] Gøtzsche PC. Deadly medicines and organised crime: How big pharma has corrupted healthcare", New York: Radcliffe, 2013.

[41] Gøtzsche PC. Deadly psychiatry and organised denial. Copenhagen: People Press, 2015.

[42] IMS Health. URL: http://www.annualreports.com/Company/ims-health/Annual rapport 2017.

Chapter 12

THE STRENGTHS AND WEAKNESSES OF TEN MAJOR MEDICAL SYSTEMS

The aim is to find the ideal type(s) of medicine, by comparing ten major medical systems with regard to: 1) range of clinical conditions helped, 2) effectivity, 3) safety, 4) cost, and 5) sustainability. Method: All medical systems are organized in 10 major classes for analysis. For each type the literature was searched for best metadata on range of clinical conditions helped, effectivity, safety, cost, and sustainability. Combined measures were calculated: cost-benefit, cost-effectiveness, Number Needed to Treat (NNT), Number Needed to Harm (NNH), Therapeutic Value (TV = Total number needed to harm (NNH_{total})/Number needed to treat (NNT)), cost per cured patient (treatment year 1–50), environmental impact per cured patient, QALYs and HALYs. Results: To be useful for a society, medicine must be generally useful, have significant therapeutic value (good benefit-to-harm ratio: TV $\geq$ 1), a documented long-term effect, safety, and sustainability. We found biomedicine (drugs) to be ineffective for most clinical conditions, harmful, expensive and very damaging to the environment. We found most CAM types harmless but ineffective. We found the most effective CAM-types (mind–body medicine, holistic medicine, Shamanism) to be effective for most clinical conditions, safe, cheap and sustainable; we found them to be 100 times more cost-effective, 1,000 times more effective, 10,000 times less harmful and 100,000 times less burdensome to the global environment compared to pharmaceutical drugs. Recommendation: Comparative studies of all types of medicine must be introduced in the curriculums of all medical schools, so all future doctors know the value of the alternatives when they choose to practice medicine.

Introduction

The aim of this study was to find the types of medicine that can serve as the medicine for a future, global, sustainable, healthy, and happy culture. The world is getting small, and cultural exchange, global trade, global media coverage, and traveling, causes all cultures to slowly merge into one global culture, "the global village". At the same time, our planetary environment is seriously challenged; a new rapport from IPBES (1) has documented the decay of nature and the coming extinction of 1,000,000 species in the near future. The concept of sustainability has therefore also come to medicine. This study includes for the first time a comparative analysis of the sustainability of all the world's different types of medicine.

We have analyzed all known types of medicine with regards to 1) range of clinical conditions helped, 2) effectivity, 3) safety, 4) cost, and 5) sustainability. The types of medicine, and the estimated number of patients using them are the following ((2), for Denmark see (3)):

- Chemical biomedicine (drugs, bioactive molecules), used by 1 billion people.
- Chemical CAM (symbolic and experiential medicine, i.e., flower medicine, herbal medicine, diets, minerals, etc.) used by 100 million people.
- Body-medicine: (a) low-energy types of massage, reflexology, physical therapy, physiotherapy, spa, sauna etc. used by 100 million people; b) high-energy types: chiropractic etc.) used by one million people.
- Mind-medicine: psychotherapy, i.e., psychodynamic, cognitive, gestalt, psychoanalysis, mindfulness and meditation, no-touch sexology etc. used by 10 million people,
- Spirit-medicine: philosophical interventions, energy medicine, prayers, spiritual healing (i.e., Reiki), Shamanism, healing music, spiritual CAM (i.e., crystal healing) etc. 5) used by 1 billion people.

- Mind–Body Medicine: Acupuncture, acupressure, homeopathy, manual sexology, body-psychotherapy, Reichian bodywork, Rosen therapy, ergo therapy etc. used by one billion people.
- Body–Spirit Medicine: Prayer involving physical activity like in Tibetan Buddhist-style meditation, pilgrimage etc. (unknown number of users).
- Holistic body-mind-spirit medicine and existential therapy: Holistic medicine, clinical medicine, clinical holistic medicine, holistic body-psychotherapy, holistic bodywork, the sexological examination, holistic mind–body medicine, biodynamic body-psychotherapy, tantric bodywork and massage, holistic sexology, Native American rituals etc. used by 10 million people.
- Chemical body-mind-spirit medicine: Traditional shamanism with Peyote and San Pedro cactus (mescaline), Ayahuasca, scopolamine, magic mushrooms; modern forms of this are Grof's LSD psychotherapy, MMDA psychotherapy etc. We estimate this is used by 10 million people. The collective use of MMDA and similar emotionally releasing drugs by young people at dance parties can also be seen as a modern practice of this kind of medicine, as the aim almost always in an improvement of the user's personal psyche, and social or sexual relations. If you include this the estimated number of users are 20 million people.
- Social and environmental medicine: Coaching, work-related personal development programs, stress management, leadership training, couching, gardening, aesthetic architecture, Feng Shui etc. used by 1 billion people.

We have used the criteria from evidence-based medicine (see below) and applied them on the body of articles (reviews, meta-analyses) using global QOL and self-assessed mental and physical health as the main outcome. We have searched in the largest medical databases:

1. PubMed. PubMed, a service of the National Library of Medicine, provides access to MEDLINE citations back to the mid-1960s to present.
2. CINAHL Plus with Full Text.
3. EMBASE: Excerpta Medica Database.
4. Cochrane Library.
5. PopLine.
6. TOXNET.
7. Agricola on herbs and medicinal plants. From the National Agricultural Library.
8. CAM on PubMed. Subset of PubMed linking to specific subjects in complementary and alternative medicine. On UM campus or for UM affiliates searching remotely, use the SFX-linked site.
9. Dr. Duke's Phytochemical and Ethnobotanical Database. Allows keyword searches for plants, chemicals, biological activity, and ethnobotanical areas and links to other databases of interest. Produced by the Agricultural Research Service of the U.S. Department of Agriculture.
10. Facts and Comparisons. Composed of a number of subsets including Herbal Interaction Facts, Off-label Drug Facts, Drug Identifier, and Review of Natural Products.
11. Alternative Medicine - Health & Wellness Resource Center From the Gale Encyclopedia of Alternative Medicine.
12. HerbMed. Published information on contraindications, toxicity and adverse effects. An evidence-based resource providing scientific data underlying the use of herbs for health. Maintained by the Alternative Medicine Foundation.
13. Micromedex Subscription databases covering herbal medicines and dietary supplements, clinical protocols, patient education and herbal-dietary supplement interactions. Addresses toxicology, pharmacology, acute care, chemical safety and regulatory compliance.
14. Natural Medicines. Subscription database presenting up to date clinical data on natural medicines, herbal medicines and dietary

supplements used in the western world. Compiled by pharmacists and physicians.

15. Review of Natural Products; See Facts and Comparisons. Composed of a number of subsets including Herbal Interaction Facts, Off-label Drug Facts, Drug Identifier, and Review of Natural Products.
16. RXList-Alternatives. Contains categories of herbal medicines comprising Western herbs, Chinese herbal remedies and homeopathic remedies, offered both through FAQ's and complete monographs.

This paper contains a revised, combined, and extended version of the analyses we have done earlier (2, 4-17). To keep the present paper so short that it can be published as an article, and not a book, we refer to these papers for references and detailed description of method.

We believe that we have covered the most relevant sources in our research. At the same time we encourage other researchers to reproduce the present study, in the aim to include more data, to carry out a more detailed analysis, and to increase the accuracy of estimates and calculations.

INTRODUCTION: WHAT IS EVIDENCE-BASED MEDICINE?

Evidence-based medicine is medicine based on scientific evidence of high quality. Medicine is anything that is intended for healing or the prevention of physical and mental disease, discomfort, suffering, pour sexual, social, work etc. functioning, general unhappiness, or any other aspect of our "global quality of life" (18-22). With global quality of life (global QOL) we mean the total, or absolute, quality of a human beings life, including all subjective, objective and existential dimensions (see the IQOL theory (18). Other theories for global QOL are as inclusive but us a different point of view (23-28); to truly understand the field you need to compare the different theories of global quality of life and see their individual strengths and weaknesses. There is no perfect theory today. What quality of life

(QOL) truly is, remains a deep mystery for science, in spite of many good theories - as does "happiness", "life", and "consciousness" in general (see our list of unexplained phenomena and concepts in biology, medicine and life science (29-51).

In spite of the severe scientific and philosophical problems regarding life and existence (52-62), we find that efforts of reducing the global QOL concept to something practical and measurable have been very successful (see, i.e., our own SEQOL, QOL1, QOL5 and QOL10 questionnaires (63-66)). People know how they are; they can sense it. Therefore a human being can easily rate his or her quality of life on a given scale; mental and physical health can also easily be rated, if you ask a cooperative person to do so (63-66). Therefore global QOL as well as self-rated health are both good outcome measures in medicine, and the improvement of *global QOL* (measuring the patients´ total well-being(66)) is a good and practical goal for future medicine. We must warn against the use of the often-used very unclear measure "health-related QOL" which are not build on any clear QOL theory; there are so many examples of these un-informative and misleading "ad hoc" scales, which are developed to document treatment success in a single aspect of the patients' life (67), but if global QOL is not improved the patient is not truly benefitting from the intervention.

WHAT IS MEDICINE?

Medicine comes in hundreds of different forms; every single culture on the planet has developed its own kind and style of medicine (68-87). Medicine can be fragrant flowers and herbs, healing touch, analytic talk, emotional support, magical rites, behavioral advices, magical amulets or potions, chemical drugs, physical interventions, like surgery or radiation therapy, physical therapy like massage and acupressure, and many different kinds and styles of therapy for body, mind, and spirit, for positive thinking, social and sexual health, understanding of self, and philosophical position. Even religious interventions like prayers, healings, meditation, and religious and philosophical teachings must be classified as medicine in the broadest meaning of this word, as the aim is to improve happiness.

Box 1. Classification of medicine (Including CAM and biomedicine) into 10 principal classes: Classes 1 and 2 are chemical medicines; 3–10 are consciousness-based/informational medicines (they often use tools, including herbs, minerals, amulets, massage oils etc., but the effect of these are experiential, often ritual or symbolic, not chemical or physical)

1. Chemical medicine (biomedicine with bioactive molecules).
2. Chemical CAM (symbolic and experiential medicine, i.e., flower medicine, herbal medicine, diets, minerals, vitamins etc.).
3. Body-medicine: a) Low-energy types: massage, reflexology, physical therapy, physiotherapy, spa, sauna etc. b) High-energy types: chiropractic, Thai style massage (i.e., walking on the body) etc.
4. Mind-medicine: a) Psychotherapy: psychodynamic, cognitive, gestalt etc. b) Psychoanalysis. c) Mindfulness and meditation. d) No-touch sexology, e) Healing music etc.
5. Spirit-medicine: Philosophical interventions, energy medicine, prayers, spiritual healing (i.e., Reichi), Shamanism, spiritual CAM (i.e., crystal healing), symbolic healing etc.
6. Mind–body medicine (acupuncture, acupressure, homeopathy, manual sexology, body-psychotherapy, Reichian bodywork, Rosen therapy, ergo therapy etc.).
7. Body–spirit medicine (prayer involving physical activity like in Tibetan Buddhist-style meditation, pilgrimage etc.).
8. Holistic body-mind-spirit medicine: Existential therapy (holistic medicine, clinical medicine, clinical holistic medicine, holistic body-psychotherapy, holistic bodywork, the sexological examination, holistic mind–body medicine, biodynamic body-psychotherapy, tantric bodywork and massage, holistic sexology, Native American rituals etc.
9. Chemical body-mind-spirit medicine: Shamanism with hallucinogenic drugs (Peyote, San Pedro, Ayahuasca, "magic" psilocybin mushrooms, Datura stramonium plants etc.), Grof's LSD-25 existential psychotherapy, MMDA psychotherapy, etc.
10. Social and environmental medicine (coaching, work-related personal development programs, stress management, leadership training, gardening, aesthetic architecture, Feng Shui etc.)

The root of our scientific and philosophical problems in medicine is that we do not, in scientific terms, understand consciousness itself (88, 89), which gives rise to all our experiences, good and bad. But even without total and deep understanding of consciousness, all cultures have old medical traditions that address the problems of poor physical, mental, sexual, and spiritual health, low quality of life, and suffering in all its human forms.

Box 1 gives a classification of medicines (including complementary and alternative medicine (CAM) and biomedicine) into 10 principal classes, which covers an estimated 95% of the medical interventions done on about 3 billion patients on this planet every year (the last 5% being Woo Do, pornography intended to help women, developing book programs, problem oriented TV shows etc., intended to raise consciousness, and similar interactions with some healing and/or damaging effects we have not yet been able to classify). While the presented system might not be complete, it definitely embraces a vast majority of the treatment types there exist today. Therefore we find it satisfactory for our purpose. Yet, we encourage other research teams to try to improve this categorization.

WHAT IS SCIENTIFIC EVIDENCE?

The next important question we must ask is: What is scientific evidence? (90). In spite of the relevance of this questions, it is almost as difficult to give a final answer to this question, as to the question about what medicine is.

All sciences use axioms which cannot be proven. Therefore, all sciences are from a philosophical point of view basically religion (readers unfamiliar with this thinking might benefit from reading (52)). That is even the case with pure mathematics, and much more the case with chemistry and physics, and even more with the life sciences like biology and medicine, where *life, consciousness, and happiness* becomes core issues, in spite of our almost total lack of scientific understanding of these subjects.

A massive body of science has pointed to the fact, that happiness seems causal to future health, to a much larger extent than other factors like our living- and working environment (91).

In science, the concept of true and false is essential, but how can any statement based on mind be absolutely true (52-62)? It can only be relatively true, so the art of science is to make it so simple and so directly related to reality, that we can be certain that our conclusions are at least true in a relative sense.

If you consider a given type of medicine and ask if such a cure is helpful to a specific clinical condition, we need to test this cure on a group of patients with this condition, and the group must be big enough to statistically determine, if the patient's condition has improved by this intervention (92). This is lovely simple. If you have a simple measure like pain, we can make the patient suffering from chronic pain rate his or her level of pain before and after treatment, and we can immediately see if we help this patients. If we test the cure on 20 patients with chronic pain, we can calculate a mean for the improvement, and say that our cure is so and so helpful for this kind of pain, with this certainty (P-value). We can even compare it to a control group of similar patients we do not give the cure. Do we need a control group for such a study? No, we actually don't, if the problem is chronic – meaning it doesn't go away by itself (92, 93). If it is not chronic, we actually do not even need medicine – the condition will correct itself, because of our self-healing nature. Many doctors believe that intervention in this situation is counterproductive, as it diminishes the patient's natural trust in the body's own healing potentials, and create an unhealthy dependency on doctors (94-97).

So, simple before-and-after studies using simple measures for simple and well-defined states of chronic illness and suffering – like low global QOL - gives us relatively true measures for effectivity and safety of medicine. We have used this simple tools to document the effect of holistic medical treatment in our own clinic (see 98-104). Done this way a scientific documentation of a medical intervention can be done in a hospital or medical clinic in 10 working hours and for a cost of around 1000 EURO. It is a simple, effective, affordable, and reliable test. You can say that we, in spite of philosophical problems, in the end have found a practical way to document any type of medicine.

But, the methods used for testing medicines today are mostly not like that. They are highly complex procedures where many things can be adjusted, until the wished-for results are created (105). The famous randomized clinical trial (RCT) is an example of such a method, which is not even relatively true (105-107). According to the many critiques of the RCT method, it allows pharmacological companies to market poisonous, harmful and ineffective chemicals as effective and safe medicine (108, 109, 110). We have ourselves made a thorough analyses of the RCT method, and even published a book warning the public against the faulty results is almost always gives (105).

In general, the more complex a procedure is made, the less transparent it is, and the less it has to do with reality, the easier it is to manipulate, and the less true it is.

TWO MAJOR COMPONENTS OF GOOD SCIENTIFIC MEDICINE: GOOD THEORY AND GOOD CLINICAL DOCUMENTATION

Human beings are bio-psycho-social beings (18-20, 27, 28, 30-51, 53-62, 88-89, 110-123)); you might even to this add a spiritual dimension taking into consideration the unfathomable depth of human consciousness. While science is quite clear and simple when it comes to chemistry and physics, and fair when it comes to biology, it gets quite unclear and flimsy when it comes to psychology, and really messy when it comes to the social and spiritual dimensions of man. You need to focus on self-rated physical, mental and sexual health, and preferably on global QOL (18, 27, 28) as a general, integrative measure of health and happiness, when you want to measure outcome of a treatment; else you are in deep trouble, because you don't know what you measure.

Good medicine-theory is of course interdisciplinary; it describes man as a bio-psycho-social-spiritual being, and disease is thus seen as a disturbance in the wholeness, not in one of its parts(68-91) and with this understanding most clinical conditions can be treated and helped (116-174). This is very important, as all dimensions of man are intimately interrelated. When you get sick, the symptoms are often in your body, but the cause is often elsewhere, i.e., in your genes, your environment, or (more likely) in your own mind and psyche – or the cause is a combination of all these factors (163-189).

If you explore your mental dimensions, you will find that your thinking, your interpretation of reality, and your experience of life, is highly dependent on your philosophy of life, your past, your present relations, your work, and your social reality, and your own conscious and unconscious intentions (in Buddhist philosophy often called "desires", in Hindu philosophy often explained with the concept of inborn irrational tendencies called "Karma") (91, 163-174). Is it so complicated, really? Yes it is!

Your disease is born out of the wholeness impacted by the quality of your genes, your inborn mental weaknesses, your social and cultural conditioning - including the misunderstandings of the world you inherited from your parents. Even more factors might be in the equation, like the information you carry from your own biological line, combined with your own early spiritual decisions (163-172). Wow, it is really complicated!

If you look at the immune system, its immunological defense power comes from the inner balance of the organism (175); but this balance is hard to describe in scientific terms. We know that staying healthy is closely related to the intensity and quality of your feelings, your life style, and your general happiness (or global QOL if you will). You can even say that it is scientifically proven that happiness is the best medicine. Even heart patients (94, 95, 176, 198-200) and cancer patients that find joy and happiness can spontaneously heal (175-180).

Immunological weakness is often found to be related to difficult feelings that are oppressed to different places in the body, most often the muscles (179-193). When the feelings are met and integrated, the chronic infection of the gingiva, the bladder, the intestines, the vulva etc. disappears (190-197). Can we understand it on a physical, mechanical level? No, we cannot. Our science it not developed enough for that. Can we use the understanding we have to help patents? Yes we can, and it works almost every time... There is no reason to cry over our present state of medicine; many types of medicine work wonders, also with the most serious diseases, like the quality-of-life improving psychosocial interventions for patients with prostate cancer (175) and sick hearts, i.e., coronary stenosis (198-200). The scientific documentation shows radical improvement for most patients in a few month!

The biological and cellular order is highly sensitive to the state of mind of the person; but happiness goes even deeper: happiness goes to the roots of you being (201) and influences your most remote relationships. Your happiness vibrates through you whole existence. Happiness is a mystery in itself; there is no really good science about happiness, so to include happiness in the scientific theory of medicine remains a real scientific challenge. But we must, as happiness/global QOL seems to be both the most important cause, and the most important outcome in medicine.

When it comes to scientific documentation of the clinical effect of medicine, we have big problems too, for what is a good test of clinical effect? We know now, as mentioned above, that the randomized clinical trial (RCT), which everybody 30 years ago believed to be the final solution to the problem of how to test pharmacological medicine, is so faulty and flawed that it cannot be taken as scientific documentation for the effect of medicine(105). Sadly most medical schools have close connections to the pharmaceutical industry and therefore they are not teaching students to be critical to the way drugs are tested by the industry. So the insufficiency of the RCT method is rarely known to doctors.

One major problem with the RCT test is, that the active placebo effect of a poisonous drugs in the RCT as it is designed today turn it into seemingly effective and safe medicine (105-110). All poisonous drugs tested by the RCT-method are simply "proven" to be effective medicine, with exactly the specific action the test aims to explore (105-109). What a wonderful thing, if you are in the business of making money from selling drugs! No wonder the method is popular.

This is a hopeless situation; the highly praised "blinding" is always broken by the toxic effects of the drugs, and the pharmaceutical companies are producing "medicines" which mostly only have toxic effects, as the critiques point out(108-109). A number of Cochrane studies have recently documented that many of the drug-groups we are using today worldwide as doctors are without significant beneficial effects and poisonous (202-207). Yet, one billion patients or so are taking these drugs every day, in the belief that they are helpful (108-110, 208). And because of the active placebo, they *are* really helpful - but only for a very short while. And they are also always very harmful.

The consequence of the lack of a valid test method for pharmacological drugs has been devastating. According to leading experts in the Cochrane Collaboration, hundreds of millions of patients are getting poisoned with severe consequences for their health every year (108, 109, 206); and hundreds of thousands of these patients have been killed by the poisoning effects of the drugs (108, 109, 206). Especially, the psychiatric patients are burdened by the toxic effects of drugs, which have been documented recently by the leader of the Nordic Cochrane Center, Peter Gøtzsche (109, 211). For many years Peter Gøtzsche kept a safe, low profile in the public space and media, but a few years ago he decided to share with the public what he knew. Peter is now fired from his jobs as professor and director, and expelled from the Cochrane Collaboration he himself has started; it is well-known that you cannot tell this truth and threaten the pharmaceutical industry without this having dire consequences for your whole life and carrier (211).

In evidence-based medicine, you need to look at the quality of the scientific evidence. The best scientific evidence we have today is the meta-analyses made by independent researchers. One example of this is the Cochrane reviews from year 1990-2015 or so (210) (before the pharmaceutical industry took over the Cochrane collaboration, as pointed out by Peter Gøtzsche (211)) made by 3,000 fairly independent physicians and researchers in the international Cochrane Collaboration. Their work has systematically shown that drugs are of little help for patients and almost always very harmful (108, 109, 210, 211). Even the best of pharmacological medicines has surprisingly little effect (212); if you look at how many patients you need to treat for one being helped (i.e., with an antibiotic like penicillin for a throat infection) the number needed to treat (NNT) it is normally 20 patients or more (250) - and often 100 or more for serious diseases like cancer and schizophrenia (212). And, if you talk about NNTs around 100 – i.e., 1% of the patient helped – this number is likely to be an artifact given by bias from data collection, study design, and statistical method (208). At the same time these strong drugs are harming all the patients (108, 109, 208, 210).

An NNT of 20 (250) means that if a doctor gives such a drug to a patient, the likelihood for the patient to be helped is 0.05, or only 5%! And the people who are helped are most often NOT even cured. They only have a few symptoms of the disease improved in most of the studies.

This is the situation of the pharmacological medicines we have today according to the leading editors of BMJ (250). At the same time, adverse effects are so normal that in average, every patient will have a harmful effect from taking a drug (109, 207, 208). Honestly, it is not worth being a doctor with such poor results. Therefore, many doctors burn out and loose the joy of working as they year after year see that their patients systematically are not improving.

So, how is it with evidence-based CAM ("complementary and alternative medicine", often these days called "non-drug medicine")? Today, hundreds of meta-analyses and Cochrane reviews have shown that there are no significant side effects of non-drug medicine (7, 11, 14, 212) - with high-energy manipulations (chiropractic) as a rare exception. So you can safely go to any psychotherapist or body worker. Talk and touch therapy are just safe (14). That is good to know.

But is CAM effective? Well, in general, alternative medicine is *not* effective (2, 4-17), in spite of more than 50% of the users reporting feeling helped shortly after the treatment (213). Sorry to say this, as so many people are happy for alternative medicine: If you look at all that we do to help and cure, this broad spectrum of activities we call CAM are mostly

NOT helpful. A number of scientific studies of prayers and positive thinking, diets, exercises, breathing exercises, yoga, meditation, art therapy, herbal medicine etc. have proven these types of CAM to be almost without a lasting, significant, positive effect for the patient. Therefore, in general, CAM cures are comforting the patient but they are *not* working as a cure.

With this said, there are some types of talk and touch therapy that has been proven extremely effective (68-78, 184-187, 214-218). These are methods that at the same time focus on (a) feelings and emotions including sexuality, (b) understanding and self-exploration including almost all types of self-inquiry, and (c) letting go of negative beliefs, attitudes, thoughts, philosophies, concepts etc. - that is, mind-work that empties your mind from all its mental contents and structures, and all your false identifications (82, 162-174).

Psychodynamic psychotherapy - that is, talk therapy with focus on emotions and sexuality - has been proven extremely effective (213-217); 95% have been helped in 12-24 month and the help is often a cure. Holistic medicine has recently been found extremely effective in the USA for cancer and coronary heart disease, with around 80% of the patients helped within 3–6 month (198-200). These are amazing results.

Similar results have been found for a number of existentially oriented talk-and-touch therapies (2, 4-17, 68-78). Methods that combine talk-and-touch therapy to help the patient FEEL, UNDERSTAND, and LET GO of negative beliefs have in general been found very effective, with amazing NNT numbers (1 or 2) and totally harmless. And the wonderful thing is that these methods seem to help a wide range of clinical conditions - almost all types of patients can be helped (4-17). Most of these results are found in meta-analyses made by independent researchers (210). See, this is good, evidence-based medicine. So we have after all come a long way in medicine.

Comparative Analysis of Cost, Effectiveness, Safety, and Sustainability of All Types of Evidence-Based Medicine for All Clinical Conditions

We have suggested that the five major categories of CAM used by National Center for Complementary and Alternative Medicine (NCCAM) are revised into a 10-class system for evidence-based medicine in general, as we agree to the viewpoint often presented in *Journal of the American Medical Association* (JAMA) that CAM and biomedicine must be combined into one integrated medical system of evidence-based medicine (90) (Table 1).

We are now able using simple and reliable science to examine the cost, efficiency and safety of the 10 different types of evidence-based medicine, and combine them with the data we recently got about sustainability (2). We want to look at the benefit-to-harm ratio (often called therapeutic value (202-207)), the cost of the production of quality of life and self-rated health, the cost of health in patient-damage per treatment, and the environmental burden of the medicine.

Methods

Today, there are three major population health measures permitting morbidity and mortality to be simultaneously evaluated: quality-adjusted life years (QALYs), health-adjusted life years (HALYs), and disability-adjusted life years (DALYs). In this paper, we will only estimate QALYs and HALYs, as we do not find the DALY concept clear enough for our use.

The method is estimating the general numbers from meta-analyses, preferably Cochrane reviews (208), and, when possible, meta-meta-analyses covering one or more of the different types of evidence-based medicine. We will include estimates from the leading medical journals of typical numbers of NNTs and number needed to harm (NNHs). To make such a highest level analysis where we look at all types of medicine for all clinical conditions, we will need to simplify matters.

The prize of pharmaceutical drugs will be calculated from the Danish cost of drugs to more than two million chronic patients in Denmark using biomedicine (2, 5, 13); this number might be high compared to the number in developing countries were medicine often is sold cheaper. The prize of CAM treatments are also coming from Danish circumstances, where a year of therapy often is about 20 sessions costing around €1700 (2); in developing countries the prize is often a tenth of that. The calculation of QALY and HALY is using the knowledge on normal loss of quality of life and self-rated health when people get ill in Denmark; and have a lot of social security to some extend compensating for loss of quality of life and health, the prize per QALY and HALY might be lower in less developed countries.

As our results are calculated based on estimated numbers, we must admit having an uncertainty of ±100%; we believe our results to be correct within a factor three. As the differences between the different types of medicine are often a factor 10 or 100, this large uncertainty is still acceptable.

As the biggest problem in medical research today is bias from economic interests, we have avoided sources that might be strongly biased, like RCTs from pharmaceutical industry, overoptimistic estimates in reviews from CAM-journals far from the scientific standard of the journals in MedLine/www.PubMed.gov etc.

Actually the process of limiting bias has been our biggest problem, forcing us to leaving out most of the sources often used in this type of analyses, like statistics made by public organs headed by people close to the pharmaceutical industry. Such statistics seems mostly to be extremely biased in favor of biomedicine.

There are many fundamental problems in biomedicine we could have addressed to make this study more thorough; there are problems from the practical use of drugs with low compliance, wrong diagnosis, errors in prescriptions and overmedication; there are problems with the RCTs at its very roots making the NNT and NNH numbers from industrial testing difficult to trust, and this paper is after all based on numbers coming from the pharmaceutical industries' use of the RCT in testing its products. So, we know that we are only scratching the surface of the problems in this paper.

We have wanted things to be so simple that complexity of things could not allow us to bias the paper our self; what happens in any complex procedure is that you unconsciously take things in the direction you wish or expect, and only by making things so simple that there are no steps to twist or manipulate, you can truly avoid bias. We believe that the simplicity of our calculations and estimates has lead us to trustworthy, fairly unbiased results.

Our main source of information is the Cochrane library (210). In former papers, where we have analyzed aspects of one of the 10 types of medicines, we have had several hundred references. In this paper, we are using the whole Cochrane library as reference (210). To make the reference list of acceptable length we are only listing complementary material used in the study in the reference list.

FINDINGS

The first and most important question is which physical diseases, mental disorders, sexual, existential and work-related problems can be bettered or cured with the different types of medicine. For people who are accustomed to the pharmaceutical medicine, and under the spell of the biased marketing of the drugs, it might come as a surprise, that most clinical conditions cannot be cured with drugs. When we go through the existing research the problem is, that the outcome studies we look for are often not existing: We want to know if the treatment with a type of medicine, i.e., a drug is better than no treatment, and if it is better that a placebo treatment.

A placebo treatment is a treatment where the doctor uses the placebo effect, meaning that he inspires hope and faith in a cure that has no other rationale than giving hope and faith. But there are almost no such studies made. Gøtzsche et al. (219) has shown that if you use an inert drug, i.e., a tablet of calcium carbonate (chalk) there is no placebo effect coming from it. We know on the other hand a number of drugs that gives a strong feeling of "getting a medicine" but without any specific curative effects, and these drugs always shows an amazing healing effect – they are called "active placebos" (105-109). You might expect that a large number of studies where a treatment is compared with active placebo exist, but the opposite is the case: there are almost no such studies made. In almost all randomized clinical tests (RCTs) the placebo is just the ineffective chalk pill. And why? The answer is simple: A test of a medicine – typically these days a drug – is mostly tested by the provider, the manufacturer of medicine, and his intention is to prove that his own medicine is working, so it can be sold. So the pharmaceutical industry designs the test in such a way, that it gives the wished-for result. In all countries there are "medical science-ethical committees" that are approving the studies, but these competes are filled with industry-friendly, totally uncritical people, most often without any expertise in scientific testing. They are only there to make it look like somebody is actually controlling the industrial testing.

Now, it is up to the world to call the bluff, and many independent researchers, i.e., the leading researchers in the Cochrane collaboration, have done this both clearly and effectively (108-109). But because of the corrupt state of affairs, where the industry has taken control over all the big scientific journals like Lancet, and the international medical institutions like WHO (220, 221), the critique that again and again has been directed towards the way the medicine has been tested, is simply ignored!

Of cause there have been many independent researchers doing amazing research. Let me tell you about cancer research. Ulrik Abel collected all the existing data on cytotoxic cancer drug research for all the major cancers (the epithelioid cancers like breast cancer, uterus cancer etc.) back in 1991 and analyzed them (222-224). He documented that whenever there was a study where a treatment with cytotoxic drugs were compared with no treatment, *no treatment was always better than the treatment*, both when it comes to the patients' survival and quality of life (222-224). The drugs destroyed the patients' well-being and killed them. You might think that all the doctors stopped using these drugs after learning about this study, and that all companies manufacturing these drugs stopped the production. But that did not happen, the drugs are still on the market 30 years after! Abel got scandalized, his computer sabotaged and his database destroyed, he almost lost his job, and he was forced to give up his cancer research. And since then the companies only tested "new drugs against the old drugs" – using a pseudo-ethical argument, that you cannot not treat a cancer patient, because that would be unethical to not give the patients a working cure!

So when we are doing this metaanalyses, we look at the good and valid studies that shows us the real world, not the nice illusion created by the pharmaceutical industry. Therefore we end up with the surprising result that drugs are good only for a few clinical conditions, while non-drug medicine can help for a huge number of clinical conditions. Drugs, i.e., antibiotics are effective for infectious diseases like syphilis, pain killers like morphine for acute pains i.e., from traffic traumas, insulin for diabetes etc. But drugs are almost always working on the *symptoms*, not the cause of a disease, which you notice if you are careful in your scientific analysis. Most infections come because your immunize system is week, not because bacteria are dangerous - and antibiotics cannot make the immune system stronger, but by attacking the infecting organism it can tip the balance in favor of the immune system. Balancing the whole human being can on the other hand radically improve the immune system status (176), which is the rationale for the psychosomatic, effective cure for chronic diseases used since Hippocrates (121).

When it comes to mental and sexual disorders, drugs simply has no curative role here. Even the praised drug Viagra that is said to help couples to overcome sexual problems are most likely giving more problems than it solves (194).

Table 1. Estimated NNT-numbers for the outcome "patient cured" for pharmaceutical drugs (biomedicine) and non-drug medicine (CAM) treatments of physical diseases, mental disorders, existential problems, sexual health issues, and working disability (primarily based on clinical studies using chronic patients as their own control, see text)

	Pharmaceutical drugs	**Non-drug medicine (CAM) for physical health**
Subjectively poor physical health	No curative drug exists	NNT=1-2
Coronary heart disease	No curative drug exists	NNT=1-3
Cancer (QOL/survival/pain)	NNT=100	NNT=1-3/1-10/1-3
Chronic pain	No curative drug exists	NNT=2-3
Chronic infections	NNT=20	NNT=2-3
CAM for mental health		
Subjectively poor mental health	No curative drug exists	NNT=1-2
Schizophrenia	No curative drug exists	NNT=2-5
Borderline	No curative drug exists	NNT=1-3
Major depression	No curative drug exists	NNT=1-3
Anorexia Nervosa	No curative drug exists	NNT=1-3
Anxiety	No curative drug exists	NNT=1-3
Social phobia	No curative drug exists	NNT=1-3
CAM for sexual dysfunctions		
Subjectively poor sexual functioning	No curative drug exists	NNT=2
Male erectile dysfunction	No curative drug exists	NNT=2
Female orgasmic dysfunction	No curative drug exists	NNT=1
Female lack of desire	No curative drug exists	NNT=2
Female dyspareunia	No curative drug exists NNT=2	
Vaginismus	No curative drug exists	NNT=2
Vulvodynia	No curative drug exists NNT=2	
Infertility (close ovarian tubes)	No curative drug exists	NNT=6
CAM for psychological and existential problems		
Subjectively poor quality of life	No curative drug exists	NNT=1-2
Sense of coherence	No curative drug exists	NNT=1-3
Suicidal prevention (with decisions)	No curative drug exists	NNT=1
Low self esteem	No curative drug exists	NNT=1-2
CAM for low working ability		
Subjectively poor working ability	No curative drug exists	NNT=1-2

(Data is taken from the Cochrane collaboration (208), complemented with data on CAM taken from sources presented in the reviews (2, 4-17)).

Table 2. Typical numbers for effect and harm, and the *Benefit-to-Harm* Ratio for ten classes of evidence-Based medicine (NNTs, NNHs, NNH_{total} and TVs) (estimated from Cochrane reviews of RCTs and from clinical studies with chronic patients) (2, 4-17, 202-207)

CAM class	**Short-term effect**	**Long-term effect**	**Side effects/ adverse events**	**Total risk of harm**	**Therapeutic value**
	(0–6 months)	(6–24 months)			TV = NNH_{total}/NNT
	NNT	NNT	NNH	NNH_{total}	TV (6–24 months)
Class 1 - Biomedicine (pharmaceuticals)	20 (5–50)	50 (5–100)	1–5	1–3	1–0.01
Class 2 - CAM (Chemical CAM)	≥20	≥50	25 (allergy)	25	0.5
Class 3a - CAM (Physical therapy, low-energy, i.e., massage, therapeutic touch)	2–4	6	>1,000,000	>1,000,000	167,000
Class 3b - CAM (Physical therapy, high-energy i.e., chiropractic treatment)	2–4	6	1000 (fractures)	1000	167
Class 4 - CAM (psychotherapy)*	3	6	>1,000,000	>1,000,000	167,000
Class 5 - CAM (spiritual therapy)	>10	>20	>1,000,000	>1,000,000	50,000
Class 6 - CAM (mind–body medicine)	2	4	>1,000,000	>1,000,000	250,000
Class 7 - CAM (body–spirit medicine)	Not known	Not known	>1,000,000	>1,000,000	Not known
Class 8 - CAM (holistic mind–body medicine)	2	1–2**	>1,000,000	>1,000,000	500,000–1,000,000
Class 9 - CAM (Shamanism with drugs etc.)***	1	1	>1000	>1000	>1000
Class 10 - CAM (Social medicine)	1	10	>1,000,000	>1,000,000	100,000

* Some types of psychotherapy have short-term NNTs of 2–3 (short-term psychodynamic *psychotherapy* (STPP)) and long term NNTs of 1–2 (long-term psychodynamic *psychotherapy* (LTPP)) for mental, somatic and sexual health problems (2, 4-17).The effect of clinical holistic medicine and similar medical systems seem to continue to increase though time. NNT: number needed to treat. NNH: number needed to harm, NNH_{total}: total likelihood of getting one side effect/adverse effect or adverse event. TV: therapeutic value, which here means benefit-to-harm ratio. For a treatment to be of true value to patients, it must be efficient, with a low NNT, and a high TV. ***Adverse effects: Brief reactive psychoses are only seen with mentally ill patients.

Consciousness-based holistic medicine can cure the most severe physical and mental disorders (Table 1). And the curative rate is impressive, often 9 out of 10 patients are cured. Sexual dysfunctions are also most often cured, if the patient manage to cooperate with the therapy (225-231). Existential and work problems are also most often cured with holistic medicine. So we have medicine that can help most clinical conditions. That is remarkable. What is surprising is that this safe, cheap and effective medicine, which was the reason European medicine got its unique status 2,500 years ago (121), is almost not used anymore by modern doctors of the western world.

And more than that: consciousness-based medicine is often today not even considered a real possibility to use, often it is look down on by "scientifically trained" doctors, and labeled as old-fashioned and outdated. This attitude comes from the universities´ medical faculties, which systematically have been taken over by industry-friendly powers.

Table 1 gives a comparison of the effectivity of biomedicine (pharmaceutical drugs) and non-drug medicine; notice the wide range of clinical conditions help non-drug medicine compared to drugs, and notice the high effectivity of non-drug medicine compared to drugs.

Based on primarily the Cochrane library and the other sources we have found reliable, we have evaluated the benefit and harm from pharmaceutical drugs and the different non-drug (CAM) medical systems. We have looked at the likelihood to benefit a patient (using NNT), the likelihood to harm a patient by the different adverse effects/side effects (using NNH), and the total likelihood to get one side effect/adverse reaction or adverse event (calculating the NNH_{total}) and from this we have calculated the ratio "benefit to harm" called the therapeutic value of the treatment ($TV = NNH_{total}/NNT$) (2, 4-17, 202-207) for the 10 different types of medicine, see Table 2.

While for a long time, thanks to the many Cochrane reviews, it has been easy to find NNT and NNH for most pharmaceutical drugs, it has been more difficult to establish these for the many different types of holistic and alternative medicine (CAM), and the relative harm of non-drug medicine had to be estimated from the number of reported cases in the literature. Recently, more than hundred Cochrane reviews have been made on a large number of CAM types for a large number of clinical conditions, and NCCAM, the US research center for CAM, has published a number of reports on five major categories of CAM, allowing us for a far better estimate of NNHs and NNTs (231-233) (see Table 3). For example, NCCAM has evaluated the number of patients treated every year in the USA with massage therapy (therapeutic touch) and the number of patients experiencing significant side effects from such treatments; NCCAM found that 20,000,000 adults and 700,000 children are treated every year in USA with very few patients harmed, allowing us to estimate NNH > 1,000,000 for massage and similar types of therapeutic touch (232-234). Of the 145 Cochrane reviews of CAM analyzed by "Committee on the Use of Complementary and Alternative Medicine by the American Public" (212), 38.4% of the reviews showed a positive or possibly positive (12.4%) effect. These Cochrane reviews documented typical NNTs of 2–30, depending on CAM type, and typical NNHs of 1000–1,000,000. Typical NNTs and NNHs for the 10 types of evidence-based medicine are presented in Table 3.

Two things are especially interesting for a patient: (a) How efficient is the medicine? This is best known from NNT telling how likely it is that the patient will benefit from the treatment. (b) How harmful is the medicine? The absolute harm (the sum of all harmful effect: NNH_{total}) is important but even more important is the benefit-to-harm ratio. Many patients will feel that a treatment is of therapeutic value if its advantages (statistically) dominate its disadvantages. The benefit-to-harm ratio is simplest expressed by the ratio $TV = NNH_{total}/NNT$, where NNH_{total} is the total likelihood of getting a side/adverse effect or adverse event (202-207). Typical values of NNH_{total} and TV can also be found in Table 3.

In general, chemical medicine, whether biomedical drugs (pharmaceutical drugs) or CAM drugs (herbs, aromatic oils, diet changes etc.) have high NNH_{total} and low TVs. The effect of chemical CAM seems to be less than pharmaceutical drugs, but it is a lot safer.

If you manipulate the biological informational system of the patient (for the scientific concept of biological information, see (29-51)) instead of body chemistry, you seem to avoid side/adverse effects and adverse events. Some types of CAM have a low efficacy, but still the TV is high because of the relative safeness. Some types of CAM are both efficient and safe. Holistic mind–body medicine seems to be as safe as other kinds of CAM but more efficient and they have the highest TV. Interestingly, there are adverse effects of the drugs traditionally used in Shamanism (79-87), giving shamanistic medicine the lowest TV of all CAM treatments; if you look at the cost during a 50-year life span, Shamanism ends up looking the best of all known treatments (see Table 7). As we do not want to return to Shamanism, we would like to pay respect and give our tribute to the pre-modern medicine. Indigenous people often know much about medicine.

The cost of different medical drugs and different non-drug CAM treatments varies a great deal. Within every class of evidence-based medicine, there are expensive and cheap alternatives. We have found it fair to set both a pharmaceutical and a CAM treatment to €2000 per year, knowing that praying is cheaper and cancer-chemotherapy is more expensive. If you know the NNT-number and the cost of one patient treated, you can find the cost for one patient cured (or at least treated successfully) by multiplying these numbers (Cost of one patient cured = NNT × yearly treatment cost) (see Table 3). The next year, the cured patients will not cost anything but the patient not cured will still cost the yearly treatment cost. In this way, we can estimate the 10 and 50 years' cost of one patient cured (see Table 3). If the NNT is very high, very few patients get cured and most become chronic patient. This is the case for pharmaceutical drugs, so here the calculation is simple: The cost as times goes by is calculated as *yearly cost × time*. If all or most patients are cured in one or a few years, the calculation is similarly simple: The total treatment cost is the one-year treatment cost. When patients get better little by little, as in psychotherapy, a more complicated estimate must be made, accounting for the current recovery of patients. Our estimates of all ten classes are found in Table 3. Due to lack of data, we could not make good estimates for Classes 5 and 7.

If there are many adverse effects and events, they cost sick days, hospitalization etc. We know that drugs are always poisonous to some extent, and that it is estimated that there are now 100,000 deaths a year in US hospitals directly caused by pharmaceutical drugs (235) and many more patients are harmed. This is a huge prize to pay but hard to put into numbers; we have only in this study included the direct cost to the drugs in our estimate. The true cost is likely to be several times larger.

Table 3. Accumulated cost (number of patients with side effects/adverse effects and adverse events) for one patient cured through time (Year 1, 10 and 50) for ten classes of evidence-based medicine

Continuous treatment (only stopped if the patients gets cured)	**Cost per patient-year**	**Accumulated cost (€)**		
	per treated patient	per cured patient	per cured patient	per cured patient
	First year	First year	Year 10	Year 50
Medicine with drugs (chemical medicine)				
Class 1 - chemical medicine*	2000	≥100,000	≥200,000	≥ 1,000,000
Class 2 - CAM (chemical CAM)	2000	>100,000	>200,000	>1,000,000
Non-drug CAM (informational medicine)				
Class 3 - CAM (physical therapy)	2000	12,000	60,000	100,000
Class 4 - CAM (psychotherapy)	2000	12,000	60,000	100,000
Class 5 - CAM (spiritual therapy)	Not known	Not known	Not known	Not known
Class 6 - CAM (mind–body medicine)	2000	8000	30,000	50,000
Class 7 - body–spirit medicine	Not known	Not known	Not known	Not known
Class 8 - CAM (holistic mind–body medicine)	2000	5000	10,000	20,000
Class 9 - CAM (Shamanism with drugs)	500	600	800	2000
Class 10 - CAM (social/environmental medicine)	5,000	50,000	350,000	500,000

* Cost of biomedical examination, hospitalization, and treatment of adverse effects and events not included (estimated round numbers, see text).

Table 4. Accumulated cost of one quality-adjusted life year (QALY) through time (Year 1, 10 and 50) for ten classes of evidence-based medicine

Continuous treatment (only stopped if the patients gets cured)	**QOL improvement from treatment (%) if successful**	**Prize of one QALY calculated from NNT (Table 1) and accumulated cost (Table 3)**		
	Global QOL	per cured patient	per cured patient	per cured patient
		First year	Year 10	Year 50
Medicine with drugs (chemical medicine)				
Class 1 - Chemical medicine*	20%	500,000	≥1,000,000	≥5,000,000
Class 2: CAM (chemical CAM)	20%	>500,000	>1,000,000	>5,000,000
Non-drug CAM (informational medicine)				
Class 3: CAM (physical therapy)	20%	60,000	300,000	60,000
Class 4: CAM (psychotherapy)	20%	60,000	300,000	60,000
Class 5: CAM (spiritual therapy)	20%	Not known	Not known	Not known
Class 6: CAM (mind–body medicine)	20%	40,000	180,000	40,000
Class 7: CAM body–spirit medicine	20%	Not known	Not known	Not known
Class 8: CAM (holistic mind–body medicine)	20%	25,000	50,000	10,000
Class 9: CAM (Shamanism with drugs)	20%	3000	4000	800
Class 10: CAM (social/environmental medicine)	20%	250,000	1,750,000	2,500,000

* Cost of biomedical examination, hospitalization, and treatment of adverse effects and events not included (estimated round numbers, see text).

A popular effect measure is QALY, or quality-adjusted life years. The idea is simple: Survival has in itself no value; if you survive but suffer to an extreme extent, it might be better if the doctor had not saved your life in the first place. To secure that the patient gets value for money, the cost per QALY must be calculated. As (global) quality of life in general is 20% lower for ill people than for healthy (236-239), we can make a simple estimate of cost/QALY, presented in Table 4. The principles of the estimate are simple: If a patient is cured right away and stays healthy, and would have become a chronic patient without treatment, the cost for one cured patient is multiplied with the time the patient's health is improved. As very few patients are cured with biomedicine (see Table 1), the cost of one QALY becomes astronomic as the treatment continues for life without results - which is normally the case in Denmark where we have socialized biomedicine, free or very cheap for all chronic patients. On the other hand, QALY-unit with an efficient CAM cure, which normally has an extra plus that patients not only stays healthy but also improves health through time (as they have learned the basic principles for human development), will as times go by be relatively cheaper. For every past year, the quality of life and health is already paid, as shown in Table 4. Interestingly one-session shamanistic healing is far the cheapest kind of medicine, presumably explaining its great popularity in almost all pre-modern cultures. In one-session healing, you are normally taken unto a daylong journey of guided self-exploration where you come to understand how you make yourself ill by the way you live and look at things (240, 241). It is thus a life-style and philosophy of life intervention. From a theoretical point of view, it might actually work. See our paper on the Peruvian use of Ayahuasca to learn more about this (241).

Instead of QALYs, WHO often recommends the use of HALYs (and DALYs), which is exactly the same, only with health (most often self-rated health) instead of quality of life. We know that the strongest measure of health is self-rated health (241-244), and we also know that sick people experience there health very much the same way as they experience their quality of life allowing us again to use a difference of 20% between healthy and ill people. This gives us Table 5, showing that mind–body medicine gives lots of health for the money, while chemical medicine and social medicine does not.

The harm caused by the 10 different types of evidence-based medicine as times goes by has been estimated in Table 6. Patients using biomedicine for years without being cured, as is normally the case, are accumulating the harmful adverse effects and events caused by the pharmaceutical drugs. Non-drug CAM does not cause significant harm. The hallucinogenic drugs have some rare but significant adverse effects but, as shamanistic medicine is often very efficient with result that lasts for life due to increase self-awareness and self-insight, the harm inflicted over a life-span becomes similar to the level of harm inflicted by the other CAM systems, indicating that we might be more open to the potential benefits of pre-modern medicine (239, 240) and drug-induced one session healing, like Grof's LSD therapy (246-248).

Table 5. Accumulated cost of one health-adjusted life year (HALY) through time (Year 1, 10 and 50) for ten classes of evidence-Based medicine

	Health improvement from treatment (%) if successful	**Prize of one HALY calculated from NNT and accumulated cost (Table 3)**		
	Self-rated health	per cured patient	per cured patient	per cured patient
		First year	Year 10	Year 50
Medicine with drugs				
Class 1: chemical medicine*	20%	500,000	≥1,000,000	≥ 5,000,000
Class 2: CAM (chemical CAM)	20%	>500,000	>1,000,000	>5,000,000
Non-drug CAM				
Class 3: CAM (physical therapy)	20%	60,000	300,000	60,000
Class 4: CAM (psychotherapy)	20%	60,000	300,000	60,000
Class 5: CAM (spiritual therapy)	20%	Not known	Not known	Not known
Class 6: CAM (mind–body medicine)	20%	40,000	180,000	40,000
Class 7: CAM body–spirit medicine	20%	Not known	Not known	Not known
Class 8: CAM (holistic mind–body medicine)	20%	25,000	50,000	10,000
Class 9: CAM (Shamanism with drugs)	20%	3000	4000	800
Class 10: CAM (social/environmental medicine)	20%	250,000	1,750,000	2,500,000

* Cost of biomedical examination, hospitalization, and treatment of adverse effects and events not included (estimated round numbers, see text).

Table 6. Accumulated harm through time (Year 1, 10 and 50) for ten classes of evidence-based medicine: Prize for one patient cured

Continuous treatment (only stopped if the patient gets cured)	**Number of patients harmed for one patient cured**	**Accumulated harm (number of patients harmed per patient cured)**		
	Self-rated health	per cured patient	per cured patient	per cured patient
	NNH_{total}	First year	Year 10	Year 50
Medicine with drugs				
Class 1: chemical medicine	3	17	25	50
Class 2: CAM (chemical CAM)	25	2	4	5
Non-drug CAM				
Class 3a: CAM (physical therapy, Low E)	1,000,000	0.00001	0.0001	0.001
Class 3b: CAM (physical therapy, high efficacy)	1000	0.002	0.01	0.1
Class 4: CAM (psychotherapy)	1,000,000	0.00001	0.0001	0.001
Class 5: CAM (spiritual therapy)	1,000,000	Not known	Not known	Not known
Class 6: CAM (mind–body medicine)	1,000,000	0.00001	0.0001	0.001
Class 7: CAM body–spirit medicine	1,000,000	Not known	Not known	Not known
Class 8: CAM (holistic mind–body medicine)	1,000,000	0.00001	0.0001	0.001
Class 9: CAM (Shamanism with drugs)	1000	0.001	0.001	0.001
Class 10: CAM (social/environmental medicine)	1,000,000	0.00001	0.0001	0.001

THE PRESENT DESTRUCTIVE IMPACT ON THE GLOBAL ENVIRONMENT OF THE TEN TYPES OF MEDICINE, USED BY THREE BILLION PEOPLE

As discussed in length in our new paper on the association between medicine and environment, the only type of medicine that courses real damage to the environment is pharmaceutical drugs (2). The damage comes from the direct burden on the planet from the pharmaceutical industry with a yearly turnover of 1,4 trillion dollars, and from the philosophical impact from drugs on the patient, making the patient less conscious and more into a consumer (see Table 7). Please notice that while the numbers in Tables 1-6 are based on the cost in a developed economy, table 7 takes into consideration the local economy of the world. It is therefore a more accurate expression of the real burden on the global environment of the different types of medicine than the Tables 1 6. We refer to (2) for details of the analysis. Chemical CAM and social/ environmental medicine are used so little that we estimate the environmental impact to be without significance.

How is the pharmaceutical industry polluting and affecting the environment? It does it three times. First when the pharmaceuticals are made. Here is an almost unimaginable use of resources, as it must be when a large chemical industry produces, for example, vaccines or antidepressants enough to treat almost the entire population of the earth. Think of a large chemical industry that produces the most toxic substances in the world, namely fat-soluble, complex organic molecules. When I read chemistry at the university back in 1979, these substances were classified as the most toxic drugs, because they penetrate all living tissue and affect all cells of the organism. And that, of course, is the purpose of chemical medicine.

Next, there is contamination of all the human bodies that ingest it, because the substances are poisonous. Few people seem to realize this, but we apply (with very few exceptions) the pharmacological drugs to use their toxic effects. They have no beneficial effects, from a biological (cellular) point of view. Whether we are talking painkillers, tranquilizers, invigorating, immune-system-soothing (e.g., anti-histamines) or immune-system-provoking (e.g., vaccines) drugs, they all work through their toxic effects, either disabling the normal function of our cells, or irritating the cells, so that they react more actively. Toxic chemicals into the body is the definition of chemical pollution; we pay a big price for using these toxic drugs as "medicine": a poorer quality of life, impaired physical and mental health, reduced mental clarity and acuity, reduced ability to work, etc. These adverse effects usually follows the use of pharmaceutical medicine.

Table 7. Accumulated destructive impact of medicine on the planets environment, expressed as cost for all patient using biomedicine and the nine CAM classes, in their actual culture (while we know the number for pharmaceutical medicine, the data regarding the nine CAM-classes are based on qualified guesses) (2)

Treatment/medicine type	Number of patients (estimated global number)	Yearly cost/treated patient (€)*	Accumulated yearly cost (total global cost) (€, estimated for CAM)
Class 1. Drugs (biomedicine)	1,000,000,000	1700	1,700,000,000,000
Class 2. Chemical CAM (medical herbs, flower medicine etc).	100,000,000	10	1,000,000,000
Class 3a-CAM (Physical therapy, low energy)	100,000,000	100	10,000,000,000
Class 3b-CAM (Physical therapy, high energy)	1,000,000	100	100,000,000
Class 4-CAM (mind medicine, i.e., psychotherapy)	10,000,000	6,000	60,000,000,000
Class 5-CAM (Spiritual therapy)	1,000,000,000	10	10,000,000,000
Class 6-CAM (Mind-Body medicine)	1,000,000,000	10	10,000,000,000
Class-7-CAM (Body-spirit medicine)	Not known	Not known	Not known
Class 8-CAM (Holistic medicine)	1,000,000	2,000	2,000,000,000
Class 9-CAM (Shamanism w. drugs)	10.000.000	50	50,000,000
Class 10-CAM (social and environmental medicine)	1,000,000,000	100**)	100,000,000,000

* Notice the big difference in the price for a medical treatment in rural Asia (10 Euro/year for healing massages) and central Europe or USA 1700 Euro/year in average for a treatment with drugs).

** 10-10.000 Euro/year, a highly diverse group of interventions.

Finally, we often excrete a large fraction of the drugs we consume, along with active metabolites with similar chemical properties. Most water cleaning facilities taking care of the black water are not very effective in removing complex organic chemicals from the water. In this way, the highly biologically active pharmaceutical molecules are spread directly into the vulnerable biological marine environment. A significant part of the chemical substances that end up in the sea are entering the living organisms that live there, which disturbs the marine ecosystems known to be very sensitive. When we consume fish, shellfish, shrimps, seaweed, etc. these organisms are already somewhat biologically disturbed from the contamination, and may also contain the pollution itself in measurable concentrations.

THE FUTURE DESTRUCTIVE IMPACT ON THE GLOBAL ENVIRONMENT OF THE 10 TYPES OF MEDICINE

Biomedicine, the drugs, are becoming increasingly popular in the third world, and the pharmaceutical industry is targeting that market strongly. The industrial influence on academic medicine is enormous, making doctors more likely to prefer drugs as medicine in the future. The industrial take-over of WHO and recently also the Cochrane Collaboration gives the pharmaceutical industry power over almost all national leading health institutions. If the corruption is not effectively dealt with, we must assume that the present development continues and even accelerates. The last decade we have seen a four-doubling in the revenues of the pharmaceutical industry (208), and if we assume this will continue, we can predict the development. Table 8 shows this calculation, predicting a 500 trillion Euros spend on pharmaceutical drugs in 2050. If this development continues, the pharmaceutical will be the leading course of environmental problems on the planet.

Table 8. Estimated future destructive impact of medicine on the planets environment, expressed as cost for all patient using biomedicine and the nine CAM classes, in their actual culture (while we know the number for pharmaceutical medicine, the data regarding the nine CAM-classes are based on qualified guesses (2)

Treatment/medicine type	**Number of patients (estimated global number)**	**Accumulated yearly cost (total global cost) (€, estimated for CAM)**		
	Year 2019	Year 2019	Year 2030 *)	Year 2050 *)
Medicine with drugs				
Class 1: chemical medicine	1.000.000.000	1.700.000.000.000	6.800.000.000.000	544.000.000.000.000
Class 2: CAM (chemical CAM)	10.000.000	1.000.000.000	4.000.000.000	32.000.000.000
Non-drug CAM				
Class 3a: CAM (physical therapy, Low Energy)	100,000,000	10.000.000.000	40.000.000.000	320.000.000.000
Class 3b: CAM (physical therapy, high energy)	1,000,000	100.000.000	400.000.000	3.200.000.000
Class 4: CAM (psychotherapy)	1,000,000	60.000.000.000	240.000.000.000	1.920.000.000.000
Class 5: CAM (spiritual therapy)	1,000,000,000	10.000.000.000	40.000.000.000	320.000.000.000
Class 6: CAM (mind–body medicine)	1,000,000	10.000.000.000	40.000.000.000	320.000.000.000
Class 7: CAM body–spirit medicine	1,000,000	Not known	Not known	Not known
Class 8: CAM (holistic mind–body medicine)	1,000,000	2.000.000.000	8.000.000.000	64.000.000.000
Class 9: CAM (Shamanism with drugs)	1,000,000	50.000.000	200.000.000	1.600.000.000
Class 10: CAM (social/environmental medicine)	1,000,000,000	100.000.000.000	400.000.000.000	3.200.000.000.000

In the estimate we have assumed that the present doubling rate with a doubling every five years continues.

DISCUSSION

Until now, the most important thing when you are choosing a medicine has been that it is affordable, and that it benefits the patients, without harming them. In practice the choice of medicine in the industrialized world has often been a drug. But the new dimension of sustainability has now entered the equation. More and more people realize that our culture in all its aspects MUST be sustainable. This also goes for medicine. And pharmaceutical medicine is clearly not sustainable (2). It is not even the most effective medicine, definitely not the safest, and if you look at the price for a healing it is hopelessly expensive!

So pharmaceutical drugs lose the race and I believe it cannot be the medicine for mankind in the future. Holistic, conscious-based medicine is the medicine we need in my opinion.

Table 7 shows the sad consequences of the large NNH and NNH_{total} numbers of the chemical medicine in the long run. As one of three patients are harmed every year with pharmaceutical drugs, and treatment often continues for life when the patient is not cured, the consequence is that almost every patient is harmed in the end, and 50 patients are harmed for every single, chronic patient helped or cured. In Denmark, over 2 million chronic patients out of a population of five million use drugs for about €6 billion per year (or €2–3000 per chronically ill patient, confirming the prize of drugs used in Table 3). It is clear for us that the same money spent on the most efficient types of non-drug CAM (group 3, 4, 6, and 8) would do immensely more for the populations' health. But even more important for the world in the future: it will not destroy the planet.

What do we need to make holistic medicine the choice of medicine in the future? The close connection between pharmaceutical industry, the physicians, and the public health system in many countries - often called the "medico-industrial complex" - must be broken. This system is often seen to actively work against CAM and holistic medicine, oppressing CAM researchers, and effectively by all means keeping CAM and holistic medicine out of the political stage (209).

Drugs obviously turn patients into chronic patients instead of curing them. Half the population of the Western world today is chronically ill, seemingly because of strong political and financial interests in biomedicine, leading to massive oppression of CAM in favor of drugs.

The shift from drugs to consciousness-based medicine (holistic medicine, CAM) would stop the burden on the environment from medicine, improve health radically in the society, and reduce the cost of healthcare to a small fraction.

CONCLUSION

Strong economic and political interests seem to control medicine in Europe, USA and Japan, making the pharmaceutical drugs often used, in spite of better and safer alternative for almost all clinical conditions. As these regions are economically strong the use of pharmaceutical drugs creates a monstrous burden on the global eco-system. A burden the planet cannot take in the long run.

People who still doubt the reality of the low cost, high efficacy and safety of consciousness-based medicine (CAM) presented in this review are encouraged to study Dean Ornish's cure for coronary heart disease. It was this well-documented CAM cure for a serious disease that made us believe in its potentials (196-198).

We have seen that the 10 different types of evidence-based medicine have very different profiles when it comes to efficacy, cost per cured patient, cost per QALY, cost per HALY, and cost per harmed patients. In general, chemical medicine is expensive and harmful both for people and for the environment, while consciousness-based CAM, that is a combination of massage therapy and psychotherapy, is safe.

The best types of CAM, like mind–body medicine, holistic mind–body medicine (i.e., the classical Hippocratic medicine, often called clinical holistic medicine/CHM) are 50.000 times less harmful and 100 times more efficient in producing health and happiness (quality of life). The cost of one cured chronic patient is about €1,000,000 with pharmaceutical drugs and much less with the efficient types of CAM.

Surprisingly, we found pre-modern medicine - Shamanism - to win the race in the end. While the drugs used often have some rare adverse effects, the efficacy of traditional one-session healing might make shamanistic medicine the cheapest, safest, and most effective in the end. While we do not advocate the back-propagation to pre-modern times, we find it very interesting that such a medicine exists, inspiring us all to continue our quest for a still better medicine.

RECOMMENDATIONS

Comparative studies of all the different types of medicine must be introduced in all medical schools all over the world, so all future doctors knows the alternatives when they choose to practice. Environmental consequences of the different types of medicine must be thought also, so the doctors can perform informed choices. It is important that this is taught in the beginning of the education, not in the end, so the students during their time as students can use their energy to study the type of medicine they choose to practice.

It takes many years to become a good holistic doctor, and it is not like that you will learn it if you first are trained to be a doctor only using pharmaceuticals – as is the case these days in most western universities. The introduction to medicine should therefore put great emphasis to traditional Hippocratic, Asian, and Native American holistic medicine, and all students should learn to practice consciousness-based (informational) medicine with focus on emotional healing (249) before they learn about the drugs.

All types of medicines must have the same legal status, so they can be practiced with the same right in all countries and districts of the world.

We need to set medicine free of the tyranny of the medico-industrial complex, which is the well-established collaboration between the pharmaceutical industry and the doctors strongly criticized by leaders of the Cochrane Collaboration. This can be done by the following: All types of medicine that does not harm – i.e., all kinds of CAM – should be allowed for everybody to practice, in all countries, without any restrictions.

Strict laws should be introduced immediately in all countries to stop the pharmaceutical industry and its collaborates from promoting drugs without evidence of therapeutic value (the ratio benefits:harm being no less than 1), without well-documented long-term effect, and without patient safety.

We also recommend the establishment of a new, independent international organization with the sole purpose to investigate and end the massive corruption of WHO and other national and supranational organizations that have allowed the pharmaceutical industry to dominate on an unscientific basis (250).

SUMMARY

This chapter has the following aim: To find the ideal type(s) of medicine for mankind in the future, by comparing the ten major medical systems of the world with regard to 1) range of clinical conditions helped, 2) effectivity, 3) safety, 4) cost, and 5) sustainability. The types of medicine, and the number of patients using them are found to be as follows:

1) Chemical biomedicine (drugs, bioactive molecules), used by 1 billion people.
2) Chemical CAM (symbolic and experiential medicine, i.e., flower medicine, herbal medicine, diets, minerals, vitamins etc.) used by 100 million people.
3) Body-medicine: (a) low-energy types of massage, reflexology, physical therapy, physiotherapy, spa, sauna etc. used by 100 million people; b) high-energy types: chiropractic etc.) used by one million people.

4) Mind-medicine: psychotherapy, i.e., psychodynamic, cognitive, gestalt, psychoanalysis, mindfulness and meditation, no-touch sexology etc. used by 10 million people.
5) Spirit-medicine: philosophical interventions, energy medicine, prayers, spiritual healing (i.e., Reiki), Shamanism, healing music, spiritual CAM (i.e., crystal healing) etc. used by 1 billion people.
6) Mind–Body Medicine: Acupuncture, acupressure, homeopathy, manual sexology, body-psychotherapy, Reichian bodywork, Rosen therapy, ergo therapy etc. used by one billion people.
7) Body–Spirit Medicine: Prayer involving physical activity like in Tibetan Buddhist-style meditation, pilgrimage etc. (unknown number of users).
8) Holistic body-mind-spirit medicine and existential therapy: Holistic medicine, clinical medicine, clinical holistic medicine, holistic body-psychotherapy, holistic bodywork, the sexological examination, holistic mind–body medicine, biodynamic body-psychotherapy, tantric bodywork and massage, holistic sexology, Native American rituals etc. used by 10 million people.
9) Chemical body-mind-spirit medicine: Shamanism with Peyote and San Pedro cactus (mescaline), Ayahuasca, scopolamine, magic mushrooms, Grof's LSD psychotherapy, MMDA psychotherapy etc. used by 10 million people.
10) Social and environmental medicine: Coaching, work-related personal development programs, stress management, leadership training, couching, gardening, aesthetic architecture, Feng Shui etc. used by 1 billion people.

Method

All medical systems are organized in 10 major classes for analysis. For each type are the literature searched for best metadata on effectivity, safety, cost, and sustainability. Combined measures, i.e., cost-benefit, cost-effectiveness, Number needed to treat (NNT), number needed to harm

(NNH), Therapeutic Value (TV = Total number needed to harm (NNH_{total})/Number needed to treat (NNT)), cost per cured patient (treatment year 1–50), and environmental impact per cured patient are calculated. Cost is presented as EURO (€) per cured patient, EURO per quality-adjusted life year (QALY), EURO per health-adjusted life year (HALY). The difference between healthy and sick was set to 20% global quality of life (QOL), or 20% self-rated health (physical/mental/global)). The burden of the global environment was expressed as cost per cured patient (primary order effects), and impact on philosophy of life and behavior in relation to sustainability (secondary order effects).

Results

To be useful for a society in the future, medicine must have significant therapeutic value (good benefit-to-harm ratio: TV $\geq$ 1), a documented long-term effect, safety, and sustainability. We found biomedicine (drugs) to be ineffective for most clinical conditions, harmful, expensive and very damaging to the environment. We found the most effective CAM-types (mind–body medicine, holistic medicine, Shamanism) to be effective for most clinical conditions, safe, cheap and sustainable; we found them to be 100 times as cost-effective, 1000 times more effective, 10,000 times less harmful and 100,000 times less burdensome to the global environment compared to pharmaceutical drugs. The 50 years' estimated cost in a developed economy for one patient cured was for drugs €1,000,000; physical therapy €100,000; psychotherapy €100,000; mind–body medicine €50,000; holistic mind–body medicine €20,000; and one-session shamanistic-type healing with hallucinogenic drugs only €2000.

Interpretation

The best types of CAM are much more efficient than pharmaceutical drugs and has no side effects and adverse events, whereas treatment with drugs always has adverse effects and events. Holistic mind–body medicine seems to be the cheapest, the safest, the most effective, and the most sustainable of all types of medicine for almost all clinical conditions. The shift from pharmaceutical drugs to non-drug medicine would improve health and quality of life radically in the developed world and dramatically reduce harm to patients and environment globally, and at the same time reduce the cost of healthcare to a small fraction.

Recommendation

Comparative studies of all types of medicine must be introduced in the curriculums of all medical schools, so all future doctors know the alternatives when they choose to practice medicine. All types of medicines must have the same legal and scientific status, so they can be practiced with the same right in all countries and districts of the world, and it must be free for all doctors to practice the medicine he or she chooses to practice, based on his or her knowledge and personal preference. Strict laws should be introduced immediately in all countries to stop the pharmaceutical industry from promoting drugs without therapeutic value, and from repressing consciousness-based, non-drug medicine types (CAMs like holistic medicine, mind-body medicine, and other types of alternative and complementary medicines). We also recommend the establishment of a new, independent international organization parallel to Interpol with the sole purpose to investigate and end the massive corruption of WHO and other national and supranational organizations, that have allowed the pharmaceutical industry to dominate the world on an unscientific basis.

REFERENCES

[1] The Intergovernmental Science-Policy Platform on Biodiversity and Ecosystem Services (IPBES). Yearly Rapport 2019: Nature's Dangerous Decline

'Unprecedented'. Species Extinction Rates 'Accelerating'. URL: https://www.ipbes.net/

[2] Ventegodt S. A comparative analysis of the environmental consequences of the world's different types of medicine: Consciousness-based, holistic medicine versus pharmaceutical medicine. J Altern Med Res 2019;11(1):00-00.

[3] Folkesundhedsrapporten Danmark 2018. Copenhagen, Statens Institut for Folkesundhed, 2018. [Danish]

[4] Allmer C, Ventegodt S, Kandel I, Merrick J. Positive effects, side effects, and adverse events of clinical holistic medicine. A review of Gerda Boyesen's nonpharmaceutical mind-body medicine (biodynamic body-psychotherapy) at two centers in the United Kingdom and Germany. Int J Adolesc Med Health 2009;21(3):281-97.

[5] Ventegodt S, Andersen NJ, Kandel I, Merrick J. Comparative analysis of cost-effectiveness of non-drug medicine (nonpharmaceutical holistic, complementary and alternative medicine/CAM) and biomedicine (pharmaceutical drugs) for all clinical conditions. Int J Disabil Hum Dev 2009;8(3):243-58.

[6] Zuzak TJ, Bosková J, Careddu D, Garami M, Hadjipanayis A, Jazbec J, et al. Use of complementary and alternative medicine by children in Europe: published data and expert perspectives. Complement Ther Med 2013;21(Suppl 1):S34-47. doi: 10.1016/j.ctim.2012.01.001.

[7] Ventegodt S, Andersen NJ, Kandel I, Merrick J. Effect, side effects and adverse events of non-pharmaceutical medicine. A review. Int J Disabil Hum Dev 2009;8(3):227-35.

[8] Ventegodt S, Andersen NJ, Merrick J, Greydanus DE. Effectiveness of traditional pharmaceutical biomedicine versus complementary and alternative medicine in a physician's general practice. J Altern Med Res 2010;2(2),

[9] Ventegodt S, Kandel I, Merrick J. Quality of life and philosophy of life determines physical and mental health: Status over research findings from the Quality of Life Research Center, Copenhagen, 1991-2007. ScientificWorldJournal 2007;7:1743–51.

[10] Ventegodt S, Merrick J. Reflections from a study tour to Hippocrates' Asklepieion on the island of Kos. J Altern Med Res 2012;4(2):221-3.

[11] Ventegodt S, Merrick J. Meta-analysis of positive effects, side effects and adverse events of holistic mind-body medicine (clinical holistic medicine): experience from Denmark, Sweden, United Kingdom and Germany. Int J Adolesc Med Health 2009;21(4):441-56.

[12] Ventegodt S, Thegler S, Andreasen T, Struve F, Enevoldsen L, Bassaine L, et al. Clinical holistic medicine: psychodynamic short-time therapy complemented with bodywork. A clinical follow-up study of 109 patients. ScientificWorldJournal 2006;6:2220–38.

[13] Ventegodt S. How Should Medicine Develop? A Comparative Analysis of Cost-Benefit and Cost-Effectiveness of All Types of Evidence-Based Medicine for All

Clinical Conditions (Report from Work-In-Progress). Altern Integr Med 2013. 2:e108. doi: 10.4172/2327-5162.1000e108.

[14] Ventegodt S, Merrick J. A review of side effects and adverse events of non-drug medicine (nonpharmaceutical complementary and alternative medicine): Psychotherapy, mind-body medicine and clinical holistic medicine. J Complement Integr Med 2009;6(1):16.

[15] Ventegodt S, Merrick J. Meta-analysis of positive effects, side effects and adverse events of holistic mind-body medicine (clinical holistic medicine): Experience from Denmark, Sweden, United Kingdom andGermany. Int J Adolesc Med Health 2009;21(4):441-56.

[16] Ventegodt S, MerrickJ. Metaanalysis of positive effects, side effects, and adverse events of holistic mind-body medicine, subtype holistic, clinical medicine: “clinical holistic medicine” (Denmark, Israel) “mindful mind-body medicine” (Sweden), “biodynamic body psychotherapy” (UK), and “biodynamishe körperpsychotherapie” (Germany). A review. Int J Disabil Hum Dev 2009: 243-258.

[17] Ventegodt S, Flensborg-Madsen T, Andersen NJ, Merrick J. Which factors determine our quality of life, health and ability? Results from a Danish population sample and the Copenhagen perinatal cohort. J Coll Physicians Surg Pak 2008;18(7):445-50. doi: 07.2008/JCPSP.445450.

[18] Ventegodt S, Andersen NJ, Merrick J. Quality of life theory I. The IQOL theory: An integrative theory of the global quality of life concept. ScientificWorldJournal 2003;3:1030-40.

[19] Jensen S, Ventegodt S. State-of-life theory. J Altern Med Res 2014;6(1):39-42.

[20] Ventegodt S, Hilden J, Merrick J. Measurement of quality of life I: A Methodological Framework. ScientificWorldJournal 2003;3:950-61.

[21] Ventegodt S, Merrick J, Andersen NJ. Measurement of quality of life II. From philosophy of life to science. ScientificWorldJournal 2003;3:962-71.

[22] Ventegodt S, Merrick J, Andersen NJ. Measurement of quality of life III: From the IQOL theory to the global, generic SEQOL questionnaire. ScientificWorldJournal 2003;3:972-91.

[23] Ventegodt S, Merrick J, Andersen NJ. Measurement of quality of life IV: Use of the SEQOL, QOL5, QOL1 and other global and generic questionnaires. ScientificWorldJournal 2003;3:992-1001.

[24] Ventegodt S, Merrick J, Andersen NJ. Measurement of quality of life V: How to use the SEQOL, QOL5, QOL1 and other and generic questionnaires for research. ScientificWorldJournal 2003;3:1002-14.

[25] Ventegodt S, Merrick J, Andersen NJ. Measurement of quality of life VI: Quality-adjusted life years (QALY) is an unfortunate use of quality of life concept. ScientificWorldJournal 2003;3:1015-9.

[26] Ventegodt S, Merrick J. Measurement of quality of life VII: Statistical covariation and global quality of life data. The method of weight-modified linear regression. ScientificWorldJournal 2003;3:1020-29.

[27] Ventegodt S, Merrick J, Andersen NJ. Quality of life theory II. Quality of life as the realization of life potential: A biological theory of human being. ScientificWorldJournal 2003;3:1041-9.

[28] Ventegodt S, Merrick J, Andersen NJ. Quality of life theory III. Maslow revisited. ScientificWorldJournal 2003;3:1050-7.

[29] Ventegodt S, Merrick J. Philosophy of science: how to identify the potential research for the day after tomorrow? ScientificWorldJournal 2004;4:483-9.

[30] Ventegodt S, Hermansen TD, Nielsen ML, Clausen B, Merrick J. Human development I: twenty fundamental problems of biology, medicine, and neuro-psychology related to biological information. ScientificWorldJournal 2006;6:747-59.

[31] Ventegodt S, Hermansen TD, Nielsen ML, Clausen B, Merrick J. Human development II: we need an integrated theory for matter, life and consciousness to understand life and healing. ScientificWorldJournal 2006;6:760-6.

[32] Ventegodt S, Hermansen TD, Rald E, Flensborg-Madsen T, Nielsen ML, Clausen B, Merrick J. Human development III: bridging brain-mind and body-mind. introduction to "deep" (fractal, poly-ray) cosmology. ScientificWorldJournal 2006;6:767-76.

[33] Ventegodt S, Hermansen TD, Flensborg-Madsen T, Nielsen ML, Clausen B, Merrick J. Human development IV: the living cell has information-directed self-organisation. ScientificWorldJournal 2006;6:1132-8.

[34] Ventegodt S, Hermansen TD, Flensborg-Madsen T, Nielsen ML, Clausen B, Merrick J. Human development V: biochemistry unable to explain the emergence of biological form (morphogenesis) and therefore a new principle as source of biological information is needed. ScientificWorldJournal 2006;6:1359-67.

[35] Ventegodt S, Hermansen TD, Flensborg-Madsen T, Nielsen M, Merrick J. Human development VI: Supracellular morphogenesis. The origin of biological and cellular order. ScientificWorldJournal 2006;6:1424-33.

[36] Ventegodt S, Hermansen TD, Flensborg-Madsen T, Rald E, Nielsen ML, Merrick J. Human development VII: A spiral fractal model of fine structure of physical energy could explain central aspects of biological information, biological organization and biological creativity. ScientificWorldJournal 2006;6:1434-40.

[37] Ventegodt S, Hermansen TD, Flensborg-Madsen T, Nielsen ML, Merrick J. Human development VIII: A theory of "deep" quantum chemistry and cell consciousness: Quantum chemistry controls genes and biochemistry to give cells and higher organisms consciousness and complex behavior. ScientificWorldJournal 2006;6:1441-53.

[38] Ventegodt S, Hermansen TD, Flensborg-Madsen T, Rald E, Nielsen ML, Merrick J. Human development IX: A model of the wholeness of man, his consciousness and collective consciousness. ScientificWorldJournal 2006;6:1454-9.

[39] Hermansen TD, Ventegodt S, Merrick J. Human development X: Explanation of macroevolution: top-down evolution materializes consciousness. The origin of metamorphosis. ScientificWorldJournal 2006;6:1656-66.

[40] Hermansen TD, Ventegodt S, Kandel I. Human development XI: the structure of the cerebral cortex. Are there really modules in the brain? ScientificWorldJournal 2007;7:1922-9.

[41] Ventegodt S, Hermansen TD, Kandel I, Merrick J. Human development XII: a theory for the structure and function of the human brain. ScientificWorldJournal 2008;8:621-42.

[42] Ventegodt S, Hermansen TD, Kandel I, Merrick J. Human development XIII: the connection between the structure of the overtone system and the tone language of music. Some implications for our understanding of the human brain. ScientificWorldJournal 2008;8:643-57.

[43] Ventegodt S, Hermansen TD, Kandel I, Merrick J. Human development XIV: Degeneration and regeneration of existence. Metamorphosis changes the purpose of life, the level of existential responsibility, and the depth of consciousness (the ray-number of the cosmology). J Altern Med Res 2009;1(4):409-18.

[44] Ventegodt S, Hermansen TD, Kandel I, Merrick J. Human development XV: The biochemical hypothesis for the etiology of the mental diseases is not substantiated. J Altern Med Res 2009;1(4):419-32.

[45] Ventegodt S, Hermansen TD, Kandel I, Merrick J. Human development XVI: General etiology of mental diseases and the role of re-metamorphosis in spontaneous recovery ("Monster theory"). J Altern Med Res 2009;1(4):433-8.

[46] Ventegodt S, Hermansen TD, Kandel I, Merrick J. Human development XVII: Jerne's anti-idiotypic network theory cannot explain self-nonself discrimination. J Altern Med Res 2009;1(4):439-44.

[47] Hermansen TD, Ventegodt S, Kandel I, Merrick J. Human development XVIII: A theory for immune system regulation ("the self-nonself discrimination"). J Altern Med Res 2009;1(4):445-52.

[48] Ventegodt S, Hermansen TD, Kandel I, Merrick J. Human development XIX: The aetiology of somatic diseases. The energetic healing crisis ("kidney-crisis") of patients in Antonovsku-salutogenesis with clinical holistic medicine and holistic sexology. J Altern Med Res 2009;1(4):453-64.

[49] Ventegodt S, Hermansen TD, Kandel I, Merrick J. Human development XX: A theory for accelerated, spontaneous existential healing (salutogenesis): Human adult metamorphosis. J Altern Med Res 2009;1(4):465-74.

[50] Hermansen TD, Ventegodt S, Kandel I, Merrick J. Human development XXI: A theory of top-down macro-evolution and metamorphosis: How the fly got its wings and how an organism's conscious intent can materialize biological order and body-form. J Altern Med Res 2009;1(4):475-80.

[51] Hermansen TD, Ventegodt S, Kandel I, Merrick J. Human development XXII: Holistic therapy induces Antonovsky salutogenesis and spontaneous healing and

recovery. Human genes for metamorphosis might control salutogenesis. If the expression of such genes are controlled by our (sub)consciousness this explains the placebo effect and possibly also spontaneous remission from cancer. J Altern Med Res 2009;1(4):481-90.

[52] Chalmers AF. What is this thing called science? 2 ed. London: Open University Press, 1982.

[53] Bateson G. Mind and nature: A necessary unity. New York: Ballantine, 1972.

[54] Gadamer H. Truth and method. New York: Continuum, 2003.

[55] Heidegger, M. Being and time. New York: Suny Press, 1996.

[56] Kierkegaard S. In vino veritas. Copenhagen: Finn Suenson, 1981. [Danish].

[57] Kierkegaard SA. The sickness unto death. Princeton, NJ: Princeton Univ Press, 1983.

[58] Endler PC. Working and writing scientifically in complementary medicine and integrated health sciences. Graz: Interuniversity College, 2004.

[59] Kuhn TS. The structure of scientific revolutions. Chicago, IL: Univ Chicago Press, 1962.

[60] Popper KR. Objective knowledge: An evolutionary approach. Oxford: Clarendon Press, 1972.

[61] Sartre JP Being and nothingness. London: Routledge, London, 2002.

[62] Schopenhauer, A. The world as will and idea. New York: Everyman Books, 1995.

[63] Lindholt JS, Ventegodt S, Henneberg EW. Development and validation of QoL5 for clinical databases. A short, global and generic questionnaire based on an integrated theory of the quality of life. Eur J Surg 2002;168:103–7.

[64] Ventegodt S, Andersen NJ, Merrick J. QOL10 for clinical quality-assurance and research in treatment-efficacy: Ten key questions for measuring the global quality of life, self-rated physical and mental health, and self-rated social-, sexual and working ability. J Altern Med Res 2009;1(2):113-22.

[65] Ventegodt S, Henneberg EW, Merrick J, Lindholt JS. Validation of two global and generic quality of life questionnaires for population screening: SCREENQOL and SEQOL. ScientificWorldJournal 2003;3:412-21.

[66] Ventegodt S. Measuring the quality of life. From theory to practice. Copenhagen: Forskningscenterets Forlag, 1996.

[67] McDowell I, Newell C. Measuring health: A guide to rating scales and questionnaires. Oxford: Oxford University Press, 1987.

[68] Ventegodt S, Merrick J. Principles of holistic psychiatry. A textbook on evidence-based holistic medicine for mental disorders. New York: Nova Science, 2011.

[69] Ventegodt S, Merrick J. Sexology from a holistic point of view. A textbook of classic and modern sexology. New York: Nova Science, 2011.

[70] Ventegodt S, Merrick J. Textbook on evidence-based holistic mind-body medicine: Basic philosophy and ethics of traditional Hippocratic medicine. New York: Nova Science, 2012.

[71] Ventegodt S, Merrick J. Textbook on evidence-based holistic mind-body medicine: Basic principles of healing in traditional Hippocratic medicine. New York: Nova Science, 2012.
[72] Ventegodt S, Merrick J. Textbook on evidence-based holistic mind-body medicine: Healing the mind in Traditional Hippocratic Medicine. New York: Nova Science, 2012.
[73] Ventegodt S, Merrick J. Textbook on evidence-based holistic mind-body medicine: Holistic practice of traditional Hippocratic medicine. New York: Nova Science, 2013.
[74] Ventegodt S, Merrick J. Textbook on evidence-based holistic mind-body medicine: Research, philosophy, economy and politics of traditional Hippocratic medicine. New York: Nova Science, 2013.
[75] Ventegodt S, Merrick J. Textbook on evidence-based holistic mind-body medicine: Sexology and traditional Hippocratic medicine. New York: Nova Science, 2013.
[76] Ventegodt S, Kandel I, Merrick J. Principles of holistic medicine. Philosophy behind quality of life. Victoria, BC: Trafford, 2005.
[77] Ventegodt S, Kandel I, Merrick J. Principles of holistic medicine. Quality of life and health. New York: Hippocrates Sci Publ, 2005.
[78] Ventegodt S, Kandel I, Merrick J. Principles of holistic medicine. Global quality of life. Theory, research and methodology. New York: Hippocrates Sci Publ, 2005.
[79] Achterberg J. Imagery in healing: Shamanism and modern medicine. Boston, MA: Shambala/New Science Library, 1985.
[80] Anderson EF. Peyote. The divine cactus. Tucson, AZ: University of Arizona Press, 1980.
[81] Baker D. Esoteric healing (I). London: Essendon, 1975.
[82] Besant A. The ancient wisdom. London: Theosophical Publishing House, 2001.
[83] Bruhn JG, De Smet PA, El-Seedi HR, Beck O. Mescaline use for 5700 years. Lancet 2002;359(9320):1866.
[84] Evans-Wentz WY. The Tibetan book of the dead. Oxford: Oxford University Press, 1980.
[85] Mann, F. The meridians of acupuncture. London: Heinemann, 1964.
[86] Mumey N. The peyote ceremony among the American Indians. Bull Med Libr Assoc 1951;39(3):182-8.
[87] Narby J. Shamans through time. London: Thacher/Putnam, 2002.
[88] Penrose R. Shadows of the mind: A search for the missing science of consciousness. New York: Oxford University Press, 1994.
[89] Hameroff SR, Kaszniak AW, Scott AC. Toward a science of consciousness II. The second Tucson discussions and debates. Tucson, AZ: Bradford Book, 1998.
[90] Fontanarosa P, Lundberg G. Alternative medicine meets science. JAMA 1998;280:1618–9.
[91] Ventegodt S, Flensborg-Madsen T, Andersen NJ, Nielsen M, Morad M, Merrick J. Global quality of life (QOL), health and ability are primarily determined by our

consciousness. Research findings from Denmark 1991-2004. Soc Indicator Res 2005;71;87-122.

[92] Ventegodt S, Andersen NJ, Merrick J. The square curve paradigm for research in alternative, complementary and holistic medicine: A cost-effectice, easy and scientifically valid design for evidence-based medicine and quality improvement. ScientificWorldJournal 2003;3:1117-27.

[93] Ventegodt S, Andersen NJ, Kandel I, Merrick J. The open source protocol of clinical holistic medicine. J Altern Med Res 2009;1(2):129-44.

[94] Chopra D. Quantum healing. Exploring the frontiers of mind body medicine. New York: Bantam Books, 1990.

[95] Deepak Chopra D, Ornish D, Roy R, Weil A. Alternative medicine is mainstream. The evidence is mounting that diet and lifestyle are the best cures for our worst afflictions. Wall Street J 2010 Sep 01. URL: http://online.wsj.com/article/SB123146318996466585.html.

[96] Goleman D. Healing emotions: Conversations with the Dalai Lama on the mindfulness, emotions, and health. Boston, MA: Mind Life Institute, 1997.

[97] Weil A. Spontaneous healing. New York: Ballantine Books, 1995.

[98] Ventegodt S, Thegler S, Andreasen T, Struve F, Enevoldsen L, Bassaine L, et al. Clinical holistic medicine (mindful, short-term psychodynamic psychotherapy complemented with bodywork) improves quality of life, health, and ability by induction of Antonovsky-salutogenesis. ScientificWorldJournal 2007;7:317-23.

[99] Ventegodt S, Clausen B, Merrick J. Clinical holistic medicine: Pilot study on the effect of vaginal acupressure (Hippocratic pelvic massage). TSW Holistic Health Medicine 2006;1:136-52.

[100] Ventegodt S, Thegler S, Andreasen T, Struve F, Enevoldsen L, Bassaine L, et al. Clinical holistic medicine: Psychodynamic short-time therapy complemented with bodywork. A clinical follow-up study of 109 patients. TSW Holistic Health Medicine 2006;1:256-7.

Ventegodt S, Thegler S, Andreasen T, Struve F, Enevoldsen L, Bassaine L, et al. Clinical holistic medicine (mindful, short-term psychodynamic psychotherapy complemented with bodywork) in the treatment of experienced impaired sexual functioning. ScientificWorldJournal 2007;7:324-9.

[101] Ventegodt S, Thegler S, Andreasen T, Struve F, Enevoldsen L, Bassaine L, et al. Clinical holistic medicine (mindful, short-term psychodynamic psychotherapy complemented with bodywork) in the treatment of experienced physical illness and chronic pain. ScientificWorldJournal 2007;7:310-6.

[102] Ventegodt S, Thegler S, Andreasen T, Struve F, Enevoldsen L, Bassaine L, et al. Clinical holistic medicine (mindful, short-term psychodynamic psychotherapy complemented with bodywork) in the treatment of experienced mental illness. ScientificWorldJournal 2007;7:306-9.

[103] Ventegodt S, Thegler S, Andreasen T, Struve F, Enevoldsen L, Bassaine L, et al.. Self-reported low self-esteem. Intervention and follow-up in a clinical setting. ScientificWorldJournal 2007;7: 299-305.

[104] Ventegodt S, Merrick J. Randomized clinical trials and placebo. Can you trust the drugs are working and safe? New York: Nova Science, 2018.

[105] Moncrieff J, Wessely S, Hardy R. Active placebos versus antidepressants for depression. Cochrane Database Syst Rev 2004;1:CD003012.

[106] Boutron I, Estellat C, Guittet L, Dechartres A, Sackett DL, Hróbjartsson A, et al. Methods of blinding in reports of randomized controlled trials assessing pharmacologic treatments: a systematic review. PLoS Med 2006;3(10):e425.

[107] Gøtzsche PC. Deadly medicines and organised crime: How big pharma has corrupted healthcare. New York: Radcliffe, 2013.

[108] Gøtzsche PC. Deadly psychiatry and organised denial. Copenhagen: People Press, 2015.

[109] Whitaker R. Mad in America. New York: Basic Books, 2002.

[110] Swinburne R. The problem of evil. Oxford: Oxford Univ Press, 1998.

[111] Sanford JA. Evil: The shadow of reality. New York: Crossroad Publ, 1981.

[112] Abrams J, Zweig C. Meeting the shadow. The hidden power of the dark side of human nature. Los Angeles, CA: JP Tarcher, 1991.

[113] Bly R. A little handbook on the human shadow. Memphis, TN: Raccoon, 1986.

[114] Yalom I. Existential psychotherapy. New York: Basic Books, 1980.

[115] Ventegodt S, Andersen NJ, Merrick J. QOL philosophy I: Quality of life, happiness, and meaning of life. ScientificWorldJournal 2003;3:1164-75.

[116] Ventegodt S, Andersen NJ, Merrick J. QOL philosophy II: What is a human being? ScientificWorldJournal 2003;3:1176-85.

[117] Ventegodt S, Andersen NJ, Merrick J. QOL philosophy IV: The brain and consciousness. ScientificWorldJournal 2003;3:1199-1209.

[118] Ventegodt S, Andersen NJ, Merrick J. QOL philosophy V: Seizing the meaning of life and getting well again. ScientificWorldJournal 2003;3:1210-29.

[119] Ventegodt S, Andersen NJ, Merrick J. QOL philosophy VI: The concepts. ScientificWorldJournal 2003;3:1230-40.

[120] Jones WHS. Hippocrates. Vol. I–IV. London: William Heinemann, 1923-1931.

[121] Ventegodt S, Andersen NJ, Merrick J. Holistic Medicine III: The holistic process theory of healing. ScientificWorldJournal 2003;3:1138-46.

[122] Ventegodt S, Andersen NJ, Merrick J. Holistic Medicine IV: Principles of existential holistic group therapy and the holistic process of healing in a group setting. ScientificWorldJournal 2003;3:1388-400.

[123] Ventegodt S, Morad M, Merrick J. Clinical holistic medicine: Prevention through healthy lifestyle and Quality of life. Oral Health Prev Dent 2004;1:239-45.

[124] Ventegodt, S. Every contact with the patient must be therapeutic. J Pediatr Adolesc Gynecol 2007;20(6):323-4.

[125] Ventegodt S, Merrick J. Clinical holistic medicine: Applied consciousness-based medicine. ScientificWorldJournal 2004;4:96-9.

[126] Ventegodt S, Merrick J. Clinical holistic medicine: Chronic pain in internal organs. ScientificWorldJournal 2005;5:205-10.

[127] Ventegodt S, Merrick J. Clinical holistic medicine: Chronic infections and autoimmune diseases. ScientificWorldJournal 2005;5:155-64.

[128] Ventegodt S, Merrick J. Clinical holistic medicine: The patient with multiple diseases ScientificWorldJournal 2005;5:324-39.

[129] Ventegodt S, Merrick J. Psychosomatic reasons for chronic pains. South Med J 2005;98(11):1063.

[130] Ventegodt S, Merrick J. Suicide from a holistic point of view. ScientificWorldJournal 2005;5:759-66.

[131] Ventegodt S, Kandel I, Neikrug S, Merrick J. Clinical holistic medicine: The existential crisis – life crisis, stress and burnout. ScientificWorldJournal 2005;5:300-12.

[132] Ventegodt S, Andersen NJ, Merrick J. Holistic Medicine IV: Principles of the holistic process of healing in a group setting. ScientificWorldJournal 2003;3:1294-1301.

[133] Ventegodt S, Andersen NJ, Merrick J. Quality of life as medicine. A pilot study of patients with chronic illness and pain. ScientificWorldJournal 2003;3:520-32.

[134] Ventegodt S, Andersen NJ, Merrick J. Quality of life as medicine II. A pilot study of a five-day "Quality of Life and Health" cure for patients with alcoholism. ScientificWorldJournal 2003;3:842-52.

[135] Ventegodt S, Andersen NJ, Neikrug S, Kandel I, Merrick J. Clinical holistic medicine: Holistic treatment of mental disorders. ScientificWorldJournal 2005; 5:427-45.

[136] Ventegodt S, Andersen NJ, Neikrug S, Kandel I, Merrick J. Clinical holistic medicine: Mental disorders in a holistic perspective. ScientificWorldJournal 2005;5:313-23.

[137] Ventegodt S, Clausen B, Merrick J. Clinical holistic medicine: The case story of Anna: I. Long term effect of child sexual abuse and incest with a treatment approach. TSW Holistic Health Medicine 2006;1:1-12.

[138] Ventegodt S, Clausen B, Langhorn M, Kroman M, Andersen NJ, Merrick J. Quality of Life as Medicine III. A qualitative analysis of the effect of a five days intervention with existential holistic group therapy or a quality of life course as a modern rite of passage. ScientificWorldJournal 2004;4: 124-33.

[139] Ventegodt S, Clausen B, Nielsen ML, Merrick J. Advanced tools for holistic medicine. TSW Holistic Health Medicine 2006;1:84–101. DOI 10.1100/tswhhm.2006.31.

[140] Ventegodt S, Flensborg-Madsen T, Andersen NJ, Morad M, Merrick J. Clinical holistic medicine: A pilot on HIV and quality of life and a suggested treatment of HIV and AIDS. ScientificWorldJournal 2004;4:264-72.

[141] Ventegodt S, Gringols G, Merrick J. Clinical holistic medicine: Holistic rehabilitation. ScientificWorldJournal 2005;5:280-7.

[142] Ventegod, S, Kandel I, Neikrug S, Merrick J. Clinical holistic medicine: Holistic treatment of rape and incest traumas. ScientificWorldJournal 2005;5:288-97.

[143] Ventegodt S, Morad M, Merrick J. Clinical holistic medicine: Classic art of healing or the therapeutic touch. ScientificWorldJournal 2004;4:134-47.

[144] Ventegodt S, Morad M, Merrick J. Clinical holistic medicine: The "new medicine", the multiparadigmatic physician and the medical record. ScientificWorldJournal 2004;4:273-85.

[145] Ventegodt S, Morad M, Merrick J. Clinical holistic medicine: Holistic pelvic examination and holistic treatment of infertility. ScientificWorldJournal 2004;4:148-58.

[146] Ventegodt S, Morad M, Merrick J. Clinical holistic medicine: Holistic treatment of children. ScientificWorldJournal 2004;4:581-8.

[147] Ventegodt S, Morad M, Merrick J. Clinical holistic medicine: Problems in sex and living together. ScientificWorldJournal 2004;4:562-70.

[148] Ventegodt S, Morad M, Merrick J. Clinical holistic medicine: Induction of spontaneous remission of cancer by recovery of the human character and the purpose of life (the life mission). ScientificWorldJournal 2004;4:362-77.

[149] Ventegodt S, Morad M, Merrick J. Clinical holistic medicine: Developing from asthma, allergy and eczema. ScientificWorldJournal 2004;4:936-42.

[150] Ventegodt S, Morad M, Merrick J. Clinical holistic medicine: Chronic pain in the locomotor system. ScientificWorldJournal 2005;5:165-72.

[151] Ventegodt S, Morad M, Merrick J. Clinical holistic medicine: the case story of Anna. II. Patient diary as a tool in treatment. TSW Holistic Health Medicine 2006;1:42-70.

[152] Ventegodt S, Morad M, Merrick J. Clinical holistic medicine: The case story of Anna. III. Rehabilitation of philosophy of life during holistic existential therapy for childhood sexual abuse. TSW Holistic Health Medicine 2006;1:102-13.

[153] Ventegodt S, Morad M, Andersen NJ, Merrick J. Clinical holistic medicine Tools for a medical science based on consciousness. ScientificWorldJournal 2004;4:347-61.

[154] Ventegodt S, Morad M, Hyam E, Merrick J. Clinical holistic medicine: Use and limitations of the biomedical paradigm. ScientificWorldJournal 2004;4:295-306.

[155] Ventegodt S, Morad M, Hyam E, Merrick J. Clinical holistic medicine: When biomedicine is inadequate. ScientificWorldJournal 2004;4:333-46.

[156] Ventegodt S, Morad M, Hyam E, Merrick J. Clinical holistic medicine: Holistic sexology and treatment of vulvodynia through existential therapy and acceptance through touch. ScientificWorldJournal 2004;4:571-80.

[157] Ventegod, S, Morad M, Kandel I, Merrick J. Clinical holistic medicine: Social problems disguised as illness. ScientificWorldJournal 2004;4:286-94.

[158] Ventegodt S, Morad M, Kandel I, Merrick J. Clinical holistic medicine: Treatment of physical health problems without a known cause, exemplified by hypertension and tinnitus. ScientificWorldJournal 2004;4:716-24.

[159] Ventegodt S, Morad M, Kandel I, Merrick J. Clinical holistic medicine: a psychological theory of dependency to improve quality of life. ScientificWorld Journal 2004;4:638-48.

[160] Ventegodt S, Morad M, Press J, Merrick J, Shek D. Clinical holistic medicine: Holistic adolescent medicine. ScientificWorldJournal 2004;4:551-61.

[161] Ventegodt S, Solheim E, Saunte ME, Morad M, Kandel I, Merrick J. Clinical holistic medicine: Metastatic cancer. ScientificWorldJournal 2004;4:913-35.

[162] Ventegodt S. The life mission theory: A theory for a consciousness-based medicine. In. J Adolesc Med Health 2003;15(1):89-91.

[163] Ventegodt S. The life mission theory: A theory for a consciousness-based medicine. Int J Adolesc Med Health 2003; 15(1): 89-91.

[164] Ventegodt S, Andersen NJ, Merrick J. The life mission theory II: The structure of the life purpose and the ego. ScientificWorldJournal 2003;3:1277-85.

[165] Ventegodt S, Andersen NJ, Merrick J. The life mission theory III: Theory of talent. ScientificWorldJournal 2003;3:1286-93.

[166] Ventegodt S, Merrick J. The life mission theory IV. A theory of child development. ScientificWorldJournal 2003;3:1294-1301.

[167] Ventegodt S, Andersen NJ, Merrick J. The life mission theory V. A theory of the anti-self and explaining the evil side of man. ScientificWorldJournal 2003;3:1302-13.

[168] Ventegodt S, Andersen NJ, Merrick J. The life mission theory VI: A theory for the human character. ScientificWorldJournal 2004;4: 859-80.

[169] Ventegodt S, Flensborg-Madsen T, Andersen NJ, Merrick J. Life Mission Theory VII: Theory of existential (Antonovsky) coherence: a theory of quality of life, health and ability for use in holistic medicine. ScientificWorldJournal 2005;5:377-89.

[170] Ventegodt S, Merrick J. Life mission theory VIII: A theory for pain. J Pain Manage 2008;1(1):5-10.

[171] Ventegodt S. Life mission theory IX: Integrative, ethical theory. J Altern Med Res 2009;1(3):301-12.

[172] Ventegodt S, Merrick J. Life mission theory X: Theory of humiliation and pain. J Pain Manage 2011;4(4):361-7.

[173] Ventegodt S. The life mission theory XI: Origin of the human thought. J Altern Med Res 2019;11(1):00-00.

[174] Ader R. Psychoneuroimmunology. Academic Press. 1981.

[175] Ornish D. Love and survival. The scientific basis for the healing power of intimacy. New York: Harper Collins, 1999.

[176] Frattaroli J, Weidner G, Dnistrian AM, Kemp C, Daubenmier JJ, Marlin RO, et al. Clinical events in prostate cancer lifestyle trial: Results from two years of follow-up. Urology 2008;72(6):1319-23.

[177] Spiegel D, Bloom JR, Kraemer HC, Gottheil E. Effect of psychosocial treatment on survival of patients with metastatic breast cancer. Lancet 1989;2(8668):888-91.

[178] Levenson FB, Levenson MD, Ventegodt S, Merrick, J. Psychodynamic psychotherapy, therapeutic touch and cancer. A review of the method of intervention and study of 75 cases. J Altern Med Res 2009;1:313-8.

[179] Ventegodt S, Andersen NJ, Merrick J. Rationality and irrationality in Ryke Geerd Hamer's System for holistic treatment of metastatic cancer. ScientificWorldJournal 2005;5:93–102.

[180] Lowen A. Honoring the body (The autobiography of Alexander Lowen, MD) Alachua, FL: Bioenergetics Press, 2004.

[181] Perls F, Hefferline R, Goodman P. Gestalt therapy. New York: Julian Press, 1951.

[182] Röhricht F, Papadopoulos N, Suzuki I, Priebe S. Ego-pathology, body experience, and body psychotherapy in chronic schizophrenia. Psychol Psychother 2009;82(Pt 1):19-30.

[183] Rosen M, Brenner S. Rosen method bodywork. Accesing the unconscious through touch. Berkeley, CA: North Atlantic Books, 2003.

[184] Rothschild B. The body remembers. The psychophysiology of trauma and trauma treatment. New York: WW Norton, 2000.

[185] Sobel DS. Mind matters, money matters: The cost-effectiveness of mind/body medicine. JAMA 2000;284(13):1704.

[186] Sobel DS. The cost-effectiveness of mind-body medicine interventions. In: Mayer EA, Saber CB, eds. The biological basis for mind body interactions. Progr Brain Res 2000;122:393-412.

[187] Ventegodt S, Kandel I, Merrick J. Clinical holistic medicine (mindful short term psychodynamic psychotherapy complimented with bodywork) in the treatment of schizophrenia (ICD10-F20) and other psychotic mental diseases (ICD10-F2/DSM-IV-code 295). ScientificWorldJournal 2007;7:1987-2008.

[188] Ventegodt S, Kandel I, Merrick J. Positive effects, side effects and negative events of intensive, clinical, holistic therapy. A review of the program "meet yourself" characterized by intensive body-psychotherapy combined with mindfulness meditation at Mullingstorp in Sweden. J Altern Med Res 2009;1(3):275-86.

[189] Grafenberg E. The role of urethra in female orgasm. Int J Sexology 1950;3(3):145-8.

[190] Hamilton WH. The therapeutic role of the sexological examination. Dissertation. Los Angeles, CA: Calif School Professional Psychol, 1978.

[191] Ventegodt S, Braga K, Nielsen TK, Merrick J. Clinical holistic medicine: Holistic sexology and female quality of life. J Alternative Med Res 2008;1(3):321-30.

[192] Ventegodt S, Merrick J. Clinical holistic medicine: Holistic sexology, sexual healing, and treatment of vulvodynia through existential therapy and acceptance through touch. ScientificWorldJournal 2004; 4:571-80.

[193] Ventegodt S, Merrick J. Mechanical and holistic paradigms in sexology: Viagra® represents a mechanical worldview and may cause female sexual pain. J Pain Manage 2009;2(2):77-88.

[194] Ventegodt S, Struck P. Five tools for manual sexological examination: Efficient treatment of genital and pelvic pains and sexual dysfunction without side effects. J Altern Med Res 2009;1(3):247-56.

[195] Ventegodt S, Vardi G, Merrick J. Holistic adolescent sexology: How to counsel and treat young people to alleviate and prevent sexual problems. BMJ 2005 Jan 15 online athttp://bmj.bmjjournals.com/cgi/eletters/330/7483/107#92872.

[196] Ventegodt S, Clausen B, Merrick J. Clinical holistic medicine: Holistic sexology and acupressure through the vagina (Hippocratic pelvic massage). TSW Holistic Health Medicine 2006;1:104-27.

[197] Ornish D. Can lifestyle changes reverse coronary heart disease? Lancet 1990;336:129-33.

[198] Ornish D. Avoiding revascularization with lifestyle changes: The Multicenter Lifestyle Demonstration Project. Am J Cardiol 1998;82(10B):72T-76T.

[199] Ornish D, Scherwitz LW, Billings JH, Brown SE, Gould KL, et al. Intensive lifestyle changes for reversal of coronary heart disease. JAMA 1998;280(23):2001-7.

[200] Rossi EL. The psychobiology of gene expression: Neuroscience and neurogenesis in hypnosis and the healing arts. New York: WW Norton, 2002.

[201] Ventegodt S, Merrick J. The therapeutic value (TV: the ratio benefit to harm) of holistic medicine is 1,000,000,000 times larger than the therapeutic value of pharmaceutical drugs for cancer, coronary heart disorder, depression and schizophrenia. BMJ 2010 Dec 12. URL: http://www.bmj.com/content/341/bmj.c5715.full/reply#bmj_el_246274.

[202] Ventegodt S, Merrick J. Therapeutic value (TV) of alternative medicine (non-drug CAM). Rough estimates for all clinical conditions based on Cochrane reviews and the ratio: Number needed to harm/number needed to treat (TV=NNHtotal/NNT). BMJ 2000 Nov 15. URL: http://www.bmj.com/content/341/bmj.c5715.full/reply#bmj_el_244740.

[203] Ventegodt S, Merrick J. Therapeutic value (TV) of alternative medicine (non-drug CAM). Rough estimates for all clinical conditions based on Cochrane reviews and the ratio: Number needed to harm/Number Needed to Treat (TV=NNHtotal/NNT). BMJ, Nov 15, 2010. (Accessed 2010-11-16)

[204] Ventegodt S, Merrick J. Therapeutic value (TV) of treatments with pharmaceutical drugs. Rough estimates for all clinical conditions based on Cochrane reviews and the ratio: Number needed to harm/number needed to treat (TV=NNHtotal/NNT).

BMJ 2010 Nov 15, 2010. URL: http://www.bmj.com/content/341/bmj.c5715.full/reply#bmj_el_244738.

[205] Ventegodt S, Merrick J. Which types of drugs can be used in evidence-based medicine? A review of metaanalyses and reviews of positive effect, adverse effects, and therapeutic value of whole groups of pharmaceutical drugs. BMJ 2010 Dec 7. URL: http://www.bmj.com/content/341/bmj.c5715.full/reply#bmj_el_246044.

[206] Ventegodt S, Greydanus DE, Merrick J. Evidence-based medicine at a crossroad. Is the therapeutic value (TV) of complementary and alternative medicine (CAM) really larger than the therapeutic value of pharmaceutical drugs? Int J Child Adolesc Health 2011;4(2):1-2.

[207] IMS Health. URL: http://www.annualreports.com/Company/ims health/Annual rapport 2017.

[208] Ventegodt S, Andersen NJ, Kandel I. Bio- and alternative medicine in conflict. Human rights protection of the alternative therapist. J Altern Med Res 2009;1(2):189-202.

[209] Cochrane Library. URL: https://www.cochranelibrary.com/

[210] Gøtzsche PC. Cochrane - no longer a collaboration. BMJ 2003;327(7428):0-h.

[211] Ventegodt S, Kandel, I Merrick J. The therapeutic value of antipsychotic drugs: A critical analysis of Cochrane meta-analyses of the therapeutic value of anti-psychotic drugs used in Denmark. J Altern Med Res 2009;1(1):63-9.

[212] Committee on the Use of Complementary and Alternative Medicine by the American Public. Complementary and Alternative Medicine (CAM) in the United States. Washington, DC: National Academies Press, 2005.

[213] Leichsenring F, Leibing E. Psychodynamic psychotherapy: a systematic review of techniques, indications and empirical evidence. Psychol Psychother 2007;80(Pt 2):217-28.

[214] Leichsenring F, Rabung S, Leibing E. The efficacy of short-term psychodynamic psychotherapy in specific psychiatric disorders: a meta-analysis. Arch Gen Psychiatry 2004;61(12):1208-16.

[215] Leichsenring F, Rabung S, Leibing E. The efficacy of short-term psychodynamic psychotherapy in specific psychiatric disorders: a meta-analysis. Arch Gen Psychiatry 2004;61(12):1208–16.

[216] Leichsenring F, Rabung S. Effectiveness of long-term psychodynamic psychotherapy: A meta-analysis. JAMA 2008;300(13):1551-65.

[217] Leichsenring F. Are psychodynamic and psychoanalytic therapies effective?: A review of empirical data. Int J Psychoanal 2005;86(Pt 3):841-68.

[218] Hròbjartsson A, Gøtzsche PC. Placebo interventions for all clinical conditions. Cochrane Database Syst Rev 2004;3:CD003974.

[219] Ventegodt S. Why the corruption of the World Health Organization (WHO) is the biggest threat to the world's public health of our time. J Integr Med Ther 2015;2(1):5.

[220] Ventegodt S. A review of World Health Organization's recommendations in "WHO's model list of essential medicines": Who provides the data for the drug register? Altern Med Res 2016;8(4):00-00.

[221] Abel U. Chemotherapy of advanced epithelial cancer - a critical review. Biomed Pharmacother 1992;46:439-52.

[222] Abel U. [Chemotherapy of advanced epithelial cancer.] Stuttgart: Hippokrates Verlag, 1990. [German]

[223] Abel U. [Chemotherapie fortgeschrittener Karzi-nome. Eine kritische Bestandsaufnahme.] Berlin: Hippokrates, 1995. [German]

[224] Bø K, Berghmans B, Mørkved S, Van Kampen, M. Evidence-based physical physical therapy for the pelvic floor. Bridging science and clinical practice. New York: Elsevier Butterworth Heinemann, 2007.

[225] Heiman JR, Meston CM. Empirically validated treatment for sexual dysfunction. Ann Rev Sex Res 1997;8:148-94.

[226] Masters WH, Johnson VE. Human sexual inadequacy. Philadelphia, PA: Lippincott Williams Wilkins, 1966.

[227] O´Donohue W, Dopke CA, Swingen DN. Psychotherapy for female sexual dysfunction: A review. Clin Psychol Rev 1997;17(5):537-66.

[228] Struck P, Ventegodt S. Clinical holistic medicine: teaching orgasm for females with chronic anorgasmia using the Betty Dodson method. ScientificWorldJournal 2008;8:883-95.

[229] Ventegodt S, Thegler S, Andreasen T, Struve F, Enevoldsen L, Bassaine L, et al. Clinical holistic medicine (mindful, short-term psychodynamic psychotherapy complemented with bodywork) in the treatment of experienced impaired sexual functioning. ScientificWorldJournal 2007;7:324-9.

[230] Ventegodt S, Thegler S, Andreasen T, Struve F, Enevoldsen L, Bassaine L, et al. Clinical holistic medicine (mindful, short-term psychodynamic psychotherapy complemented with bodywork) improves quality of life, health, and ability by induction of Antonovsky-salutogenesis. ScientificWorldJournal 2007;7:317-23.

[231] NCCAM Publication No. D327. Bethesda, MD: National Institute of Child Health and Human Development, 2008.

[232] NCCAM Clearinghourse (National Center for Complementary and Alternative Medicine, U.S. Department of Health and Human Services). Mind-body medicine: An overview. Backgrounder. August 2005. URL: www.nccam.nih.gov.

[233] NCCAM rapport Briggs JP. Clinical Essentials: XII Complementary, Alternative, and Integrative Medicine. URL: http://www.acpmedicine.com/acpmedicine/institutional/tableOfContent.action.

[234] Death in America. URL: https://www.cnbc.com/2018/02/22/medical-errors-third-leading-cause-of-death-in-america.html.

[235] Ventegodt S. [Livskvalitet i Danmark]. Quality of life in Denmark. Results from a population survey. Copenhagen: Forskningscentrets Forlag, 1995. [partly in Danish]

[236] Ventegodt S. [Livskvalitet hos 4500 31-33 årige]. The quality of life of 4500 31-33 year-olds. Result from a study of the Prospective Pediatric Cohort of persons born at the University Hospital in Copenhagen. Copenhagen: Forskningscentrets Forlag, 1996. [partly in Danish]

[237] Ventegodt S. [Livskvalitet og omstændigheder tidligt i livet]. The quality of life and factors in pregnancy, birth and infancy. Results from a follow-up study of the Prospective Pediatric Cohort of persons born at the University Hospital in Copenhagen 1959-61. Copenhagen: Forskningscentrets Forlag, 1995. [partly in Danish]

[238] Ventegodt S. [Livskvalitet og livets store begivenheder]. The quality of life and major events in life. Copenhagen: Forskningscentrets Forlag, 2000. [partly in Danish]

[239] Luna LE. Ayahuasca reader – Amazon´s sacred vine. New York: Synergetic Press, 2000.

[240] Ventegodt S and Kordova P. Contemporary strategies in Peru for medical use of the hallucinogenic tea Ayahuasca containing DMT: In search of the optimal strategy for the use of medical hallucinogens. J Altern Med Res 2016;8(4):455-470.

[241] Long MJ, McQueen DA, Banga-lore VG, Schurman JR2nd. Using self-assessed health to predict patient outcomes after total knee replacement. Clin Orthop Relat Res 2005;434:189-92.

[242] Burström B, Fredlund P. Self rated health: Is it as good a predictor of subsequent mortality among adults in lower as well as in higher social classes. J Epidemiol Commun Health 2001;55(11):836-40.

[243] Idler EL, Kasl S. Health perceptions and survival: do global evaluations of health status really predict mortality? J Gerontol 1991;46(2):S55-65.

[244] Idler EL, Russell LB, Davis D. Survival, functional limitations, and self-rated health in the NHANES I epidemiologic follow-up study, 1992. First national health and nutrition examination survey. Am J Epidemiol 2000;152(9):874-83.

[245] Grof S. LSD psychotherapy: Exploring the frontiers of the hidden mind. Alameda, CA: Hunter House, 1980.

[246] Grof S. The cosmic game: Explorations of the frontiers of human consciousness. New York: State Univ New York Press, 1998.

[247] Grof S. Implications of modern consciousness research for psychology: Holotropic experiences and their healing and heuristic potential. Humanistic Psychol 2003;31(2-3):50-85.

[248] Goleman D. Healing emotions: Conversations with the Dalai Lama on the mindfulness, emotions, and health. Boston, MA: Mind Life Institute, 1997.

[249] Smith R. The drugs don't work. BMJ 2003;327(7428):0-h.

Chapter 13

THE AUTHORS' EPILOGUE: WHAT NOW?

Life has two sides: Either it is joyful, or it is painful. If it is joyful, we need to enjoy it the best we can. If it is painful, we need to take learning the best we can. The Corona COVID-19 pandemics has been painful for a large fraction of the planets population. The question is what there is to learn. What we see is that people are scared to stand up for themselves and speak the truth. They are scared to follow what they know. They are scared to believe in themselves and their own intuition. Therefore, people follow. People follow the media, the politicians, and each other. Better were it if we instead of following blindly started to think for ourselves. Better were it if we found courage to do what feels true to us. Better were it if we were free, autonomous beings. But what does it take to be that?

INTRODUCTION

Every single human being, who cherish the fundamental human values of freedom, happiness, independence, sustainability, happy co-existence, and human rights, needs to understand the importance of knowledge from free and unbiased science and exploration and most of all the value and necessity of wisdom and spirituality.

Most people see little need for spiritual growth and a deeper seeking into our own existence; for a well-functioning person engaged in practical life, existence is good as it is.

Have we been lucky?

The truth is that we have been very lucky in the COVID-19 pandemic. The Corona COVID-19 pandemic has shown us something of extreme importance: how fragile our whole world, our global culture, has become; how easy it is to take the power over, how vulnerable we collectively are to lies, manipulation and misinformation.

Extreme scientific and technological development during the last century has given humankind a degree of wealth and freedom, we have never known before. But we can too easily lose everything we have won. We can do that from one day to another.

We live in a common reality, which looks very much like a dream, a theater piece, or a film. Everybody is playing his or her own role in this play, and everybody is with little reflection enjoying the fun it gives. However, we need to be conscious of the role we play; we need to be deeper, and much more responsible.

Different roles

If we look at all the different roles people played so enthusiastically in the Corona-COVID-19 theater, at all the scientists, all the politicians, the doctors, the police, the people of the world helping each other, and the pharmaceutical industry ready to explore the lucrative new situation, it is easy to understand why this pandemic of a harmless common cold could spin totally out of control - until the regretful state of a harmed world economy and three billion people suffering under lock-down was a reality.

Everybody should have been more attentive, everybody should have voiced the questions he or she asked in his or her own mind. Everybody should have considered the possibility that he or she was right - and the people that blindly followed were wrong.

It takes courage to step up against the stream. However, we all know where it goes if we blindly follow authorities. So many meaningless wars have been fought; so many Stalins, Hitlers and Mussolinis of the world have ruled and done horrible things, because they were blindly followed by the masses. It all happened because of exactly this fear, we all felt during the Corona hype: Can it be that I am right and all the many that just follow blindly, are wrong? This is what we think, just before we chose to follow our self. After that, it gets easier, but the nagging worm of doubt might still peek out from its hide.

THE EMPEROR'S NEW CLOTHES

Somebody has to say it first. There is nothing new under the sun. In Hand Christian Andersen's wonderful story of The Emperor's new clothes, it is a small child. In the Corona COVID-19 pandemic, is has been a few extremely brave scientists. Many of them already suffering the dire consequences of their choice to talk. Some lost their jobs. Some their good name and reputation.

It seems that we collectively survived it this time – the big bluff, the big fraud, the big deception. We were lucky. In the future, we do not have the luxury to behave so irresponsibly, so senselessly, so mindlessly unaware of what we intuitively feel is right. In the future we all need to be more courageous.

We need to be on our marks not to fall in this trap again (but it seems we keep on doing it). We need to understand that nothing is more important than our common sense. Nothing is a better compass than our intuition. When common sense clashes with outer authority, we need to stop and think: Is something wrong here?

We all also need to know things. We cannot let it up to the experts to understand matters like chemistry and physics, biology and medicine, psychology and sociology, economics and politics. It is a lot to learn, a lot to know, a lot to study. But there is no way out. If we are to keep our freedom, our democracy, our values of love, closeness and kindness, we need to wake up and claim the power of consciousness.

WAYS TO POWER

There are many ways to claim this power. Long academic studies are ways to power, unfortunately not always to consciousness.

The path to consciousness is more about taking challenges, finding talents, about personal development of love, compassion and understanding of self and others; it can be about meditation, about studies of mind and the Self, about spiritual searches, religious revelations, artistic explorations.

Consciousness' can grow wonderfully our of relationships and deep dialogues and sharing; and nothing is growing consciousness as our one-to-one relationships, our sexuality, and our conflicts and problems with our partner and in the family, if we take them seriously, and really work un-selflessly on solving them.

Nevertheless, it is always about coming to know yourself; it is always about landing in your true being, about realizing yourself as love and truth.

Spiritual growth must be a part of our future culture on this planet, if we are to find a wise and balanced way to live, where we take care of each other and the fragile, unique planet.

> Humanity has three great enemies: fever, famine and war; of these, the greatest, by far the most terrible, is fever. Sir William Osler, MD (1849-1919)

CALL OF ELEVEN: FROM THE DOCTORS OF CHARLES UNIVERSITY TO THE PUBLIC

This statement below has just been published by physicians from the Czech Republic is now almost blocked by restrictive precaution, which was introduced to protect health of citizens during epidemic COVID-19. We need to value our government for giving the first precautions quickly and in big areas, which undoubtedly helped to manage the risks. Now it is necessary to accelerate loosening of these precautions in concern of actual epidemiological data and development of the epidemic – for health benefit of the citizens and economic and social prosperity of the country (1).

> When comparing deaths from respiratory diseases in 2019, we do not find a difference with 2020. From a statistical point of view, it should be objectively noted that coronavirus did not increase natural mortality in the Czech Republic (1)

One of the motivations of this call is to protect health of the citizens of the Czech Republic, which these long-term precautions are putting in danger. Motivating is also a worry about our medical or economic future and there is an effort to disprove the spreading myths and falsehood about the epidemic.

Precaution in the whole country will not lead to eradicating of COVID-19. Primarily it is needed to create immunity in most of the population, which will also protect the groups of residents in danger, which are defined by their diagnosis and not by their age.

We Need Now in the Czech Republic

- to end the state of emergency by 30th of April 2020,
- to resume the availability of healthcare for all citizen,
- to resume teaching in primary schools, high schools and universities during May 2020,
- to remove obstacles to free the operation of the economy, to prevent from economic collapse, which big part of small or medium companies and tradesmen is threatened by,
- to free borders in coordination with surrounding countries, especially with our neighbors who are having similar epidemic situation who are for instance Germany or Austria,
- to receive thought trough solutions instead of chaotic precautions.

Each of the items above are then discussed further and argument for returning to normal procedures and health care for all citizens and concluded.

The professionals are convinced, that the emotional charge of the current situation, which is fed by media, has to be corrected with documented facts and with regard to the facts and not fiction and the possible societal consequences and impacts of crisis measures. It is necessary to act and accelerate the state's strategy to return to normal life. All this with reasonable observance of hygienic measures, i.e., wearing a veil in contact with other people, washing hands and maintaining a social distance. During the coronavirus crisis, citizens have shown not only great solidarity and held together, but also discipline in complying with these rules, so there is no doubt that they will no longer follow these basic measures. In this difficult time we need more optimism and reasonable solutions, we cannot fall into fear, panic and hopelessness. We believe that our call will help also to that.

In Prague 21.4.2020 and signed in alphabet order:

Doc. MUDr. Martin Balík, PhD
Prof. MUDr. Jirina Bartunková, DrSc, MBA
Prof. MUDr. Cyril Höschl, DrSc
MUDr. Zdenek Kalvach, CSc
Prof. PaedDr. Pavel Kolár, PhD
Prof. MUDr. Robert Lischke, PhD
Prof. MUDr. Jirí Neuwirth, CSc, MBA
Prof. MUDr. Jan Pirk, DrSc
MUDr. Jaroslav Svoboda
Prof. MUDr. Julius Špicák, CSc
Prof. MUDr. Tomáš Zima, DrSc, MBA

ACKNOWLEDGEMENTS

This chapter is based on: Ventegodt S, Merrick J. A citizen's guide to survive Corona COVID-19 (SARS-CoV-2). Copenhagen: Quality-of-Life Research Center Press, 2020.

REFERENCES

[1] Call of eleven: From the Doctors of Charles University to the public. URL: https://cuni.cz/UK-6311.html?news=10013&locale=cz&fbclid=IwAR0AjONUynrPrpoCWvEIcUY5SQxdiSRvInfg8rMjX1PYwwv04zId0IsfnrM.

SECTION THREE: ACKNOWLEDGMENTS

Chapter 14

ABOUT THE AUTHORS

Søren Ventegodt, MD, MMedSci, EU-MSc is the director of the independent Quality of Life Research Center in Copenhagen, and Research Clinic for Holistic Medicine and Sexology, Copenhagen. He teaches holistic medicine, psychiatry and sexology at the Nordic School of Holistic Health and Denmark, Sweden and the Czech Republic. From 2006-2008 he was the director for and lecturer at Inter-University College, International Campus, Denmark in collaboration with Inter-University Consortium for Integrative Health Promotion, Inter-University College Graz, Austria and the Austrian Ministry of Education, Science and Culture. 2002-2012 he taught quality of life in the Danish Army. He is a popular speaker throughout Scandinavia with more than 1000 presentations. As holistic physician he has treated over 1000 chronically ill patients and given more than 20.000 hours of holistic therapy. He has published numerous scientific or popular articles and a number of books on holistic medicine, quality of life and quality of working life. He is reviewer for more than 10 scientific journals. 130 of his scientific papers on quality of life, holistic medicine and psychosomatics are listed on www.pubmed.gov making him one of the most productive scientists in these fields. His most important scientific contributions are the theory of holistic healing, the integrated quality of life (QOL) theory, the comprehensive SEQOL questionnaire, the very short

QOL5 questionnaire, the life mission theory, and the ongoing Danish Quality of Life Research Survey, 1991-94 in connection with follow-up studies of the Copenhagen Perinatal Birth Cohort 1959-61 initiated at the University Hospital of Copenhagen by the late professor of pediatrics, Bengt Zachau-Christiansen, MD, PhD. The recent years he has also done research in effectiveness, safety and sustainably of the world's different types of medicine. E-mail: ventegodt@livskvalitet.org.

Niels Jørgen Andersen, MSc, Professor, Department of Innovation and Economic Organization, Norwegian School of Management. This department conducts research and provides teaching in central topics related to innovation, business development, management of global companies, business history and economic organization. Research activities within the Department are related to four core subjects within the discipline: business history, cooperative organizations, business development, entrepreneurship and finally studies of industries with a special focus on the electricity industry. Niels Jørgen Andersen is educated as a Master of Science at the Technical University of Denmark. He was one of the first to learn about cybernetics and self-executing industrial systems in production and distribution. He was hired by an American company to participate in the development of full automation and self-learning production facilities in the US and Europe. He was early engaged in the revitalization and re-establishment of companies that were threatened by bankruptcy or were decided closed by the board or the owners. He discovered the importance of not talking about crisis or illness in such companies, but to focus on opportunities, interactions and the importance of every single one in the company. He achieved, among other things, a reduced absence from sickness (without focusing on it) from 10-20% down to 1-2%, while the company's profit changed from minus 8 million EURO over some years to a plus of more than 10 million EURO. He has served as associate professor and industrial professor at The Norwegian School of Management, with national responsibility for teaching innovation, entrepreneurship and business development. He is member of the board of the non-profit organization Nature-Culture-Health

(Na-Ku-Hel), Norway and International, which runs a property supporting development of people and their wellbeing. The project has received more than eight million Euros in donations, which are invested in a property at Sem in Asker, Oslo. Here many of Na-Ku-Hel's innovative projects in health promotion and personal growth are happening. E-mail: friisebrygga2@gmail.com.

Joav Merrick, MD, MMedSci, DMSc, born and educated in Denmark, is professor of pediatrics, Division of Pediatrics, Hadassah Hebrew University Medical Center, Mt Scopus Campus, Jerusalem, Israel and Kentucky Children's Hospital, University of Kentucky, Lexington, Kentucky United States and professor of public health at the Center for Healthy Development, School of Public Health, Georgia State University, Atlanta, United States, the former medical director of the Health Services, Division for Intellectual and Developmental Disabilities, Ministry of Social Affairs and Social Services, Jerusalem, the founder and director of the National Institute of Child Health and Human Development in Israel. Numerous publications in the field of pediatrics, child health and human development, rehabilitation, intellectual disability, disability, health, welfare, abuse, advocacy, quality of life and prevention. Received the Peter Sabroe Child Award for outstanding work on behalf of Danish Children in 1985 and the International LEGO-Prize ("The Children's Nobel Prize") for an extraordinary contribution towards improvement in child welfare and well-being in 1987. In 2017 appointed a Kentucky Colonel by the Commonwealth of Kentucky, the highest honor the governor can bestow to a person. E-mail: jmerrick@zahav.net.il.

Chapter 15

About the Quality of Life Research Center in Copenhagen, Denmark

The Quality of Life Research Center in Copenhagen was established in 1989, when the physician Søren Ventegodt succeeded in getting a collaboration started with the Department of Social Medicine at the University of Copenhagen in response to the project "Quality of life and causes of disease." An interdisciplinary "Working group for the quality of life in Copenhagen" was established, and when funds were raised in 1991, the University Hospital of Copenhagen (Rigshospitalet) opened its doors for the project.

The main task was a comprehensive follow-up of 9,006 pregnancies and the children delivered during 1959-61. This Copenhagen Perinatal Birth Cohort was established by the a gynecologist and a pediatrician, the late Aage Villumsen, MD, PhD and the late Bengt Zachau-Christiansen, MD, PhD, who had made intensive studies during pregnancy, early childhood and young adulthood. The cohort was during 1980-1989, directed by the pediatrician Joav Merrick, MD, DMSc, who established the Prospective Pediatric Research Unit at the University Hospital of Copenhagen and managed to update the cohort for further follow-up register research, until he moved to Israel. The focus was to study quality of life related to socio-economic status and health in order to compare with the data collected during pregnancy, delivery and early childhood.

The project continued to grow, and later in 1993, the work was organized into a statistics group, a software group that developed the computer programs for use in the data entry and a group responsible for analysis of the data.

Quality of Life Research Center at the University Medical Center

The Quality of Life Center at the University Hospital generated grants, publicity with research and discussions among the professionals leading to the claim that quality of life was significant for health and disease. It is obvious that a single person cannot do much about his/her own disease, if it is caused by chemical defects in the body or outside chemical-physical influences. However, if a substantial part of diseases are caused by a low quality of life, we can all prevent a lot of disease and operate as our own physicians, if we make a personal effort and work to improve our quality of life. A series of investigations showed that this was indeed possible. This view of the role of personal responsibility for illness and health would naturally lead to a radical re-consideration of the role of the physician and also influence our society.

Independent Quality of Life Research Center

In 1994, The Quality of Life Research Center became an independent institution located in the center of the old Copenhagen with a number of full-time employees. The Research Center expanded and several companies and numerous institutions made use of the resources, such as lectures, courses, consulting or contract research. The companies, which have used the competence of the research center and its tools on quality of life and quality of working life, include IBM, Lego, several banks, a number of counties, municipalities, several ministries, The National Defense Center for Leadership and many other management training institutions, along with more than 300 public and private companies. It started in Denmark but has expanded to involve the whole Scandinavian area.

The center's research on the quality of life has been through several phases from measurement of quality of life, from theory to practice over several projects on the quality of life in Denmark, which have been published and received extended public coverage and public impact in Denmark and Scandinavia. The data is now also an important part of Veenhoven's Database on Happiness at Rotterdam University in the Netherlands.

NEW RESEARCH

Since The Quality-of-Life Research Center became independent, a number of new research projects were launched. One was a project that aimed to prevent illness and social problems among the elderly in one of the municipalities by inspiring the elderly to improve their quality of life themselves. Another was a project about quality of life after apoplectic attacks at one of the major hospitals in Copenhagen, and the Danish Agency for Industry granted funds for a project about the quality of work life.

QUALITY OF LIFE OF 10,000 DANES

There is a general consensus that many of the diseases that plague the Western world (which are not the result of external factors such as starvation, microorganisms, infection or genetic defects) are lifestyle related and as such, preventable through lifestyle changes. Thus, increasing time and effort is spent on developing public health strategies to promote "healthy" lifestyles. However, it is not a simple task to identify and dispel the negative and unhealthy parts of our modern lifestyle even with numerous behavioural factors that can be readily highlighted as harmful, like the use of alcohol, use of tobacco, the lack of regular exercise and a high-fat, low-fibre diet.

However, there is more to Western culture and lifestyle than these factors, and if we only focus on them, we can risk overlooking others. We refer to other large parts of our life, for instance the way we think about and perceive life (our life attitudes, our perception of reality and our quality of life) and the degree of happiness we experience through the different dimensions of our existence. These factors or dimensions can now, to some degree, be isolated and examined. The medical sociologist Aaron Antonovsky (1923-1994) from the Faculty of Health Sciences at Ben Gurion University in Beer-Sheva, who developed the salutogenic model of health and illness, discussed the dimension, "sense of coherence", that is closely related to the dimension of "life meaning", as perhaps the deepest and most important dimension of quality of life. Typically, the clinician or researcher, when attempting to reveal a connection between health and a certain factor, sides with only one of the possible dimensions stated above. A simple, one-dimensional hypothesis is then postulated, like for instance, that cholesterol is harmful to circulation. Cholesterol levels are then measured, manipulated, and ensuing changes to circulatory function monitored. The subsequent result may show a significant, though small, connection, which supports the initial hypothesis and in turn becomes the basis for implementing preventive measures, like a change of diet. The multi-factorial dimension is, therefore, often overlooked.

In order to investigate this multifactorial dimension, a cross-sectional survey examining close to 10,000 Danes was undertaken in order to investigate the connections among lifestyle, quality of life and health status by way of a questionnaire-based survey. The questionnaire was mailed in February 1993, to 2,460 persons aged between 18-88, randomly selected from the CPR (Danish Central Register) and 7,222 persons from the Copenhagen Perinatal Birth Cohort 1959-61.

A total of 1,501 persons between the ages 18-88 years and 4,626 persons between the ages 31-33 years returned the questionnaire (response rates 61.0% and 64.1% respectively). The results showed that health had a stronger correlation to quality of life ($r = 0.5$, $p < 0.0001$), than it had to lifestyle ($r=0.2$, $p< 0.0001$).

It was concluded that preventable diseases could be more effectively handled through a concentrated effort to improve quality of life rather than through n approach that focuses solely on the factors that are traditionally seen to reflect an unhealthy lifestyle.

COLLABORATIONS ACROSS BORDERS

The project developed during several phases. The first phase, 1980-1990, was about mapping the medical systems of the pre-modern cultures of the world, understanding their philosophies and practices and merging this knowledge with Western biomedicine. A huge task seemingly successfully accomplished in the Quality of Life (QOL) theories, and the QOL philosophy, and the most recent theories of existence, explaining the human nature, and especially the hidden resources of man, their nature, their location in human existence and the way to approach them through human consciousness.

Søren Ventegodt visited several countries around the globe in the late 1980s, and analysed about ten pre-modern medical systems and a dozen of shamans, shangomas and spiritual leaders noticing most surprisingly similarities, allowing him together with about 20 colleagues at the QOL Study Group at the University of Copenhagen to model the connection between QOL and health. This model was later further developed and represented in the integrative QOL theories and a number of publications. Based on this philosophical breakthrough, the Quality of Life Research Center was established at the University hospital. Here a broad cooperation took place with many interested physicians and nurses from the hospital.

A QOL conference in 1993, with more than 100 scientific participants discussed the connection between QOL and the development of disease and its prevention. Four physicians collaborated on the QOL population survey 1993. For the next ten years, the difficult task of integrating biomedicine and the traditional medicine went on, and Søren Ventegodt again visited several centers and scientists at the Universities of New York, Berkeley, Stanford and other institutions. He also met people like David Spiegel, Dean Ornish, Louise Hay, Dalai Lama and many other leading persons in the field of holistic medicine and spirituality.

Around the year 2000, an international scientific network started to take form with an intense collaboration with the National Institute of Child Health and Human Development (NICHD) in Israel, which has now developed the concept of "Holistic Medicine". We believe that the trained physician today has three medical toolboxes: the manual medicine (traditional), the biomedicine (with drugs and pharmacology) and the consciousness-based medicine (scientific, holistic medicine). What is extremely interesting is that most diseases can be alleviated with all three sets of medical tools, but only the biomedical toolset is highly expensive. The physician, using his hands and his consciousness to improve the health of the patient by mobilising hidden resources in the patient, can use his skills in any cultural setting, rich or poor.

Another project that took many resources over two decades, from 1990-2010, were the development of a psychosomatic theory that could explain the clinical finding: that improvement of the patients' quality of life and happiness could lead to spontaneous healing of cancer and coronary heart disease. The aim was to conquer sufficient understand for this knowledge to be used in clinical holistic medicine. The project ended successfully with the conclusion that the optimal medicine is close to the traditional medicines from our different continents; we found that there is a deep wisdom in the ways the early and pre-modern cultures treated there patients.

Traditional medicine

This research led naturally to a deep exploration of the traditional medicine on the continents that happened from 2010-2018, where the best use of bodywork was studied in Asia and Australia (Aboriginal healers of the rain forest), the best used of talk-therapy/psychodynamic psychothe-rapy with focus on feelings, emotions and sexuality) was studied in the UK and USA, and the optimal use of medical hallucinogens were studied in Peru (shamanism with Ayahuasca). Studies in South Africa and Botswana shed further light into the understanding of psychosomatics and the use of traditional symbolism in healing.

From 2018 the sustainability of the world's different kinds of medicine has been the focus of research. Comprehensive comparative analyses have led to the conclusion that the traditional Hippocratic medicine, used for more than two thousand years in Europe, which is a psychosomatic medicine, might be a good alternative for our choice of medicine in the future. This kind of medicine is effective for most diseases, it is absolutely safe as it has no side and adverse effects, and is is sustainable as it is a people-to people medicine. "The doctor is medicine" could be a slogan for this traditional but great medicine.

The Native Americans, Africans and Samic people's traditional use of hallucinogenic plants and mushrooms should be an issue for further research, as there might be a great potential both for preventive medicine, and for helping the very sick and dying patients.

Contact

Director Søren Ventegodt, MD, MMedSci, EU-MSc-CAM
Quality of Life Research Center
Denmark
E-mail: ventegodt@livskvalitet.org
Websites: www.livskvalitet.org and www.qualityoflife.dk

Chapter 16

About the National Institute of Child Health and Human Development in Israel

The National Institute of Child Health and Human Development (NICHD) in Israel was established in 1998 as a virtual institute under the auspices of the Medical Director, Ministry of Social Affairs and Social Services in order to function as the research arm for the Office of the Medical Director. In 1998 the National Council for Child Health and Pediatrics, Ministry of Health and in 1999 the Director General and Deputy Director General of the Ministry of Health endorsed the establishment of the NICHD.

Mission

The mission of a National Institute for Child Health and Human Development in Israel is to provide an academic focal point for the scholarly interdisciplinary study of child life, health, public health, welfare, disability, rehabilitation, intellectual disability and related aspects of human development. This mission includes research, teaching, clinical work, information and public service activities in the field of child health and human development.

Service and Academic Activities

Over the years many activities became focused in the south of Israel due to collaboration with various professionals at the Faculty of Health Sciences (FOHS) at the Ben Gurion University of the Negev (BGU). Since 2000 an affiliation with the Zusman Child Development Center at the Pediatric Division of Soroka University Medical Center has resulted in collaboration around the establishment of the Down Syndrome Clinic at that center. In 2002 a full course on "Disability" was established at the Recanati School for Allied Professions in the Community, FOHS, BGU and in 2005 collaboration was started with the Primary Care Unit of the faculty and disability became part of the master of public health course on "Children and society". In the academic year 2005-2006 a one semester course on "Aging with disability" was started as part of the master of science program in gerontology in our collaboration with the Center for Multidisciplinary Research in Aging. In 2010 collaborations with the Division of Pediatrics, Hadassah Hebrew University Medical Center, Jerusalem, Israel around the National Down Syndrome Center and teaching students and residents about intellectual and developmental disabilities as part of their training at this campus.

Research Activities

The affiliated staff have over the years published work from projects and research activities in this national and international collaboration. In the year 2000 the International Journal of Adolescent Medicine and Health and in 2005 the International Journal on Disability and Human Development of De Gruyter Publishing House (Berlin and New York) were affiliated with the National Institute of Child Health and Human Development. From 2008 also the International Journal of Child Health and Human Development (Nova Science, New York), the International Journal of Child and Adolescent Health (Nova Science) and the Journal of Pain Management (Nova Science) affiliated and from 2009 the International Public Health Journal (Nova Science) and Journal of Alternative Medicine Research (Nova Science). All peer-reviewed international journals.

NATIONAL COLLABORATIONS

Nationally the NICHD works in collaboration with the Faculty of Health Sciences, Ben Gurion University of the Negev; Department of Physical Therapy, Sackler School of Medicine, Tel Aviv University; Autism Center, Assaf HaRofeh Medical Center; National Rett and PKU Centers at Chaim Sheba Medical Center, Tel HaShomer; Department of Physiotherapy, Haifa University; Department of Education, Bar Ilan University, Ramat Gan, Faculty of Social Sciences and Health Sciences; College of Judea and Samaria in Ariel and in 2011 affiliation with Center for Pediatric Chronic Diseases and National Center for Down Syndrome, Department of Pediatrics, Hadassah Hebrew University Medical Center, Mount Scopus Campus, Jerusalem.

INTERNATIONAL COLLABORATIONS

Internationally with the Department of Disability and Human Development, College of Applied Health Sciences, University of Illinois at Chicago; Strong Center for Developmental Disabilities, Golisano Children's Hospital at Strong, University of Rochester School of Medicine and Dentistry, New York; Centre on Intellectual Disabilities, University of Albany, New York; Centre for Chronic Disease Prevention and Control, Health Canada, Ottawa; Chandler Medical Center and Children's Hospital,

Kentucky Children's Hospital, Section of Adolescent Medicine, University of Kentucky, Lexington; Chronic Disease Prevention and Control Research Center, Baylor College of Medicine, Houston, Texas; Division of Neuroscience, Department of Psychiatry, Columbia University, New York; Institute for the Study of Disadvantage and Disability, Atlanta; Center for Autism and Related Disorders, Department Psychiatry, Children's Hospital Boston, Boston; Department of Pediatric and Adolescent Medicine, Western Michigan University Homer Stryker MD School of Medicine, Kalamazoo, Michigan, United States; Department of Paediatrics, Child Health and Adolescent Medicine, Children's Hospital at Westmead, Westmead, Australia; International Centre for the Study of Occupational and Mental Health, Düsseldorf, Germany; Centre for Advanced Studies in Nursing, Department of General Practice and Primary Care, University of Aberdeen, Aberdeen, United Kingdom; Quality of Life Research Center, Copenhagen, Denmark; Nordic School of Public Health, Gottenburg, Sweden, Scandinavian Institute of Quality of Working Life, Oslo, Norway; The Department of Applied Social Sciences (APSS) of The Hong Kong Polytechnic University Hong Kong.

TARGETS

Our focus is on research, international collaborations, clinical work, teaching and policy in health, disability and human development and to establish the NICHD as a permanent institute in Israel in order to conduct model research and policy.

CONTACT

Professor Joav Merrick, MD, MMedSci, DMSc.
Director, National Institute of Child Health and Human Development, Jerusalem, Israel.
E-mail: jmerrick@zahav.net.il.

SECTION FOUR: INDEX

INDEX

A

adverse effects, 61, 85, 111, 117, 119, 120, 121, 125, 128, 136, 139, 142, 145, 151, 154, 165, 236, 246, 255, 257, 258, 259, 260, 261, 264, 269, 273, 287, 311
adverse event, 151, 154, 158, 230, 254, 255, 256, 257, 258, 272, 274, 275
age, 23, 52, 53, 70, 88, 90, 97, 107, 165, 168, 170, 295
alternative hypothesis, 22
alternative medicine, 113, 156, 158, 165, 230, 236, 240, 246, 255, 274, 275, 286, 287
alternative treatments, 114
antibiotic resistance, 30
antisocial, xiii
antisocial ideas, xiii
artery, 7, 164, 215
authorities, xiii, xv, 5, 36, 44, 46, 55, 56, 67, 79, 81, 92, 103, 104, 109, 112, 125, 136, 137, 142, 146, 152, 154, 166, 292
autoimmune diseases, 207, 282
autopsy, 16, 40, 90, 106
awareness, 70, 182, 183, 185, 186, 187

B

bacteria, 40, 66, 195, 201, 252
bankrupt, xiii
behaviors, xiii
beneficial effect, 114, 121, 145, 245, 263
benefits, 138, 139, 166, 267, 270
bias, 31, 39, 121, 133, 137, 140, 144, 146, 147, 152, 153, 246, 249, 250
biochemistry, 205, 276
biological activity, 236
biological systems, 7, 192, 196, 197
blood vessels, 166, 170
brain, xv, 5, 7, 20, 21, 59, 175, 176, 177, 178, 179, 180, 181, 182, 183, 184, 185, 186, 187, 188, 189, 190, 191, 192, 197, 202, 205, 211, 212, 276, 277, 281
brain structure, 181
brainwashing, xiii
breast cancer, 159, 251, 285
breathing, 43, 52, 64, 98, 224, 247

C

cancer, xiv, 7, 8, 65, 114, 121, 122, 133, 141, 152, 155, 158, 159, 163, 164, 165, 172, 206, 207, 215, 223, 231, 243, 244, 246, 247, 251, 253, 257, 278, 283, 284, 285, 286, 288, 310
cardiovascular disease, 166, 167, 223
cardiovascular diseases, 223
chemical, xvi, 7, 10, 70, 76, 158, 183, 189, 198, 218, 219, 228, 236, 238, 239, 256, 258, 259, 260, 261, 262, 263, 265, 266, 267, 268, 306
chemical industry, 263
chemical properties, 265
chemotherapy, 114, 121, 133, 143, 152
child development, 284
childhood, 81, 207, 211, 213, 283, 305
childhood sexual abuse, 207, 283
children, 5, 56, 65, 73, 123, 158, 206, 256, 274, 283, 305
China, xiii, 27, 28, 35, 68, 82, 97, 113, 120
chronic illness, 193, 241, 282
citizens, xiii, 8, 37, 44, 56, 63, 117, 137, 165, 294, 295, 296
clinical holistic medicine, 163, 230, 235, 239, 254, 268, 271, 274, 275, 277, 280, 310
clinical symptoms, 49
clinical trials, 142, 164, 281
closeness, xiii, xiv, 163, 166, 214, 217, 218, 293
coherence, 141, 172, 202, 208, 209, 253, 284, 308
collaboration, 130, 133, 245, 251, 253, 269, 287, 301, 305, 310, 314, 315
common cold, ix, xii, xiv, 3, 6, 15, 16, 17, 18, 20, 21, 25, 30, 33, 41, 42, 45, 46, 48, 49, 50, 51, 53, 56, 57, 58, 59, 60, 61, 62, 66, 67, 71, 72, 73, 76, 80, 81, 85, 86, 88, 89, 99, 105, 106, 108, 115, 120, 195, 292
common sense, xv, 24, 58, 67, 79, 81, 293
communication, 74, 87, 183
comparative analysis, 101, 231, 234, 274
computer, 175, 178, 181, 182, 252, 306
confused, xii, 6, 107, 146
consciousness, x, xi, xiv, 4, 7, 60, 100, 167, 169, 172, 175, 176, 177, 178, 179, 180, 181, 182, 183, 185, 186, 188, 189, 190, 191, 192, 197, 198, 201, 202, 203, 205, 206, 215, 223, 224, 228, 238, 239, 240, 242, 255, 268, 269, 273, 276, 277, 278, 279, 280, 281, 282, 283, 284, 289, 293, 294, 309, 310
conspiracy, 27, 96, 97, 124, 132, 156
contagious, xiii
contamination, 263, 265
control group, 167, 241
controlled studies, 42
cooperation, 19, 23, 48, 57, 77, 86, 120, 309
corona pandemic, ix, xi, xvi, 4, 34, 44, 45, 56, 57, 73, 101, 103, 104
corona whistleblowers, 1, ii, vii, xi
coronary artery disease, 168, 170, 172
coronary heart disease, 155, 159, 171, 172, 231, 247, 268, 286, 310
coronavirus, 38, 40, 41, 52, 93, 94, 97, 98, 99, 100, 101, 295, 296
corruption, xv, 19, 68, 86, 87, 97, 122, 125, 131, 265, 270, 273, 287
cost, 25, 127, 128, 135, 165, 168, 230, 233, 234, 241, 248, 249, 257, 258, 259, 261, 263, 264, 266, 268, 270, 271, 272, 273, 274, 280, 285
COVID-19 pandemic, vii, ix, xi, xii, xiii, xiv, 3, 4, 5, 9, 18, 22, 23, 25, 27, 29, 31, 44, 45, 47, 48, 58, 59, 60, 66, 69, 70, 71, 74, 77, 83, 85, 87, 103, 105, 106, 109, 291, 292, 293
culture, xiii, xv, 8, 10, 56, 57, 71, 78, 80, 81, 86, 228, 234, 238, 264, 266, 267, 292, 294, 308

cure, 8, 22, 163, 164, 169, 170, 193, 202, 223, 227, 241, 246, 247, 251, 252, 255, 260, 268, 282
Czech Republic, xii, 20, 63, 294, 295, 301

D

danger, xiii, xiv, 9, 28, 30, 35, 42, 43, 45, 50, 67, 71, 75, 80, 114, 295
death rate, 94
deaths, 35, 36, 39, 40, 54, 97, 116, 165, 258, 295
democracy, 5, 25, 47, 48, 57, 67, 68, 69, 77, 82, 101, 293
denial, 101, 118, 231, 281
Denmark, x, xii, 20, 43, 44, 45, 54, 57, 63, 88, 89, 97, 98, 99, 100, 101, 137, 139, 140, 147, 153, 157, 159, 205, 230, 234, 249, 260, 267, 274, 275, 280, 287, 288, 301, 302, 303, 305, 307, 311, 316
Department of Education, 315
Department of Health and Human Services, 288
depressants, 139
depression, 123, 141, 158, 215, 253, 281, 286
depth, 182, 183, 187, 242, 277
destruction, 10, 19, 71, 75, 116
diet, 157, 163, 167, 170, 256, 280, 308
disability, 141, 180, 248, 253, 303, 313, 314, 316
disaster, xii, xvi, 15, 70, 71, 72, 75, 83, 107, 115, 116, 154
discrimination, 7, 99, 196, 197, 198, 199, 200, 201, 203, 204, 205, 277
disease model, 38
diseases, xiv, 7, 15, 23, 27, 30, 35, 43, 60, 65, 80, 83, 87, 90, 99, 139, 150, 154, 164, 196, 197, 200, 201, 202, 204, 207, 212, 215, 223, 226, 227, 244, 246, 250, 252, 253, 277, 282, 285, 295, 306, 307, 309, 310, 311
disinfection, xiii, 63
doctors, xv, 23, 24, 25, 45, 46, 56, 57, 59, 60, 74, 78, 80, 90, 98, 105, 106, 111, 128, 136, 142, 164, 166, 211, 213, 220, 222, 223, 225, 228, 233, 241, 244, 245, 246, 252, 255, 265, 269, 273, 292
drug treatment, 136, 140, 141, 147
drugs, 7, 10, 15, 66, 74, 80, 84, 85, 86, 95, 106, 111, 113, 114, 115, 116, 117, 118, 121, 123, 127, 128, 129, 131, 133, 134, 135, 136, 137, 138, 139, 140, 141, 142, 143, 144, 145, 146, 147, 148, 149, 151, 152, 153, 154, 155, 158, 165, 167, 170, 218, 219, 223, 227, 230, 231, 233, 234, 235, 238, 239, 244, 245, 246, 249, 250, 251, 252, 253, 254, 255, 256, 257, 258, 259, 260, 261, 262, 263, 264, 265, 266, 267, 268, 269, 270, 272, 273, 274, 281, 286, 287, 289, 310
dyspareunia, 141, 253

E

economic status, 306
economics, 26, 293
ecosystem, xv, 215, 228, 273
emergency, 25, 29, 36, 61, 63, 116
emergency rule, 63
energy, 3, 6, 164, 186, 187, 190, 205, 227, 234, 239, 246, 254, 264, 266, 269, 270, 271, 276
environment, 10, 47, 52, 63, 70, 190, 228, 233, 234, 241, 243, 262, 263, 264, 265, 266, 268, 272, 273
environmental impact, 233, 263, 272
epidemic, 28, 38, 43, 44, 57, 98, 99, 100, 116, 119, 294, 295
evidence, 17, 29, 38, 39, 128, 130, 131, 134, 135, 136, 140, 141, 143, 146, 147, 155,

156, 157, 158, 229, 230, 231, 235, 236, 237, 240, 245, 246, 247, 248, 254, 256, 257, 258, 259, 260, 261, 262, 268, 270, 278, 279, 280, 287
exhausted, xii, 6
existential healing, 205, 277

F

fear, xiii, xiv, 3, 4, 5, 6, 10, 15, 21, 23, 24, 35, 44, 47, 56, 57, 59, 60, 62, 66, 72, 73, 80, 82, 84, 90, 107, 119, 126, 196, 293, 296
feelings, 168, 169, 171, 243, 247, 311
financial, 39, 113, 137, 268
freedom, 8, 9, 16, 17, 47, 67, 69, 71, 82, 291, 292, 293
funding, 22, 42, 81, 86, 87, 94, 113, 122
funds, 113, 305, 307

G

gene expression, 196, 204, 286
genes, 205, 243, 276, 278
global economy, xiii, 63
global scale, 85
global trade, 234
global village, 234
governments, 38, 68, 75, 77, 101, 116, 117, 118, 120, 134
group therapy, 281, 282
growth, 140, 291, 294, 303
guidance, ix, 48, 68, 74, 124, 127, 131, 156, 212

H

happiness, xiii, 5, 68, 142, 166, 192, 211, 213, 238, 239, 240, 242, 243, 244, 268, 281, 291, 308, 310
healing, xiv, 130, 156, 163, 164, 170, 171, 172, 187, 192, 202, 205, 206, 217, 220, 221, 223, 227, 229, 231, 234, 237, 238, 239, 240, 241, 251, 260, 261, 264, 267, 269, 271, 272, 276, 277, 279, 280, 281, 282, 283, 284, 286, 289, 301, 310, 311
health care, 8, 16, 21, 43, 47, 104, 105, 108, 296
health care sector, 16, 21, 43, 105
health care system, 104, 108
health problems, 141, 202, 212
health promotion, 303
health status, 289, 308
heart attack, 168
heart disease, xiv, 7, 141, 164, 166, 167, 172, 253, 268
herbal medicine, 234, 236, 237, 239, 247, 270
history, xv, 24, 43, 50, 80, 86, 87, 99, 108, 118, 127, 302
holistic medicine, 101, 140, 164, 165, 166, 167, 168, 169, 206, 207, 208, 209, 212, 217, 219, 229, 230, 231, 233, 239, 255, 267, 268, 269, 272, 273, 274, 278, 279, 280, 281, 282, 283, 284, 285, 286, 288, 301, 310
hospitalization, 21, 61, 66, 257, 258, 259, 261
human body, 197, 198, 199, 200, 204
human brain, 4, 7, 175, 176, 178, 181, 182, 183, 277
human development, 260, 303, 313, 316
human existence, 172, 309
human health, 201
human nature, 225, 281, 309
human right, 28, 291
human values, 291
hypertension, 206, 284
hypothesis, 3, 6, 20, 22, 23, 30, 200, 204, 277, 308

hysteria, xiii, xv, 24, 62, 68, 80, 82, 85, 94, 97, 122, 131

I

illusion, 9, 15, 72, 81, 82, 85, 183, 193, 252
immune defense, 197
immune response, 119, 195, 201, 202
immune system, x, xiv, xv, 6, 7, 16, 32, 49, 52, 59, 61, 62, 65, 66, 85, 109, 175, 195, 196, 197, 199, 202, 203, 204, 211, 212, 243, 252, 277
immunity, 16, 22, 42, 52, 65, 100, 195, 203, 295
individuals, 4, 77, 176, 179, 190, 211, 213
industry, xv, 10, 19, 22, 23, 24, 47, 70, 72, 74, 75, 76, 77, 78, 79, 81, 82, 83, 87, 96, 97, 112, 113, 114, 115, 116, 117, 118, 119, 120, 121, 125, 126, 129, 130, 133, 135, 136, 137, 141, 142, 143, 144, 146, 147, 149, 152, 153, 155, 228, 244, 245, 249, 251, 252, 255, 263, 265, 267, 269, 270, 273, 292, 302
infected people, xii, 22, 36, 43, 46, 52, 54, 65, 79, 84
infection, xii, xiv, 3, 6, 15, 17, 21, 30, 33, 44, 46, 47, 51, 52, 53, 54, 55, 58, 59, 60, 62, 63, 64, 65, 66, 71, 75, 80, 84, 85, 88, 97, 99, 100, 107, 116, 244, 246, 307
influenza, 18, 29, 40, 95, 99, 108, 114, 115, 116, 117, 118, 119, 120, 121, 123, 124, 126, 127, 129, 131, 132, 133, 135, 139, 143, 152, 156, 157, 158
influenza vaccine, 114, 116, 121, 133, 139, 143, 152
institutions, 77, 144, 251, 265, 306, 310
intervention, 44, 150, 164, 165, 167, 168, 238, 241, 260, 282, 285
intimacy, xiii, xiv, 163, 166, 167, 171, 218, 231, 284
Israel, ii, x, 100, 275, 303, 305, 310, 313, 314, 316
issues, xv, 26, 141, 240, 253
Italy, 18, 20, 23, 27, 29, 30, 35, 40, 53, 66, 70, 93, 94, 104, 107, 108

K

kill, xii, 17, 30, 36, 80, 90, 127, 129, 135

L

laws, xii, 17, 65, 131, 137, 140, 142, 270, 273
leadership, ii, iii, iv, vi, 235, 239, 271
learning, xiv, xvi, 52, 102, 192, 204, 252, 291, 302
life expectancy, 16, 37, 63, 166
life quality, 154
life sciences, 240
lifestyle changes, 159, 168, 171, 231, 286, 307
love, xiii, 5, 8, 23, 66, 107, 163, 164, 166, 167, 218, 220, 224, 293, 294

M

manipulation, 5, 79, 80, 107, 292
marketing, 23, 72, 77, 137, 138, 152, 250
mass, xiii, xv, 24, 62, 70, 80, 85, 94, 97, 112, 122, 131, 181
mass-hysteria, xiii, xv, 85, 122, 131
mathematics, 79, 179, 212, 240
matter, viii, xv, 7, 19, 65, 76, 84, 87, 144, 176, 178, 180, 185, 189, 190, 202, 205, 276
media, ix, xii, 5, 17, 20, 31, 46, 47, 54, 55, 56, 57, 59, 63, 66, 67, 72, 75, 81, 85, 86, 103, 104, 105, 106, 107, 108, 109, 116, 117, 118, 130, 136, 234, 245, 291, 296

medical, x, 18, 26, 32, 35, 37, 42, 43, 58, 60, 63, 64, 74, 75, 79, 106, 111, 113, 116, 118, 130, 134, 136, 138, 140, 143, 147, 154, 155, 158, 163, 165, 168, 169, 170, 171, 172, 176, 177, 190, 191, 206, 211, 212, 213, 214, 216, 217, 218, 219, 222, 223, 224, 228, 230, 233, 235, 240, 241, 244, 248, 249, 251, 254, 255, 257, 264, 269, 270, 271, 273, 283, 288, 289, 295, 303, 308, 309, 310, 311
mental disorder, 207, 223, 229, 250, 253, 255, 278, 282
mental health, 9, 109, 141, 145, 146, 212, 253, 264, 274, 278
mental illness, 208, 215, 226, 230, 280
meta-analysis, 119, 143, 144, 147, 152, 154, 157, 231, 287
metamorphosis, 199, 200, 201, 204, 205, 277, 278
mind-body, x, 130, 131, 140, 156, 165, 214, 215, 222, 223, 228, 229, 230, 273, 274, 275, 278, 279, 285
mission, 172, 192, 200, 204, 209, 283, 284, 302, 313
molecules, 119, 182, 192, 234, 239, 263, 265, 270
mortality, xii, 15, 16, 17, 18, 19, 20, 22, 24, 29, 30, 31, 35, 36, 41, 42, 46, 47, 48, 50, 51, 52, 53, 54, 55, 56, 57, 58, 59, 61, 62, 63, 64, 66, 68, 74, 75, 79, 83, 84, 85, 86, 87, 88, 89, 90, 94, 97, 104, 105, 107, 168, 248, 289, 295
mortality rate, xii, 16, 18, 19, 20, 24, 31, 35, 36, 41, 42, 46, 54, 55, 58, 66, 68, 79, 84, 86, 87, 88, 90, 104, 105, 107

N

narcolepsy, 96, 117, 119, 125
national borders, 63, 115
negative effects, 114, 119, 128, 129, 133, 134, 135, 139, 143, 144, 146, 148, 149, 151, 153, 155
negative emotions, 5, 60
negative outcomes, 145, 146
nerve, 117, 175, 178, 180, 181, 183, 187
nerve fibers, 175, 178, 187
no closeness, xiii
no-going-out, xiii
no-touch, xiii, 234, 239, 271
no-visits, xiii

O

organ, 176, 178, 183, 188, 202, 226
organic chemicals, 265
organised crime, 101, 122, 131, 157, 231, 281
organism, 7, 182, 183, 184, 185, 186, 187, 196, 198, 203, 243, 252, 263, 277
organs, 184, 198, 207, 211, 249, 282

P

pain, 68, 81, 82, 117, 119, 141, 164, 169, 193, 207, 208, 220, 230, 241, 252, 253, 280, 282, 283, 284, 286
personal development, 169, 235, 239, 271, 294
pharmaceutical, xv, xvi, 10, 19, 22, 23, 24, 25, 47, 70, 72, 74, 75, 76, 77, 78, 79, 81, 82, 86, 87, 96, 101, 112, 113, 114, 115, 116, 117, 118, 120, 121, 124, 128, 129, 131, 133, 134, 135, 137, 138, 139, 140, 141, 142, 143, 144, 145, 146, 147, 148, 149, 152, 153, 155, 156, 158, 215, 217, 223, 227, 228, 230, 231, 233, 244, 245, 249, 250, 251, 252, 253, 255, 256, 257, 258, 260, 263, 264, 265, 266, 267, 268, 269, 270, 272, 273, 274, 286, 287, 292

pharmaceutical industry, xv, 10, 19, 22, 23, 24, 47, 70, 72, 74, 75, 76, 77, 78, 79, 81, 82, 87, 96, 112, 113, 114, 115, 116, 117, 120, 121, 125, 129, 133, 135, 137, 141, 142, 143, 144, 146, 147, 149, 152, 153, 155, 228, 244, 245, 249, 251, 252, 263, 265, 267, 269, 270, 273, 292
physical activity, 235, 239, 271
physical exercise, 169
physical health, 5, 141, 142, 150, 151, 206, 208, 209, 235, 238, 253, 284
physical therapy, 113, 136, 157, 234, 238, 239, 258, 259, 261, 262, 266, 270, 272, 288
physical well-being, 172
physicians, 114, 116, 126, 128, 134, 136, 137, 140, 144, 145, 150, 152, 153, 155, 164, 237, 245, 267, 294, 306, 309, 310
placebo, 61, 122, 134, 145, 146, 147, 150, 151, 158, 244, 245, 250, 251, 278, 281
political interventions, xiii, 69
political system, 63
politics, xi, 4, 24, 26, 28, 43, 87, 101, 124, 131, 156, 189, 229, 279, 293
pollution, 35, 228, 263, 265
population, 15, 24, 37, 39, 50, 51, 54, 66, 67, 70, 71, 72, 73, 84, 87, 98, 101, 103, 113, 119, 136, 140, 154, 166, 202, 248, 263, 267, 268, 275, 278, 288, 291, 295, 310
positive feedback, 201
principles, 47, 67, 130, 133, 151, 155, 156, 163, 172, 180, 189, 212, 214, 222, 225, 228, 229, 259, 279
professionals, 44, 64, 87, 296, 306, 314
project, 87, 171, 177, 303, 305, 306, 307, 309, 310
prostate cancer, 164, 172, 231, 244, 285
psychiatric disorder, 157, 231, 287
psychiatric patients, 245
psychiatry, 101, 111, 229, 231, 278, 281, 301
psycho-immunology, x, xiv, xv, 6, 60, 62, 161, 211, 212, 213
psychology, xi, 4, 172, 193, 205, 242, 276, 289, 293
psychosomatic, x, xiv, xv, 3, 6, 8, 15, 20, 45, 46, 59, 60, 62, 66, 80, 84, 87, 163, 166, 167, 211, 213, 228, 252, 310, 311
psychosomatic medicine, xiv, 8, 62, 167, 211, 213, 228, 311
psychosomatics, xiv, xv, 60, 85, 213, 301, 311
psychotherapy, 113, 136, 157, 208, 229, 230, 231, 234, 235, 239, 247, 254, 257, 258, 259, 261, 262, 264, 266, 268, 271, 272, 274, 275, 280, 281, 285, 287, 288, 289
public health, 8, 44, 57, 68, 95, 100, 112, 113, 117, 122, 127, 129, 131, 135, 154, 267, 287, 303, 308, 313, 314
public opinion, 57
public service, 314

Q

quality improvement, 280
quality of life, 16, 63, 65, 71, 100, 101, 114, 141, 142, 143, 145, 150, 151, 153, 158, 166, 169, 170, 172, 173, 176, 190, 192, 193, 202, 206, 207, 208, 209, 229, 237, 238, 240, 248, 249, 252, 253, 259, 260, 263, 268, 272, 273, 275, 278, 279, 280, 282, 283, 284, 285, 288, 289, 301, 303, 305, 306, 307, 308, 309, 310
quantum chemistry, 205, 276
quantum mechanics, 179
questionnaire, 142, 158, 275, 278, 301, 308, 309

R

reality, 4, 8, 25, 72, 79, 81, 96, 109, 124, 176, 177, 179, 184, 185, 186, 188, 189, 190, 212, 224, 225, 241, 242, 243, 268, 281, 292, 308
recommendations, viii, ix, 86, 101, 111, 112, 113, 114, 128, 129, 133, 134, 135, 136, 137, 139, 153, 155, 288
relevance, 127, 129, 135, 240
researchers, xv, 17, 31, 32, 38, 49, 53, 62, 67, 74, 75, 111, 114, 117, 129, 130, 133, 135, 136, 143, 144, 152, 187, 237, 245, 247, 251, 267
resources, 10, 47, 70, 263, 306, 309, 310
response, 119, 126, 132, 146, 157, 166, 221, 305, 309

S

safety, 64, 138, 153, 166, 215, 233, 234, 236, 241, 248, 268, 270, 271, 272, 302
school, 17, 85, 140, 158, 219, 222, 233, 244, 269, 273
science, 7, 17, 23, 24, 26, 31, 37, 41, 48, 60, 62, 67, 78, 80, 84, 87, 99, 113, 128, 129, 134, 135, 157, 176, 177, 178, 179, 191, 197, 212, 222, 223, 225, 238, 241, 242, 244, 248, 275, 276, 278, 279, 288, 291, 314
scientific knowledge, 58
scientific method, 87
scientific papers, 177, 301
scientific theory, 244
scientific understanding, 240
scientists, xii, xiv, 25, 35, 46, 57, 65, 72, 84, 87, 95, 123, 124, 131, 156, 182, 183, 197, 292, 293, 301, 310
sexological examination, 235, 239, 271, 285, 286
sexology, 206, 207, 229, 234, 235, 239, 271, 277, 278, 283, 285, 286, 301
sexual abuse, 207, 282
sexual dysfunctions, 141, 253
sexual healing, 286
sexual health, 141, 238, 242, 253, 254
sexual problems, 215, 252, 286
sexuality, 164, 166, 167, 170, 212, 218, 223, 247, 294, 311
side effects, 15, 66, 80, 85, 119, 140, 158, 165, 166, 227, 230, 246, 255, 256, 258, 272, 274, 275, 285, 286
social beings, xiii, 242
social class, 289
social contact, xiii, xiv, 37, 63
social distance, 296
social distancing, xiii, 38, 101
social events, 37, 63
social problems, 307
social reality, 243
social resources, 70
social rules, 178
social security, 249
social skills, 6
social support, 163, 170
society, 5, 8, 24, 28, 31, 37, 44, 46, 63, 78, 79, 85, 106, 125, 189, 233, 268, 272, 306, 314
sociology, xi, xv, 4, 293
spirituality, 9, 164, 225, 226, 291, 310
sterilization, xiii
strangers, xiii
stress, 45, 61, 66, 87, 99, 100, 106, 117, 163, 167, 170, 172, 193, 196, 207, 235, 239, 271, 282
stress management, 163, 167, 170, 172, 235, 239, 271
survival, 5, 114, 141, 143, 154, 159, 171, 198, 199, 200, 201, 203, 204, 231, 252, 253, 284, 285, 289

sustainability, x, xv, 10, 70, 81, 161, 233, 234, 248, 267, 270, 271, 272, 291, 311
swine flu pandemic, xv, 20, 43, 75, 79, 95, 96, 123, 124, 127, 129, 132, 135, 157
symptoms, xiv, 3, 6, 15, 16, 20, 21, 24, 35, 36, 39, 46, 52, 53, 59, 60, 62, 65, 66, 84, 88, 97, 105, 142, 243, 246, 252
syphilis, 128, 139, 252

T

testing, 38, 39, 51, 60, 223, 242, 250, 251
therapeutic effect, 138
therapeutic touch, 206, 219, 254, 256, 283, 285
therapist, 168, 170, 201, 287
therapy, 8, 136, 169, 200, 201, 204, 206, 207, 208, 223, 229, 235, 238, 239, 247, 249, 254, 255, 256, 258, 259, 261, 262, 264, 266, 268, 271, 274, 277, 280, 283, 285, 286, 301, 311
tissue, 49, 108, 180, 187, 192, 202, 263
touch, xiii, xiv, 140, 206, 219, 238, 246, 247, 254, 256, 283, 285, 286
touch therapy, 140, 246, 247
training, 57, 167, 169, 172, 235, 239, 271, 307, 314
transparency, 74, 97, 126, 132, 157
treatment, ix, 21, 66, 113, 127, 128, 129, 134, 135, 136, 138, 139, 140, 147, 149, 150, 151, 154, 155, 159, 163, 164, 166, 167, 168, 169, 206, 207, 208, 212, 216, 219, 221, 222, 223, 227, 229, 230, 233, 238, 240, 241, 242, 246, 248, 250, 251, 254, 255, 256, 257, 258, 259, 260, 261, 262, 264, 267, 272, 278, 280, 282, 283, 285, 286, 288
trial, 115, 144, 147, 158, 159, 164, 172, 231, 242, 244, 285

U

United Kingdom, 49, 230, 274, 275, 316
United States, 8, 23, 26, 32, 87, 122, 130, 156, 163, 164, 287, 303, 316
United States of America, xiii, 8, 20, 38, 39, 40, 54, 58, 136, 158, 165, 247, 256, 258, 264, 268, 302, 311
universe, xiv, 175, 178, 202, 225
universities, 26, 140, 255, 269, 295

V

vaccines, xvi, 10, 22, 48, 72, 74, 75, 76, 77, 79, 85, 86, 96, 101, 111, 113, 114, 116, 117, 118, 120, 121, 123, 124, 125, 127, 128, 129, 130, 133, 134, 135, 139, 143, 147, 152, 153, 158, 263
viral infection, 54, 59, 60, 61, 84
virology, xi, xv, 9, 25
virus, ix, xii, xiii, 3, 6, 9, 15, 16, 17, 18, 20, 22, 23, 25, 30, 31, 35, 36, 39, 40, 41, 42, 43, 44, 45, 46, 47, 48, 49, 50, 51, 52, 53, 54, 55, 58, 59, 60, 62, 64, 65, 66, 69, 70, 71, 72, 73, 75, 77, 80, 83, 85, 87, 88, 89, 90, 92, 94, 98, 103, 104, 105, 106, 107, 108, 109, 112, 119, 195, 203

W

whistle-blowing experts, xii
World Health Organization (WHO), ix, xi, xii, xv, xvi, 10, 15, 16, 18, 19, 20, 22, 23, 24, 25, 27, 29, 30, 31, 39, 42, 46, 47, 48, 51, 53, 54, 55, 56, 64, 67, 68, 70, 71, 72, 74, 75, 76, 77, 78, 79, 80, 82, 83, 84, 85, 86, 87, 89, 90, 92, 94, 95, 96, 97, 99, 101, 102, 104, 105, 107, 109, 111, 112, 113, 114, 115, 116, 117, 118, 120, 121, 122, 123, 124, 125, 126, 127, 128, 129,

130, 131, 132, 133, 134, 135, 136, 137, 140, 141, 142, 143, 147, 149, 151, 152, 153, 154, 155, 156, 157, 158, 166, 251, 260, 265, 270, 273, 287, 288
worldwide, 17, 23, 25, 39, 63, 73, 85, 111, 116, 128, 134, 154, 155, 245

Y

young people, 36, 56, 106, 108, 235, 286